IMMUNOLOGICAL ASPECTS OF ALLERGY AND ALLERGIC DISEASES

VOLUME 3

Clinical Aspects of Autoimmune Diseases

IMMUNOLOGICAL ASPECTS OF ALLERGY AND ALLERGIC DISEASES

Edited by E. Rajka and S. Korossy

VOLUME 1
Basic Concepts in Experimental Immunology

VOLUME 2
Methods in Experimental Immunology

VOLUME 3
Clinical Aspects of Autoimmune Diseases

VOLUME 4
Clinical Aspects of Immune Pathology

VOLUME 5
Clinical Aspects of Allergic Diseases

VOLUME 6
Antigen–Antibody Reactions in Different Organs

VOLUME 7
Allergic Diseases of the Skin

VOLUME 8
Allergic Responses to Infectious Agents

IMMUNOLOGICAL ASPECTS OF ALLERGY AND ALLERGIC DISEASES

Edited by

E. RAJKA

and

S. KOROSSY

Department of Dermatology
István Municipal Hospital
Budapest, Hungary

VOLUME 3

Clinical Aspects of Autoimmune Diseases

Springer Science+Business Media, LLC

Originally published by Akedémiai Kiadó, Budapest in 1975.
Softcover reprint of the hardcover 1st edition 1975

ISBN 978-1-4615-7236-7 ISBN 978-1-4615-7234-3 (eBook)
DOI 10.1007/978-1-4615-7234-3

Library of Congress Catalog Card Number 75-34966

LIST OF CONTRIBUTORS TO VOLUME 3

LÁSZLÓ BAKOS, M. D.

Head of Department, National Institute of Rheumatology and Physiotherapy, Frankel L. út 17–19., 1027 Budapest, Hungary

SÁNDOR BOZSÓKY, M. D., D. Sc. (med.)

Professor and Head, Department of Rheumatology and Physiotherapy, Postgraduate Medical School, Frankel L. út 25–27, 1023 Budapest, Hungary

SÁNDOR KOROSSY, M. D., C. Sc. (med.)

Head, Department of Dermatology, Municipal István Hospital, Nagyvárad tér 1., 1096 Budapest, Hungary

GYULA LUGOSSY, M. D., C. Sc. (med.)

Associate Professor of Ophthalmology, Head, Department of Ophthalmology, National Institute of Rheumatology and Physiotherapy, Frankel L. út 17–19., 1027 Budapest, Hungary

JENŐ MOLNÁR, M. D., C. Sc. (med.)

Assistant Professor, Department of Urology, Semmelweis University Medical School, Üllői út 78/b., 1082 Budapest, Hungary

GYULA PETRÁNYI, M. D.

Corresponding Member of the Hungarian Academy of Sciences
Professor and Head, 2nd Department of Medicine, Semmelweis University Medical School, Szentkirályi u. 46., 1088 Budapest, Hungary

BÉLA STEINER, M. D., C. Sc. (med.)

Late Professor of Paediatrics, 2nd Department of Paediatrics, Postgraduate Medical School, Budapest, Hungary

CONTENTS OF VOLUME 3

CHAPTER 34

THE CONCEPT OF AUTOIMMUNE DISEASES

by

GY. PETRÁNYI

Several comprehensive surveys have already been published on the pathogenesis of autoimmune diseases [2, 10*b*, 16, 33, 80, 81, 85, 87]; however, based on experimental data and clinical experiences, each investigator tends to form more or less different ideas about autoimmunity. On the other hand, our knowledge in this field is constantly widening as a consequence of intensive research, outdating earlier views. This holds also for the present review.

In the strict sense autoimmune disease is a clinical disorder resulting from structural and functional damage produced by the pathologic action of the immune system in one or more normal constituents of the body's own tissues. It is supposed that autoimmune reactions arise as special disorders in autoimmune tolerance, an inability to differentiate between 'self' and 'not-self' antigens. The disorder in self recognition may cause diseases *by* autoantibodies, whereas in conditions associated rather with cell-mediated autoimmunity the presence of such antibodies may be defined as diseases *with* autoantibodies. It is important to distinguish carefully between *cause* and *effect*. In contrast with the allergic diseases elicited by exogenous antigens, or haptens, autoimmune diseases are caused by an immune response against normal, unaltered 'self' autoantigens.

Autoimmune lesions may be classified into two groups: (*i*) The *'organ-specific'*, e.g. thyroiditis, pernicious anaemia, adrenalitis, aspermatogenesis, etc. characterized by high titres of autoantibodies reacting with antigens of the diseased organ *in vitro* and *in vivo*; the disorder can be elicited experimentally by 'autoimmunization', e.g. by sensitization with the respective tissue antigens in complete Freund's adjuvant. (*ii*) The *'non-organ-specific'* group is characterized by the presence of auto-antibodies which are not directed against constituents of a specific organ but against antigens which are present in various organs and tissues, e.g. anti-nuclear antibodies, anti-γ-globulin antibodies, etc. Systemic lupus erythematosus (SLE) and perhaps rheumatoid arthritis are the most important prototypes of this group. SLE cannot be induced by autoimmunization. The two forms of autoimmune diseases may occur in the same patient, either simultaneously or during different periods of his history (see Chapter 35). In principle, autoimmune inflammation may persist until either the autologous antigen is eliminated (self-perpetuation) or the special self-intolerance ceases.

Although in theory the autoimmune disease or reaction is easily defined as an immune response to some unaltered autoantigen in consequence of a disorder in self-tolerance, to prove this is not an easy matter. The clinical evidence is mostly insufficient and equivocal; thus, for the time being, it is more proper to speak about immunopathogenic hypotheses in connection with the various diseases grouped under the term of 'autoimmunity'.

HISTORY OF THE AUTOIMMUNE CONCEPT

A common pathogenesis might be presumed on the basis of identical characteristics even when the aetiology is unknown. All diseases which are characterized by fibrinoid alterations in the connective tissue show striking similarities with serum disease and certain allergic disorders observed in animal experiments. These have been classified by Klinge [49] as 'allergic-hyperergic' or 'rheumatic' diseases as far back as in 1930. Based on the assumption that fibrinoid is the degeneration product of the collagen fibres of the connective tissue, Klemperer [47, 48] coined the term 'collagen diseases' for a group of diseases in which he included SLE, rheumatoid arthritis, rheumatic fever, subacute and chronic glomerulonephritis, dermatomyositis, progressive systemic sclerosis and several other diseases all of which had well defined symptomatology but unknown aetiopathogenesis.

Systemic lupus erythematosus, which proved to be of increasingly variable appearance, attracted numerous investigators. The discovery of the LE cell phenomenon [36*a*,*b*, 37] by Hargraves and the recognition that it was the result of an *in vitro* immune reaction [63, 64] caused by a γ-globulin fraction, a 7S antibody against leukocyte nuclei denominated as LE factor [38*a*, *b*], gave considerable impetus to research work in this field. An increasing number of autoantibodies was discovered, and evidence had accumulated indicating that SLE as well as its various monosystemic manifestations (see Chapter 35) occurring also as separate entities (as 'organ-specific' diseases) were the results of immune reactions.

The fact that, in contrast to the earlier concept of 'horror autotoxicus' proposed by Ehrlich, certain autologous substances might possess autoantigenic properties under certain experimental circumstances was recognized in the early 1930's. It was shown that injection of normal brain tissue homogenate might be encephalitogenic [7, 57, 72, 89] and that experimental allergic encephalomyelitis, a model of similar diseases of the central nervous system can, be produced in this way [28, 66]. The results of these experiments were utilized in subsequent attempts to elicit inflammatory diseases by homologous and autologous antigens in the same organs which served as the source of antigen.

Diseases in different organs could be produced experimentally by various 'allergic' or 'immune' methods, and these exhibited striking similarities with human diseases of unknown aetiopathogenesis. Much attention was devoted to the experimental immune diseases of the kidney regarded as models of human 'glomerulonephritis' and 'genuine nephrosis'. This abnormality can be induced by (*i*)

Masugi's heterologous nephrotoxic serum [45, 59], (*ii*) soluble antigen–antibody complexes [19*a*, *b*, 71, 83] and (*iii*) kidney homogenate with Freund's adjuvant.

The results of these experiments have clearly indicated that the immune mechanisms resulting in diseases of the autologous tissues are very diverse.

The possible mechanisms of production of autoantibodies have been summarized by Vaughan as follows [85]: I. With normal immune responses: (*a*) to chemically modified tissue autoantigens, (*b*) to extrinsic antigens that cross-reacted with tissue components, (*c*) to neoplastically altered tissues, (*d*) to ontogenetically late-developing tissue autoantigens, (*e*) to cloistered tissue autoantigens. II. With abnormal immunological responses: (*a*) abnormal mutant clones, (*b*) loss of normal suppressor mechanisms.

In the kidney, the simplest case is the specific binding of antibodies produced experimentally against the glomerular basement membrane as the principal antigen; an inflammatory reaction is thus directly produced through the interaction of complement. However, no self-perpetuating autoimmune process will arise in such cases if the kidney is otherwise normal [75]. Experimental animals with nephrotoxic nephritis fail to develop nephritis in a transplanted isologous kidney if the transplantation is performed after the binding of the heterologous nephrotoxic serum [84]. The mechanism responsible for certain types of glomerulo-focal nephritis induced by circulating finely precipitated antigen–antibody complexes or, in case of antigen excess, by the deposition of soluble antigen–antibody complexes in the basement membrane is basically different, because neither the antigen nor the antibody is in immunological relationship with the glomeruli or arterioles. The circulating macromolecular immune complexes seem to exert their inflammatory action by non-immunological mechanism [19*a*, *b*]. This type of glomerulonephritis may arise theoretically in all conditions where soluble immune complexes are formed, thus in various autoimmune diseases, e.g. in SLE [84] and in heteroimmune reactions, e.g. in serum sickness, virus persistence (HB_s Ag, etc.).

Autologous inflammatory reactions and specific autoantibodies can be induced experimentally in selected tissues by the depot injection of their respective antigens mixed with Freund's adjuvant. It is a remarkable finding that the disease thus produced cannot be transferred to another animal with the specific autoantibodies but only with lymphoid cells, indicating the importance of cell-mediated immunity [3, 82]. The direct pathogenicity of the majority of autoantibodies is thus uncertain [68*e*, 69], though their binding to the diseased tissues can be demonstrated *in situ* by isotope techniques. Autoantibody production against alum-precipitated thyroglobulin can be demonstrated yet the animal fails to develop thyroiditis, while administration of the antigen in Freund's adjuvant not only results in the formation of autoantibodies but also causes thyroiditis [73*a*, *b*, 74].

The mechanism of effect of Freund's adjuvant is still uncertain. It is known to produce, when given together with the specific antigen or with tissue homogenate (brain, thyroid gland, etc.), inflammatory reactions in the respective organ. This inflammation is very similar to the organic manifestations (encephalitis, thyroiditis, etc.) of human autoimmune diseases.

In relation to SLE, too, the problem had already emerged in the early phases of investigation that no previous alteration in the antigenicity of the affected organ which could provoke the reaction of a normal immune system could be proved. On the other hand, the numerous autoantibodies demonstrated in the sera of such patients usually had no direct pathogenic significance. The primary event seems to be an abnormal immune reactivity, a partial loss of self-recognizing ability, and a derangement of the mutual interactions between the cell-mediated (T cell) and humoral antibody producing (B cell) parts of the immune system. Thus the appearance of abundant autoantibodies—produced [29] perhaps because of the lack of the hitherto mysterious suppressor T cells—are only a partial manifestation of these defects. A further proof is that autoantibodies are often produced reacting *in vitro* against antigens of unaffected organs. This, of course, does not exclude that certain autoantibodies could be pathogenic, either directly, and specifically, like some of the haemolysins, enzyme inhibitors [46], inhibitors of coagulation factors [4] in arteriolar basement membranes (GBM and lung in Goodpasture's syndrome), or indirectly, through the formation and deposition of circulating soluble antigen–antibody complexes.

Of the four fundamental types of pathogenic allergic response according to Gell and Coombs' classification [23], in most cases the cell-mediated (type IV hypersensitivity) T cell actions seem to be responsible for the triggering of the autoimmune process, while the others (mainly type II and III hypersensitivity reactions) appear to be secondary. The inflammatory reaction in autoimmune diseases is characterized histologically by lymphoid cell (immunocellular) infiltration (cf. other chapters of this book) and immunologically by the demonstration of antibodies. Antibodies are supposed to react specifically with antigens of the inflamed area. In autoimmune diseases, especially in SLE there is a great chance for the formation of soluble antigen–antibody complexes, with additional binding of complement and for their deposition in the glomerular basement membrane and in the skin (causing an immune complex glomerulonephritis and the characteristic rash).

When studying these reactions, it is important to distinguish the primary events from the numerous superimposed phenomena which usually impede accurate evaluation of the basic process.

Although we are not able to prove that autologous tissue might become primarily autoantigenic in the various autoimmune diseases, the possibility cannot be excluded. It has been supposed that so-called sequestered antigens may exist within the body; these are substances to which immunological tolerance does not develop because they are secluded from the immune system in foetal life. The lens of the eye is such a tissue, the antigens of which may be released due to some damage; they may reach the lymphatic organs and induce specific autoimmune reaction. Furthermore, it is conceivable that coupling of otherwise harmless haptens, intruding virus-like particles may cause alterations in the antigenic structure of normal body constituents, provoking the normal immune system to respond. Provided it is a virus-like agent that causes SLE, it certainly must be a peculiar one to account for the protean clinical appearance of the disease and for the different manifestations variable both in localization and time.

More recently, a group of viruses has been discovered, the so-called 'slow viruses' [79*a*, *b*, *c*] which might play a role in the pathogenesis of two rare human chronic progressive diseases of the nervous system, viz. kuru and Jakob–Creutzfeld disease, in some disorders of sheep and goats, and probably in the Aleutian mink disease. The latter is in many respects similar to SLE and polyarteritis nodosa of man, all three being characterized by hepatitis, vasculitis, nephritis, hypergammaglobulinaemia and the presence of anti-nuclear antibodies [86]. The problem of viruses in autoimmune diseases is a very intricate one [26]. Virus persistence seems to be responsible for most cases of spontaneous murine glomerulonephritis, as antigens of the deposited immune complexes. The problem of virus persistence is double faced: either their antigens are not 'strong enough', or the presence of special viral antigens suppress the adequate immune reaction which would eliminate them. Until now no virus has been found to cause or promote human autoimmune disease.

It is most probable that if viruses have any role in human autoimmunity, they are rather companions than causes of autoimmune syndromes on the basis of some suppressed immunocellular reactivity.

Antigens released as a consequence of necroses act as autoantigens, e.g. in cases of the so-called postinfarction or Dressler's syndrome after myocardial infarction, and of the so-called postcardiotomy syndrome after cardiac surgery. However, these are no longer unaltered self-antigens, and the immune reaction against the necrotic tissue only causes transient symptoms by affecting the marginal zone between the intact and necrosed areas; it does not, however, affect the intact myocardium, and the process will not be perpetuated.

In certain cases when there is a striking similarity between a heterologous and an autologous antigen, the immune response provoked by the heterologous antigen may fail to distinguish between the two and cross-react with the autologous tissue. Such antigens are present in group A streptococci [44], and may induce serum antibodies which cross-react with human cardiac, renal and cutaneous antigens. These are detectable in 55 per cent of patients with rheumatic fever, 58 per cent of those with rheumatic carditis, 60 per cent of glomerulonephritis cases, and 24 per cent of healed streptococcal infections. On the other hand, such antibodies are rarely found in patients with SLE, rheumatoid arthritis and other autoimmune disorders. These findings merely indicate the post-streptococcal immunological state. The demonstration by immunofluorescence of bound anti-streptococcal antibodies in the tissues underlines the pathogenetic role of such immune complexes in some human diseases. As regards rheumatic fever, rheumatic carditis and post-streptococcal acute glomerulonephritis, it is known that streptococcal infection is the primary event in their aetiology, followed by an immunopathological process which is, in fact, heteroimmune.

Since it was not possible to demonstrate unequivocally that the body's own tissues had become antigenic for the body's own normal immune system, the possibility arose that it was not the antigen which became abnormal but rather the immune system, by losing its ability to recognize as self one or several unaltered constituents of the body. Whether self recognition is genetically determined or acquired during the intrauterine life is still open to debate. The theory of sequestered autoantigens [65] has been based on the latter assumption, claiming that autotolerance fails to develop against autoantigens which were inaccessible or secluded during foetal life; these antigens, e. g. thyroglobulin, the lens of the eye, testes, brain tissue, when encountered by the immune system at a later time during the individual's life, give rise to antibody production. As for thyroglobulin, it is frequently found in the circulating blood of healthy newborns [39], and anti-thyroid antibodies may be detected in the sera of patients with apparently no thyroid disease. The theory of sequestered antigens being the cause of autoimmune diseases is open for much criticism and has been mostly disproved.

CURRENT CONCEPTS OF AUTOIMMUNITY

Theoretically, there are two possibilities for the immune system to become abnormal. Based on his clonal selection theory, Burnet believed [10*a*, *b*, *c*, *d*, *e*] that unresponsiveness against self substances is an acquired property of the organism, and attributed autoimmune diseases to autoreactive 'forbidden clones' which have been suppressed in foetal life and which may regain activity later either spontaneously or through induced mutations. He has suggested that these clones be related to the thymus, since in autoimmune animal experiments there is abundant hyperplasia due to germinal follicles in the thymus. However, this is not present in all autoimmune diseases, and might rather be regarded as a consequence like lymphoid hyperplasia observed in the lymph nodes and spleen.

The other possibility has been based on clinical experience. Like any other organ, the immune system may also become pathological [68*a*, *c*]. Some of the infectious diseases, e.g. morbilli, infectious mononucleosis, pertussis, typhoid fever, tuberculosis, not only stimulate the immune system but also severely damage it, morphologically as well as functionally. The most common examples of diseases causing immunosuppression are morbilli and Hodgkin's disease. Different forms of congenital immune defects are also known. Various cellular elements of the immune system may proliferate to give rise to malignancies, e. g. lymphoid leukaemia, plasmocytoma, reticulosis, which often bear immunological relations (anaemia due to autoimmune haemolysis, nephropathy caused by deposited paraproteins, etc.).

In view of these considerations, certain autoimmune processes might be defined as follows: the primary event is the disorder of the immune system which, owing to some inherent metabolic defect (perhaps of viral or chemical origin), loses its ability of self recognition and turns against certain antigens which are the normal constituents of the body. This 'functional derangement' [68*a*, c] or 'homeostatic breakdown' [10*ε*] of the immune system is only partial, for in most patients with some kind of autoimmune disease, antibody production and induction are retained [6]. We have found, similarly to others, a depression of the delayed-type hypersensitivity to various exogenous test antigens in the active phases of SLE.

The diminishing of the level of circulating T cells in the peripheral blood may be explained by two opposite mechanisms: (*i*) T cell production is impaired or (*ii*) T cells are attracted and bound to the target tissues and production cannot keep pace with consumption.

Constituents of the immune system, like the different immunologically active cells [13, 14, 32], e. g. the thymus dependent (T) lymphocytes, which are responsible for cell-mediated immunity, and their subtypes, the thymus-independent bone marrow (B) lymphocytes, which are responsible for the secretion of humoral antibodies, the free macrophages and fixed histiocytes (characterized by their capacity to phagocytose), further other factors like lysosomes, receptors for cytophilic antibody, response to chemotactic agents, role of leukocytes in non-specific immunity and in transport of antigen to the lymphoid tissues for the initiation and promotion of the responses of specific immunity might be affected independently.

The various autoimmune diseases, and also the various manifestations of SLE, might be due to substantially different immune mechanisms. Thus it is not necessary to assume a uniform pathomechanism for the interpretation of the various types of reactions, the ultimate cause being nevertheless common, namely an abnormal T cell response. The complicated interaction between the cell lines involved in the specific immune aggression and others taking part in inflammatory processes might be the reason why autoimmune diseases are in some cases restricted to a single organ, tissue, cell type or antigen, appearing as a monosystemic abnormality, while in other cases the autoimmune syndrome is a complex of several monosystemic elements combining independently. The single manifestations may in the latter case appear concomitantly but also with a considerable delay between them [68*a*, *b*, *c*]. The best known of these syndromes is SLE. Autoimmune thyroid disorders have been shown to be frequently associated with autoimmune gastritis causing pernicious anaemia [20*a*, *b*, 81].

Further progress in this field has been made by the recognition of a number of clinical and experimental syndromes having immune pathomechanisms, some with underlying genetically determined immune defects.

Several animal models have been studied like the spontaneous autoimmune haemolytic anaemia and SLE-like syndrome of inbred strains of mice, particularly of the NZB strain and their F_1 hybrids [5, 40, 42]. The genetical background of the disease in the strains originating from Dunedin is beyond any doubt. The NZB inbred strain is likely to develop spontaneous autoimmune haemolytic anaemia. They show a positive direct antiglobulin test between 4 and 10 months of age, at which time glomerular and tubular renal lesions (and extra-medullary haemopoiesis) were also seen. But the LE cell phenomenon is positive in only 1 to 5 per cent and anti-nuclear antibody cannot be demonstrated much more frequently either. The various F_1 hybrids of this strain with other strains not having autoimmune diseases (e.g. NZB × NZF, NZB × NZY, NZB × CBA/T6, and the most thoroughly studied hybrids NZB × NZW) develop SLE syndrome from the 3rd to 4th month on almost invariably. The signs include leukopenia, positive LE cell phenomenon, anti-nuclear and rheumatoid factors, gross albuminuria, lupus-nephritis, oedema formation, ascites and pleural effusion, progressive uraemia, premortal duodenal ulcer, gastrointestinal bleeding and pulmonary oedema. The severity of the symptoms varies considerably even within the same population. The main difference as compared with the SLE of man is the almost equal distribution between the two sexes, although females tend to develop more severe symptoms much earlier; also, rheumatoid arthritis so commonly seen in humans with SLE is absent in mice although positivity of the rheumatoid factor may attain 50 per cent; pleurisy is also absent. These models are suitable for pathogenetic and therapeutic studies. The disease in the mouse is influenced favourably by ACTH and corticosteroids, similarly to SLE in humans.

The autoimmune pathogenesis has been put in a new light by experiments made in mice deprived of their thymus gland [42], although the results were not always reproducible and could be interpreted in quite different ways. Undoubtedly, however, in NZB mice and their F_1 hybrids neonatal thymectomy has a significant deteriorating effect on the course of the disease. Autoantibody production is not prevented but occasionally delayed by this procedure, and the inflammatory reactions are usually more severe. Exchange of the thymus gland between NZB and non-autoimmune mice in the neonatal period will not eliminate the unfavourable consequences of thymectomy in the NZB mice, but seems to transfer the autoimmune disease to the non-autoimmune animals. As an explanation, it has been suggested that the autoimmune forbidden clones might have been dispersed from the thymus prior to thymectomy, i.e. during intrauterine life, but there still remained an amount sufficient to cause the transfer of the autoimmune disease. However, the agent responsible for the transfer may also be a virus harboured in the thymus.

It is more probable, nevertheless, that the exchange transplantation of thymuses between non-isologous strains has no lasting effect; it only helps to surmount the consequences of the wasting syndrome transiently. The mice survive longer, having enough time left for the consequences of the immune deficiency caused by thymectomy to develop, which either give rise to an autoimmune disease, or, depending on the genetic background, aggravate an existing defect and promote the establishment of viral infection. It is certainly possible that a resultant infection is responsible for the triggering of the autoimmune disease in genetically determined, thymectomy-induced immune disorder. This view is supported by the observation still awaiting confirmation that if a non-autoimmune mouse can be kept alive for a sufficiently long time after thymectomy in a conventional environment, it will develop SLE signs similar to those seen in NZB $\times$ NZW F_1 hybrids, whereas these changes fail to ensue in thymectomized axenic (sterile) controls [18]. The autoantibodies are not provoked by the microorganisms of the conventional environment, since they may also occur in axenic (germ-free) NZB mice [22].

It is interesting from this point of view that nude mice (having genetically no or defective thymuses) do not show autoimmune phenomena. In summary the genetic or aquired defect which causes the development of autoimmune reactions lies essentially within the immune system but many features of the immune deficiency are still to be clarified, since the circumstances and the mechanisms responsible for the autoimmune reaction are still unknown. The relationship between the Aleutian mink disease and the 'slow virus' has already been mentioned. Germ-free breeding does not, of course, exclude the possibility of a virus passing in an inbred mouse strain; virus-like particles have, in fact, been demonstrated in NZB strain in association with alterations indicating malignancy [21, 62]. Genetic immune deficiency and the presence of a virus do by no means exclude each other, moreover, such a relationship might be mutually pathogenic. A very interesting genetic animal model of an organ-specific (monosystemic) autoimmune disease is the Obese Strain (OS) of white Leghorn chickens [87]. These display hereditary spontaneous autoimmune thyroiditis beginning within the first weeks of life and characterized by hypothyroidism, severe mononuclear cell infiltration of the thyroid gland and circulating anti-thyroglobulin antibodies. The fact that this occurs in a bird made it possible to see how it could be influenced by bursectomy and thymectomy. These investigations revealed that in contrast to most experimentally induced and genetically produced autoimmune diseases, the OS thyroiditis is not T, but B cell dependent. Early bursectomy ameliorated or almost prevented the thyroiditis, whereas thymectomy had an opposite effect.

The different observations with the OS chickens allow a new classification of autoimmune diseases into T- and B-cell dependent groups with intermediate forms. The data do not exclude the possibility of a primary thyroid alteration, but rather favour an aberration theory of the immunological self-recognition mechanism.

In certain congenital immune defects of man the incidence of malignant growths is remarkably high, furthermore, autoimmune diseases, particularly rheumatoid arthritis, are also frequently encountered in such patients [31, 35]. A genetic background of autoimmune diseases is also indicated by the association of certain manifestations of these diseases with various chromosomal abnormalities [23, 24, 25] and by the frequent experience that autoimmune diseases are discovered in other family members, particularly if looking for somewhat different manifestations and γ-globulin anomalies [8, 29, 30*a*, *b*, 34, 41, 51, 53*a*, *b*, 54, 55*a*, *b*, *c*, 58, 81, 90]. It is always worth while to screen the whole family if an autoimmune disease, immunodeficiency or malignancy in relatively young persons are discovered.

The immune response has a deteriorating effect on its antigen, and an autoimmune pathogenesis was mainly postulated in non-infective 'idiopathic' destructive processes. This concept is principally correct. Nevertheless, since the recognition that the long acting thyroid stimulator (LATS) is an IgG whose activity is related to the Fab fragment [50, 61], it seems reasonable to presume an autoimmune pathogenesis even in diseases which are characterized by hyperfunction, hypertrophy, hyperplasia and cell proliferation. Thus, for example, hypertrophy of the contralateral kidney that follows the removal of a kidney is mediated, in addition to the functional load, by immune reactions [27]; moreover, regulation of the growth and cellularity of tissues also depends on the immune system [9, 11]. All these indicate that, under certain conditions, the immune system may have a stimulating effect, both on function and cell mass, by a mechanism which has not yet been defined (transfer of information?). It is, therefore, appropriate to investigate the possibility of an immune or autoimmune pathogenesis in all diseases with hitherto unknown pathomechanism.

DIAGNOSIS OF AUTOIMMUNE PATHOGENESIS

Criteria and diagnostic methods utilized in the study of possible autoimmune pathogenesis are summarized in Table 34-I. It should be noted that none of these signs should be regarded as an exclusive proof, nevertheless, an autoimmune pathogenesis is the more likely to underlie a vague clinical picture, the more of these signs occur in the same patient. These signs can be more or less detected in the diseases listed in Table 34-II.

TABLE 34-I

Diagnosis of autoimmune pathogenesis

Family history	Genetical background	Family members should be screened even if free of complaints for diseases which may fit in the autoimmune spectrum, and for immune defects, abnormal laboratory findings of immunological significance.
Case history	Previous diseases	All autoimmune phenomena should be sought for, not only the present disease of the patient. On screening examinations, also laboratory immunoabnormalities should be considered.
Present disease	History	Suspected provocative agents (drugs, viral infection, etc.).
	Symptoms	They should fit in one of the autoimmune diseases so far known. Exclusion of other plausible aetiologies; joint presence of other diseases is however possible (infection, tumour).
	Onset	May vary from hyperacute to that of very slowly developing chronic disease.
	Course	Variable. Excitatory manifestations (inflammation, hyperfunction) being followed by cell destruction (cytopenia), parenchymal damage and consequent deterioration of function, scarring and, finally, failure of the organ to maintain its function. Associated other autoimmune diseases are frequently found not only in the history but also simultaneously.
Laboratory tests	Autoantibodies in the serum and in exudates	Only positivity can be evaluated; since positivity is waxing and waning, it is necessary to repeat the tests regularly. LE factor, anti-nuclear antibodies, rheumatoid factors and other antiglobulin tests (anti-IgG antibody), biological false positive Wassermann reaction (cardiolipin antibody), autohaemagglutinin, autohaemolysin, anti-thrombocyte factor, blocking autoantibodies, leukoagglutinins, cytotoxic antibodies, anti-coagulation-factor antibodies, anti-enzymatic globulins (anti-lactate dehydrogenase, etc.), anti-hormone antibodies, etc. Antibodies produced against tissue antigens. LATS. Paraproteins, cryoglobulins (cold-precipitation or only gelification). Search for soluble immune complexes (antigen + antibody . . . + complement) in the blood. Autoimmune pathogenesis may be suspected if any of these tests is positive without demonstrable hetero-immunization. Accelerated erythrocyte sedimentation rate. Diminishing complement titre during activation of the disease. Immunoelectrophoresis (ratio of the Ig classes and subclasses) (paraproteinaemia? dysproteinaemia?).

Biopsy, histology	Usual staining techniques	Absence of other demonstrable pathogenesis. Limphocytic-plasmocytic infiltration, indirect signs of the binding of certain antibodies or antigen–antibody complexes (fibrinoid necrosis, haematoxyphil bodies, etc.); secondary parenchymal lesion, scarring.
	Demonstration of antibodies *in situ*	Fluorescent anti-immunoglobulin and anti-complement techniques; examination of the specificity of the binding and the composition of the eluate.
Immuno-cytology	Demonstration of the autoimmune competence of the lymphoid cells *in vitro*	Number of lymphocytes in the peripheral blood. Assessment of the degree of sensitization to the antigen by: *in vitro* target-cell damage (killer cells); immunocyto-adherence with rosette techniques; absolute and relative number of RFC and SIg-cells; absolute number and ratio of B and T cells; macrophage and lymphocyte migration test (LMT) and production of lymphokine factors to antigens.
Skin tests	Assessment of the capability to delayed hyper-sensitivity	Tuberculin mumps, candida, trichophyton, etc. The immune reactivity should be tested (blood cell counts, autoantibody titres, T cell reactivity, positivity of skin tests) before and during immunosuppressive treatment.
Microbiology	Infectious agents	Cannot be cultured, although superinfection is possible.
	Antitoxic, antimicrobial antibodies	Titres are not characteristic, they might be increased or diminished.
Results of treatment	Antibiotics	No effect on fever and inflammation.
	Corticosteroid	General symptoms (fever) and exudative inflammations are rapidly controlled, depending on the dose; paraproteinaemia and antibody-titres are less quickly affected. Never give steroid in ineffective low dosage!
	Cytostatic drugs	The favourable results are restricted to certain well defined and empirically determined manifestations. Initially, a paradoxical response is often observed, leukopenia and thrombopenia being ameliorated.
Prognosis	Early	Depends on the success of treatment. Generally good.
	Late	Uncertain. Relapses are likely to occur even in various combinations with other forms of the autoimmune disease spectrum.

TABLE 34-II

Diseases with signs of autoimmune pathogenesis

Systemic lupus erythematosus (SLE)	LE cell phenomenon, anti-nuclear antibodies, and possible occurrence of almost all autoimmune phenomena listed in Table 34-I and below as organ-specific or monosystemic autoimmune diseases, often resulting in a protean polysystemic syndrome, although with great individual variations in constituents, course and time.
Rheumatoid arthritis (RA)	Rheumatoid factor (anti-IgG antibody); relations with SLE.
Autoimmune vascular diseases	Polyarteritis nodosa, Wegener's granulomatosis, vasculitis nodosa, giant cell arteritis? malignant hypertension? Schönlein–Henoch syndrome?
Autoimmune nephropathy	Chronic nephrotic nephritis, immune complex nephritis, Goodpasture's syndrome.
Autoimmune hepatitis	Chronic active hepatitis.
Autoimmune endocrine diseases	Lymphocytic thyroiditis, Hashimoto's goiter (followed by hypothyroidism), Graves' disease, adrenal atrophy (consequent Addison's disease), testicular atrophy (consequent azoospermia), hypoparathyroidism (consequent tetany), insulitis (consequent diabetes mellitus).
Autoimmune diseases of the haemopoietic system	Autoimmune haemolytic anaemia, thrombopenia, leukopenia.
Autoimmune sialadenitis	Sicca syndrome. Sjörgen's syndrome.
Autoimmune cutaneous diseases	SLE, discoid LE, dermatomyositis, progressive systemic sclerosis, part of the pemphigus group.
Autoimmune diseases of the eye	Sympathic ophthalmitis, phacogenic uveitis, iridocyclitis, scleritis-episcleritis, sicca syndrome, some forms of retinitis, papillitis, malignant exophthalmos (usually with Graves' disease).
Autoimmune heart diseases	'Idiopathic' exudative-adhesive pericarditis, cardiac manifestations of SLE and RA (Libman–Sacks endocarditis, myocarditis, aortic valve disease).
Autoimmune diseases of the lung and pleura	Pleuro-pulmonary manifestations of SLE, RA and progressive systemic sclerosis (pneumonitis, fibrositis), most cases of non-microbial pleurisy, Hamman–Rich syndrome, pulmonary haemosiderosis, (Goodpasture's syndrome), sarcoidosis?
Autoimmune gastrointestinal diseases	Ulcerative colitis, IgA-deficient sprue, scleropathy, regional enteritis (Crohn's disease)?, antibodies to gastric mucosa and intrinsic factor (consequent pernicious anaemia), some cases of peptic ulcer?
Autoimmune diseases of the nervous system	Demyelinization processes, multiple sclerosis, epilepsy (cf. SLE).
Autoimmune muscle diseases	Myasthenia gravis, polymyositis, dermatomyositis.
Autoimmune coagulopathy	Antibodies against coagulation factors (inhibitory antibodies).
Autoimmune cryopathy	Raynaud's syndrome, hyperviscosity syndrome.
Autoimmune enzymopathies	Inhibitory antibodies (lactate dehydrogenase, other enzymes?).
Autoimmune diseases not classified in any of the above groups	Moschcowitz's disease (thrombotic thrombocytopenic purpura), certain aseptic bone necroses, tendosynovitis, Dupuytren's contracture?, osteochondritis.

CONCLUSION TO AUTOIMMUNE PATHOGENESIS FROM THE EFFICIENCY OF TREATMENT

Essentially, the therapy of autoimmune diseases is empirical. If the mechanism of action of the various immunosuppressive drugs [60] were more accurately known, the type of immune pathomechanism could be deduced from the benefit of treatment. The action of cytostatic drugs can be most safely assessed by studying their effect on tumour growth in the clinical practice. Corticosteroids probably exert their action by lymphosuppression in the first place. There is no drug available at present with a definite selective action on the antibody producing plasma cell system. Most of the drugs called immunosuppressive agents have earlier been used as cytostatic drugs and have proved to be effective in lymphoid neoplasms (nitrogen, mustard and its derivatives, cyclophosphamide, chlorambucil, etc.). However, there is still controversy about the use of alkylating agents in autoimmune diseases. It is known that 6-mercaptopurine and azathioprine are purine antagonists, however, this does not explain the well-known clinical experience that they have a beneficial effect in autoimmune haemolytic anaemia [76, 77], thrombopenia and leukopenia of SLE, and in lupus nephritis with gross oedema [68*d*], but have no or only a slight effect on numerous other manifestations of SLE.

Of the immunosuppressive agents, the anti-lymphocyte serum (ALS) and anti-thymocyte globulin (ATG) seem to be the most specific. So far anti-lymphocyte serum has mainly been utilized for preventing rejection of transplanted organs. Experience is still lacking concerning their value in human autoimmune diseases. The results so far obtained [70] are difficult to evaluate since these sera cannot be sufficiently standardized and are usually produced individually. These circumstances might be responsible for the considerable differences in the reports on their therapeutic results. In view of the existence of the two types of lymphoid systems the following question must be answered: if anti-lymphocyte serum is raised against neonatal thymus cell suspension or against lymphoid cells derived from the thoracic duct, blood or various lymphoid cells [1], how specific will it be to the thymus dependent part of the immune system? Early bursectomy is insufficient for complete elimination of the antibody producing system: this is achieved only if supplemented with 650 r whole-body irradiation [15]. The anti-lymphocyte and anti-thymocyte antibody available at present also reacts with antigens which are not restricted to the thymus [78].

Despite the difficulties of interpretation and the conflicting experimental data, certain conclusions can nevertheless be drawn regarding the pathogenesis of autoimmune diseases from the results obtained with the clinical and experimental use of anti-lymphocyte serum and anti-lymphocyte globulin [17]. Anti-lymphocyte antibody is capable of preventing the sensitization following skin grafting in adult mice and consequently, the rejection of a subsequent graft is not accelerated [52, 56*a*, *b*, *c*], furthermore, the tuberculin, mumps, candida and trichophyton intracutaneous reactions can transiently be eliminated. The assumption can be made based on these findings that anti-lymphocyte globulin might in the future be used with success in some selected cases of cell-mediated immune diseases. On the other hand, the secondary immune response is not affected by the antiserum raised against small lymphocytes [43]; moreover, it is rather augmented [?], and the titre of natural antibodies also remains unchanged [67]. Results of treatment seem to support the concept of a basic T cell disorder, nevertheless, further investigations are necessary to obtain a more accurate picture of cellular co-operation, of the role of thymic hormones, lymphokines, transfer factors, etc.

Up to now the effective treatment of autoimmune diseases was thought to be immunosuppression, and the aim was to kill the cells of the autoaggressive clones. Now it seems more appropriate to think that the good results achieved with steroids, cytostatics and antimalarials are due rather to a correction of the derailed regulation of different parts of the immune system and their function. Thus, instead of non-specific general immunosuppression it would be better to stress the need for *immunocorrection*.

REFERENCES

1. Asakuma, R. and Reif, A. E.: *Cancer Res.* **28,** 707 (1968).
2. Ascherson, G. L.: *Sci. Basis of Med. Ann. Rev.* 1968, p. 109.
3. Benacerraf, B. and Green, I.: *Ann. Rev. Med.* **20,** 141 (1969).
4. Bidwell, E.: *Ann. Rev. Med.* **20,** 63 (1969).
5. Bielschowsky, M., Helyer, B. J. and Howie, J. B.: *Proc. Univ. Otago med. Sch.* **37,** 9 (1959).
6. Block, S., Gibbs, C. B., Stevens, M. B. and Shulman, L. E.: *Arthr. and Rheum.* **9,** 848 (1966).
7. Brandt, R., Guth, H. and Müller, R.: *Klin. Wschr.* **5,** 655 (1926).
8. Brunjes, S., Zike, K. and Julian, R.: *Amer. J. Med.* **30,** 529 (1961).
9. Bullough, W. S. and Rytömea, T.: *Nature (London)* **205,** 573 (1965).

10*a*. Burnet, F. M.: *Brit. med. J.* **2,** 645 (1959).

10*b*. ibid., **2,** 720 (1959).

10*c*. ibid., **2,** 807 (1962).

10*d*. id., *Proc. roy. Soc. Med.* **55,** 619 (1962).

10*e*. id., *Cellular Immunology.* Melbourne Univ. Press, Victoria and Cambridge Univ. Press, London 1969.

11. Burwell, R. G.: *Lancet* **ii,** 69 (1963).
12. Coombs, R. R. A. and Gell, P. G. H.: In *Clinical Aspects of Immunology.* 2nd ed. Ed. by Gell, P. G. H. and Coombs, R. R. A. Blackwell, Oxford 1968, p. 575.
13. Cooper, M. D., Perey, D. V., McKneally, M. F., Gabrielsen, A. E., Sutherland, D. E. R. and Good, R. A.: *Lancet* **i,** 1388 (1966).
14. Cooper, M. D., Peterson, R. D. A. and Good, R. A.: *Nature (London)* **205,** 143 (1965).
15. Cooper, M. D., Peterson, R. D. A., South, M. A. and Good, R. A.: *J. exp. Med.* **123,** 75 (1966).
16. Dameshek, W., Schwartz, R. and Oliner, H.: *Blood* **17,** 6 (1961).
17. Denman, A. M.: *Clin. exp. Immunol.* **5,** 217 (1969).
18. de Vries, M. J., van Putten, L. M., Balner, H. and van Bekkum, D. W.: *Rev. franç. Ét. clin. biol.* **9,** 381 (1964).

19*a*. Dixon, F. J.: *Harvey Lect.* **58,** 21 (1963).

19*b*. id., *Amer. J. Med.* **44,** 493 (1968).

20*a*. Doniach, D., Roitt, I. M. and Taylor, K. R.: *Brit. med. J.* **1,** 1374 (1963).

20*b*. id., *Ann. N. Y. Acad. Sci.* **124,** 605 (1965).

21. East, J. and Branca, M.: *Clin. exp. Immunol.* **4,** 624 (1969).
22. East, J., Prosser, P., Holborow, E. J. and Jacket, H.: *Lancet* **i,** 755 (1967).
23. Ferguson-Smith, M. A., Anderson, J. R., Frøland, A. and Gray, K. G.: *Lancet* **ii,** 566 (1966).
24. Fialkov, P. J.: *Amer. J. hum. Genet.* **18,** 93 (1966).
25. Fialkov, P. J., Hecht, F., Uchida, I. A. and Motulsky, A. G.: *Lancet* **ii,** 868 (1965).
26. Fifth Annual ASCP Research Symposium. Viruses and autoimmune disease. *Amer. J. clin. Path.* **56,** 259 (1971).

27. Fox, M.: *Proc. roy. Soc. Med.* **62,** 861 (1969).
28. Freund, J., Stein, E. R. and Pisani, T. M.: *J. Immunol.* **57,** 179 (1947).
29. Fundenberg, H. H.: *Clin. immunol. immunopathol.* **2,** 281 (1974).
30*a*. Fundenberg, H. H. and Franklin, E. C.: *Ann. intern. Med.* **58,** 171 (1963).
30*b*. Fundenberg, H. H., German, J. H. and Kunkel, H. S.: *Arthr. and Rheum.* **5,** 565 (1962).
31. Gitlin, D., Janeway, C. A., Apt, L. and Crays, J. M.: In *Cellular and Humoral Aspects of the Hypersensitive State*. Ed. by Lawrence, H. S., Hoeber, New York 1959, p. 375.
32. Glick, B., Chang, T. S. and Jaap, R. G.: *Poultry Sci.* **35,** 224 (1956).
33. Glynn, L. E. and Holborow, E. J.: *Autoimmunity and Disease*. Blackwell, Oxford 1965.
34. Good, R. A.: In *1st Int. Symp. on Immunopathology*. Ed. by Grabar, P. and Miescher, P. A. Schwabe, Basel 1958, p. 41.
35. Good, R. A., Rötstein, J. and Mazzitello, W. T.: *J. Lab. clin. Med.* **49,** 343 (1957).
36*a*. Hargraves, M. M.: *Proc. Mayo Clin.* **24,** 234 (1949).
36*b*. ibid., **27,** 419 (1952).
37. Hargraves, M. M., Richmond, H. and Morton, R.: *Proc. Mayo Clin.* **23,** 25 (1948).
38*a*. Haserick, J. R. and Bortz, D. W.: *J. invest. Derm.* **13,** 47 (1949).
38*b*. id., *Blood* **5,** 718 (1950).
39. Helyer, B. J. and Howie, J. B.: *Brit. J. Haemat.* **9,** 119 (1963).
40. Hjort, T. and Pederson, G.: *Lancet* **ii,** 259 (1962).
41. Holman, H. R.: *Arthr. and Rheum.* **6,** 513 (1963).
42. Howie, J. B.: In *Textbook of Immunopathology*. Ed. by Miescher, P. A. and Müller-Eberhard, H. J. Grune and Stratton, New York 1968, pp. 179–188.
43. James, K.: *Clin. exp. Immunol.* **2,** 615 (1967).
44. Kaplan, M. H.: In *Textbook of Immunopathology*. Ed. by Miescher, P. A. and Müller-Eberhard, H. J. Grune and Stratton, New York 1968, pp. 641–650.
45. Kay, C. F.: *J. exp. Med.* **72,** 559 (1940).
46. Kindmark, C. O.: *Scand. J. clin. lab. Invest.* **24,** 49 (1969).
47. Klemperer, P.: *Amer. J. Path.* **26,** 505 (1950).
48. Klemperer, P., Pollak, A. D. and Bacher, G.: *Arch. Path.* **39,** 569 (1941).
49. Klinge, F.: *Beitr. path. Anat.* **83,** 185 (1930).
50. Kriss, J. P., Pleshakow, V. and Chien, J. R.: *J. clin. Endocr.* **24,** 1005 (1964).
51. Lambie, J. A. and Duft, I. F.: *Ann. intern. Med.* **59,** 839 (1963).
52. Lance, E. M.: *Nature (London)* **217,** 557 (1968).
53*a*. Lawrence, H. S.: *Proc. roy. Soc. Med.* **53,** 522 (1960).
53*b*. id., *Arthr. and Rheum.* **6,** 166 (1963).
54. Lawrence, H. S. and Ball, J.: *Ann. rheum. Dis.* **17,** 169 (1958).
55*a*. Leonhardt, T.: *Lancet* **ii,** 1200 (1957).
55*b*. id., *Acta med. scand.* **165,** 395 (1959).
55*c*. ibid., 416 (1964).
56*a*. Levey, R. H. and Medawar, P. B.: *Proc. nat. Acad. Sci. (Wash.)* **56,** 1130 (1960).
56*b*. ibid., **58,** 470 (1967).
56*c*. id., *Ann. N. Y. Acad. Sci.* **129,** 164 (1966).
57. Lewis, J. H.: *J. Immunol.* **27,** 473 (1934).
58. Marlow, A. A., Peabody, H. D., jr. and Nickel, W. R.: *J. Amer. med. Ass.* **173,** 1641 (1960).
59. Massugi, M.: *Beitr. path. Anat.* **92,** 429 (1930).
60. Mechanisms of action of drugs affecting immune responses. Joint meeting 2. *Proc. roy. Soc. Med.* **65,** 255 (1972).
61. Meek, J. C., Jones, A. E., Lewis, U. J. and Van der Laan, W. P.: *Proc. nat. Acad. Sci. (Wash.)* **52,** 342 (1964).
62. Mellors, R. C. and Huang, C. Y.: *J. exp. Med.* **124,** 1031 (1966).
63. Miescher, P. A.: *Experientia (Basel)* **10,** 252 (1954).
64. Miescher, P. A. and Müller-Eberhard, H. J.: *Textbook of Immunopathology*. Grune and Stratton, New York 1968.
65. Milgrom, F.: In *Human Transplantation*. Ed. by Rapaport, F. T. and Dausset, J. J. Grune and Stratton, New York 1968, pp. 587–600.

66. Morgan, I.: *J. exp. Med.* **85,** 131 (1947).
67. Mushel, L. H., Gustafson, L. and Atai, M.: *Immunology* **14,** 285 (1968).
68*a*. Petrányi, Gy.: *Acta med. Acad. Sci. hung.* **12,** 85 (1958).
68*b*. id., *Magy. Belorv. Arch.* **15,** 65 (1962).
68*c*. id., *Orv. Hetil.* **102,** 1585 (1961).
68*d*. id., *Acta med. Acad. Sci. hung.* **20,** 387 (1964).
68*e*. id., *Orv. Hetil.* **106,** 1873 (1965).
68*f*. id., Unpublished data.
69. Petrányi, Gy. and Kakuk, Gy.: *Acta allerg. (Kbh.)* **22,** 57 (1967).
70. Pilchmayr, R., Brendel, W. and Zenker, R.: *Münch. med. Wschr.* **110,** 893 (1968).
71. Rich, A. R.: *Bull. Johns Hopk. Hosp.* **98,** 120 (1967).
72. Rivers, T. M. and Schwentker, F. F.: *J. exp. Med.* **61,** 689 (1935).
73*a*. Rose, N. R. and Witebsky, E. J.: *J. Immunol.* **76,** 417 (1956).
73*b*. ibid., **83,** 34 (1959).
74. Rose, N. R., Kite, J. H., jr. and Dobbler, T. K.: In *Mechanism of Cell and Tissue Damage Produced by Immune Reactions.* Ed. by Miescher, P. A. and Grabar, P. Schwabe, Basel 1962, p. 161.
75. Rother, K. and Sarre, H.: *Klin. Wschr.* **40,** 429 (1962).
76. Schwartz, R. and Dameshek, W.: *Blood* **19,** 484 (1962).
77. Schwartz, R. and Eisner, A.: *Clin. Res.* **7,** 39 (1959).
78. Shigeno, N., Hämmerling, G., Arpels, G., Boyse, E. A. and Old, L. J.: *Lancet* **ii,** 320 (1968).
79*a*. Sigurdsson, B.: *Brit. vet. J.* **110,** 255 (1954).
79*b*. ibid., **110,** 307 (1954).
79*c*. ibid., **110,** 341 (1954).
80. Stiller, A., Russel, S. and Dossetor, J. B.: *Ann. int. Med.* **82,** 405 (1975).
81. Symposium on Autoimmunity and Genetics: *Clin. exp. Immunol.* **2,** 705 (1967).
82. Turk, J. L.: *Sci. Basis of Med. Ann. Rev.* 1969, p. 278.
83. Unanue, E. R. and Dixon, F. J.: *Advanc. Immunol.* **6,** 1 (1967).
84. Unanue, E. R., Lee, S., Dixon, F. J. and Feldman, J. D.: *J. exper. Med.* **122,** 565 (1965).
85. Vaughan, J. H.: In *Immunological Diseases.* 2nd ed. Vol. II. Ed. by Samter, M. Little-Brown, Boston 1971, p. 987.
86. Wagner, B. M.: *Arthr. and Rheum.* **6,** 386 (1963).
87. Wick, G., Sundick, R. S. and Albini, B.: *Clin. immunol. immunopathol.* **3,** 272 (1974).
88. Witebsky, E.: In 1*st Int. Symp. on Immunopathology* Ed. by Grabar, P. and Miescher, P. A. Schwabe, Basel 1959, p. 1.
89. Witebsky, E. and Steinfeld, J.: *Z. Immunol. exp. Ther.* **58,** 271 (1928).
90. Ziff, M.: *Amer. J. Med.* **30,** 1 (1961).

CHAPTER 35

SYSTEMIC LUPUS ERYTHEMATOSUS

by

GY. PETRÁNYI

Systemic lupus erythematosus (SLE) is a polysystemic autoimmune syndrome with a variable pattern of signs and symptoms and changeable course, characterized by non-microbial inflammatory destructive lesions in some or many tissue-systems and organs (mainly joints, kidney, heart, serous membranes, lungs, blood vessels, nervous system, etc.), by the denominating skin eruption (lupus erythematosus), by numerous immunological abnormalities) including the presence of autoantibodies, depressed delayed hypersensitivity, but chiefly by high titre anti-nuclear antibodies, the LE factor responsible for the LE cell phenomenon and the histological picture of the affected organs.

HISTORY OF SLE

This prototype of autoimmune syndromes became known as an apparently insignificant dermatological disease. The term 'lupus erythematodes' originates from Cazenave [20], although the skin lesion was recognized and described much earlier. Kaposi [45] was the first to report in 1872 that the local skin lesions appearing in acute and subacute forms were accompanied by irregular fever and, not infrequently, by lethal 'concomitant' involvement of internal organs, e.g. enlargement of lymph nodes, rheumatic pains, oedematous swelling of the joints, purpura, pleuritis and pneumonia, cerebral manifestations, etc. Kaposi called the disease with only local skin lesion 'lupus erythematosus discoides', and the systemic form 'lupus erythematosus disseminatus'. He also noted that it was more frequent in women. After this early definition of the disease the number of organs found to be affected by lupus erythematosus disseminatus kept increasing. Libman and Sacks [57] described the atypical endocarditis named after them, then Gross [37] discovered its histological substrate, the haematoxyphil bodies. Baehr, Klemperer and Schifrin [4] studied the involvement of small peripheral vessels and described the wire-loop lesion of the kidneys. Klemperer classified SLE into the group of 'collagen diseases' [46].

Significant advance was made in learning the pathomechanism of the disease by the discovery in 1948 of the LE cell phenomenon by Hargraves [40*a*, *b*, *c*]. Earlier the diagnosis had been made on the basis of the skin eruption of lupus erythematosus. The LE cell phenomenon allowed the diagnosis of SLE even in a variety of visceral diseases without the characteristic skin lesion (SLE *sine lupo*). Soon it was recognized, however, that the LE serum factor too (which is responsible for the LE cell phenomenon) may be absent. This recognition has initiated a debate, which has not been settled so far, on the relationships (*i*) between discoid lupus erythematosus which is a dermatological disease, and 'disseminated', 'acute', 'visceral' or, as usually termed today, 'systemic' lupus erythematosus (SLE) as well as (*ii*) between SLE and those 'monosystemic' *sine lupo* autoimmune diseases which are confined to a single organ or system but are associated with positive LE cell phenomenon, e.g. lupoid hepatitis, many cases of rheumatoid arthritis, sicca syndrome, etc., and further (*iii*) between SLE and those cases which show the clinical signs of the disease but *sine lupo* and without the LE cell phenomenon (SLE *sine lupo, sine* LE). Abnormal immune reactions were also indicated by the relatively frequent biological false positive Wassermann reaction [33, 81]. Nevertheless, the most significant advance has been made by the recognition of the LE cell phenomenon as an immune reaction [43, 62*a*, *b*, 63].

AETIOLOGY

According to the present concept of autoimmune diseases, SLE has no uniform aetiology. In addition to genetically determined or acquired predisposition (lupus diathesis), it is common to attribute great significance to various precipitating agents, although most of the autoimmune diseases ensue without any demonstrable provoking factor. Emotional stress rarely precedes the disease and it seems more likely that severe emotional reactions by external impacts are evoked in the already ill patient. Cold might be a precipitating factor particularly in cases with previous cryoglobulinaemia and cold agglutinins. In discoid lupus erythematodes, sunshine has a deteriorating effect and UV-rays are also harmful in SLE both to the skin lesions and systemic manifestations, not only in the initial phase of the disease but also in its later course. It is unlikely that infection would play a causal role since microbiological affirmation is lacking. Moreover, symptoms attributed to infection, e.g. pneumonia and pleuritis as well as fever, are manifestations of the autoimmune reaction, since improvement may be attained with corticosteroids instead of antibiotics.

Many drugs seem to have a precipitating effect, although it is possible that the drug believed to have played such a role was given to control the initial manifestations of unrecognized SLE. There is no relationship, either chemical or pharmacological, between the drugs most frequently cited as possible precipitating factors in SLE, e.g. sulphonamides, penicillin and other antibiotics (streptomycin, tetracyclines, griseofulvin), isoniazide, para-aminosalicylic acid, phenylbutazone, thiouracil, procainamide, etc. It has been suggested [55, 75] that in 3 to 12 per cent of SLE cases the disease is precipitated by medicinal treatment. Careful analysis of 170 cases observed by us has revealed similar frequency; moreover, in already manifest SLE cases the incidence of drug allergy could be demonstrated in 30 per cent of the patients. This observation indicates that patients with manifest SLE are more prone to develop drug allergy and, on the basis of lupus diathesis, drug allergy might be a precipitating factor.

Anticonvulsive hydantoin derivatives used in patients with epilepsy may provoke not only SLE but also tumour-like lymphadenopathy, indicating that they probably cause SLE by interfering with the function of the immune system, although specific antibodies against the drug as hapten are usually present.

The drug most thoroughly studied from this aspect is hydralazine [24, 65, 68]; it has been shown to provoke a SLE-like syndrome in about 10 per cent of patients taking this drug over longer periods of time [74]. By continuous long-term administration it was possible to provoke LE factor which produced the LE cell phenomenon in part of the dogs [23, 32] and guinea pigs treated [56]. It should be added, however, that the LE factor and anti-hydralazine antibody titres failed to show any correlation. Experimental studies clarifying the mechanism of autoimmune defect in the experimental hydralazine syndrome are still lacking.

That a drug might have played the role of the provoking agent can be readily demonstrated if the drug is discontinued [2, 19, 48*b*, 49, 57, 58, 72, 77, 82]. In such cases the symptoms indicating drug allergy and the concomitant LE cell phenomenon with the presence of anti-nuclear antibodies, and also the SLE-like syndrome, will show rapid improvement with or without the administration of corticosteroids, and no relapse occurs.

PATHOGENESIS

There are only a few of the numerous autoantibodies detected in patients with SLE the pathogenic significance of which is readily demonstrable. It is believed that autoantibodies directed against important humoral or cell-surface antigens may be involved in the pathogenesis. Thus, circulating anticoagulant antibodies reacting against a coagulation factor of the serum may give rise to haemorrhagic diathesis [13, 30, 73]. Of the antibodies produced against cell-surface antigens haemolysin has been repeatedly proved to be of pathogenetic importance, although remarkable differences have been found between the *in vitro* titre of haemolysin and its *in vivo* effectivity as measured by the life-span of erythrocytes [26]. Complement fixing antibodies attached to the erythrocytes caused predominantly hepatic, while those not requiring complement, splenic elimination of the cells [54]. Non-specifically attached antigen–antibody complexes absorbed on the surface of leukocytes and thrombocytes may cause their lesion and depressed number in the blood. Similar non-specific immune complexes can often be detected in the vascular lesions of SLE patients, particularly in the glomerular basement membrane (GBM). The immunoglobulins eluted from the affected glomeruli have been shown to possess significant anti-nuclear activity [47]. Since anti-nuclear antibodies as well as free DNA can be readily detected in sera of patients with SLE [79], it seems reasonable to assume that circulating immune complexes are deposited in the basement membrane and give rise to an inflammatory immune-complex disease (glomerulonephritis membranacea). The activity of the immune complex might be increased by the attachment of complement: the serum complement titre is low during such episodes [38, 51, 60].

Many of the characteristic pathologic findings of autoimmune diseases may be revealed in SLE, however, the only characteristic histological feature not seen in the other conditions is the appearance of haematoxyphil body which may be regarded as the tissue equivalent of the *in vitro* formed LE cell, or the LE body released by the latter. These tissue LE bodies are presumably formed in response to anti-nuclear antibodies in the already damaged tissues, through reaction with the nuclei of injured cells. The antibodies with the highest specificity to SLE, i. e. the LE factor and the anti-nuclear antibodies, have no direct pathogenic action since they are incapable of penetrating intact cells. This is supported by the observation of our own that the activity of the disease and the titre of these antibodies failed to show a correlation during numerous relapses of 250 SLE patients. The same is indicated by the findings that the LE factor and anti-nuclear antibodies pass the placenta of mothers having SLE and can be detected in the infants for 2 to 3 months after birth without causing disease [17], further by the repeated observation that the transfusion of serum containing LE factor fails to cause SLE in the recipient [9, 11, 59]. They might, however, be pathogenic in a non-specific manner, in the form of antigen–antibody complexes; of course, this is a secondary phenomenon although it is of considerable importance in determining the fate of the patient.

It is an important feature of SLE, which might bear some importance as regards its pathogenesis, that in the majority of the cases it affects women. Various authors have found the percentage of female cases to be 78, 89 and even 96 per cent [27*a*, 41, 52]. In our material comprising 250 cases, 88 per cent were women. Although the disease may occur at any age, its onset is most frequent in the 15–40-year age group. The difference between the sexes is less marked in children and among elderly patients. The overwhelming predominance of women in the reproductive age points to the possible role of endocrine factors in the pathogenesis of SLE. It is also conceivable that lupus diathesis is linked with the X chromosome [18]. Some HL-A specificities may be more frequent in SLE patients, but the investigation of a larger number of patients is needed to prove its significance.

DIAGNOSIS AND DIFFERENTIAL DIAGNOSIS

If we see a young woman with a butterfly eruption on the malar regions overbridging the nose, or with erythematous rashes on the face, neck, fingertips, palms, etc. (on skin parts exposed to the sun, some of them healing with hyperpigmentation) and the dry brittling scalp hair getting thin, who complains of weakness, fatigability, weight-loss, fever, joint pains, etc., the diagnosis of classical SLE is made at a glance. Although the more or less typical form of SLE occurs rather frequently, the number of atypical cases is also high. It seems, therefore, reasonable to consider the symptoms and signs with regard to their frequency and importance. SLE is characterized by the simultaneous (but often consecutive) presence of several autoimmune diseases associated with more or less well defined general symptoms of inflammation (subfebrility, fever, increased erythrocyte sedimentation rate, but no leukocytosis, WBC number around 5,000–4,000). Often only these latter dominate the clinical picture. Sooner or later, and for variable lengths of time, either the LE cell phenomenon, high titre antinuclear antibodies and/or the denominating skin lesions can be demonstrated. The suspicion of SLE arises sooner if the number of autoimmune manifestations is higher; in other words, the more pronounced the polysystemic character of the disease, the more suggestive it is of SLE, even in *sine lupo, sine* LE cases (Table 35-I). This holds also for the number of autoantibodies detected in the serum of the patient. If, however, such a polysystemic autoimmune disease is not accompanied by either the skin lesion or antinuclear antibodies (with or without LE cell phenomenon), the condition can only be defined as 'unspecified autoimmune syndrome' [69*c*].

An important problem of the diagnosis of SLE is that discoid lupus erythematosus as well as the autoimmune manifestations observed in SLE (rheumatoid arthritis, pleurisy with or without effusion etc., see Table 35-I) may appear as independent diseases. However, while the association of lupus erythematosus with some other autoimmune manifestations usually justifies the diagnosis of SLE, the association of two or more unrelated autoimmune diseases without discoid lupus erythematosus cannot be diagnosed as SLE unless the patients' serum gives a positive anti-DNA or LE cell test. However, the LE factor producing the LE cell phenomenon is essentially an anti-deoxyribonucleoprotein (anti-DNP) antibody, which is only one of the signs, but not the cause of SLE; its titre is variable even in the same patient, and it might be present with low titres in other autoimmune diseases, too. Thus, the LE cell phenomenon may be regarded as a most characteristic sign of SLE which is, however, not always demonstrable. Its absence does not exclude the possibility of SLE especially in inactive periods. If SLE is diagnosed on the basis of the characteristic skin lesion, actually the LE cell phenomenon can only be demonstrated in about 70 per cent of the patients [69*b*], the frequency being somewhat higher when the test is repeated several times over a longer period. The LE cell test is positive in about 5 to 10 per cent of patients with rheumatoid arthritis (without autoimmune manifestations in other tissues), in 15 per cent of patients with Sjögren's syndrome, and occasionally also in other single autoimmune diseases which are frequently associated with SLE. Furthermore, it might be positive in chronic active hepatitis which is therefore termed lupoid hepatitis, although it is usually an independent disease and rare in SLE patients.

In terms of the above considerations it seems more appropriate to regard SLE as an autoimmune mosaic the elements of which may appear alone or in combinations with variable frequency. The individual autoimmune diseases which also occur as manifestations of SLE (see Table 35-I) should not be regarded as 'symptoms', but as independent monosystemic autoimmune abnormalities which may appear either alone, or in overlapping associations.

This opinion is supported by the follow-up studies of SLE patients (Table 35-II). There are monosystemic organ-specific autoimmune diseases (i.e. local-

TABLE 35-1

*Per cent incidence of autoimmune manifestations in SLE**

Author	Dubois [27b]	Harvey et al. [41]	Petrányi [69a]	Dubois and Tuffanelli [28]	Miescher and Paronetto [64]	Petrányi et al. [71]
Year	1953	1954	1957	1964	1968	1969
No. of cases	62	105	33	520	127	250
1. *General symptoms*						
loss of weight	82	71	70	51.3	60	—
fever	97	86	90	83.6	97	96
2. *Skin*						
all forms	84	85	63	71.5	72	73
butterfly rash	69	39	—	56.7	40	46
discoid eruption	—	—	—	—	16	6
urticaria	—	—	—	—	16	6
bullous eruption	—	—	—	6.9	6	—
purpura	—	—	9	19.8	12	27
photosensitivity	40	9	—	32.7	22	12
mucous membranes	11	—	—	9.1	20	—
3. *Joints*						
all forms	90	90	90	91.9	81	80
transient arthritis	—	—	24	—	40	66
chronic arthr. + deform.	31	27	75	26.3	20	14
4. *Kidney*						
all forms	57	65	27	46.1	61	45
nephritis	—	—	—	—	55	—
nephrosis	—	—	—	23.0	6	—
5. *Heart*						
all forms	—	52	63	—	54	43
cardiomegaly	—	15	—	15.7	30	16
pathol. auscult.	42	44	6	21.3	32	23
congest. heart failure	—	8	6	5.0	10	16
pathologic ECG	—	—	63	35.1	56	43
6. *Serous membranes*						
pericarditis	44	45	18	30.5	15	45
pleurisy	60	57	36	45.0	39	29
peritonitis	24	—	4	11.3	13	—
7. *Lungs*						
atyp. infiltr.	—	22	27	0.9	15	19

* Categories of clinical manifestations — in a somewhat modified form — have been taken from Miescher and Paronetto [64]. In our own cases we omitted the decimals because of diagnostic inaccuracies in the judgment of slighter manifestations.

(Table 35-I cont'd)

Author	Dubois [27*b*]	Harvey et al, [41]	Petrányi [69*a*]	Dubois [28]	Miescher and Paronetto [64]	Petrányi et al. [71]
Year	1953	1954	1957	1964	1968	1969
No. of cases	62	105	33	520	127	250
8. *Liver*						
hepatomegaly	34	32	15	23.2	35	25
jaundice	11	3	—	3.8	6	2
9. *Splenomegaly*	8	15	9	9.0	21	6
10. *Lymph node enlargement*	42	58	42	58.6	48	24
11. *Gastrointest. system*						
all forms	40	10	39	53.2	25	18
12. *Thyroid enlargement*	—	—	—	—	3	2
13. *Parotid enlargement*	—	—	—	—	5	2
14. *Periph. blood vessels*						
all forms	—	—	23	—	20	28
Raynaud's syndrome	26	10	—	18.4	15	5
thrombophlebitis	—	—	15	—	16	10
15. *Central nervous system*						
all forms	—	—	27	25.5	40	28
psychosis	29	19	—	12.1	22	5
convulsions	36	17	—	13.8	10	10
16. *Peripheral nerves*	—	—	—	11.7	14	2
17. *Eyes*						
all forms	32	30	9	30.4	15	16

ized only in one organ or tissue) which frequently occur as partial manifestations of the polysystemic SLE syndrome while others are rarely encountered in such a combination (see Table 35-I).

This way of looking at SLE eliminates the much debated problem of the 'specificity' of the LE cell phenomenon or of the different anti-nuclear antibodies.

Even if the physician takes into consideration the above aspects, he sometimes may be faced with serious difficulties in establishing the 'final' diagnosis. It may happen, for example, that a patient develops rheumatoid arthritis or Sjögren's syndrome and subsequently other systems and tissues may slowly become involved in a disease characterized by autoimmune pathogenesis, leading temporarily to a picture which corresponds to SLE with the classic butterfly eruption, positive LE cell phenomenon and anti-DNA antibodies in the serum. This may,

TABLE 35-II

*Examples illustrating the variability of SLE**

Case No.	Name, date of birth	Sequence of diseases					
1	Cs. J. 1906	1947–1949 DLE	1950–1951 SLE: death				
2	H. B. 1925	1944 ?	1945–1950 Ø	1951 RA	1952 SLE	1953 SLE: death	
3	K. J. 1924	1952–1953 RA	1954 nephritis	1955 SLE: death			
4	V. E. 1929	1947–1949 RA 1955–1957 ?	1950 SLE 1958 ulcus cruris	1951 purpura, RA 1959–1969 RA	1952 SLE	1953 RA	1954 SLE
5	K. K. 1910	1945 DLE	1957–1958 SLE	1959–1961 ?	1962 SLE, nephr. azotaemia	1963 Ø	1965 splenomegaly
		1967 SLE	1968–1969 hepatospleno- megaly	1971–1972 biliary cirrhosis: death			
6	Sz. A. 1929	1950 pleuritis 1963 ?	1951 Ø 1964 SLE	1952 SLE 1965 Ø	1953–1954 Ø 1967 ?	1955–1956 SLE 1969 Ø	1962 Ø
7	Sz. M. 1927	1950 – 1962 arthralgy 1965. X. thyroiditis	1963. IX. SLE 1966–1967 ?	1963. XII. Ø 1969 Ø	1964. II. SLE	1964. X. Ø	1965. V. ?
8	T. K. 1922	1953 RA 1958 ?	1954 SLE 1959–1960 Ø	1955 ? 1964 Ø	1956 SLE 1968 SLE	1957. I. SLE 1969 Ø	1957. XII. SLE, nephr.

	G. I. 1924	1956 A 1963 Hodgkin's disease	1957 Gr. D. 1968 death, post-mortem: Hodgkin's disease	1958 DLE	1959 SLE	1960 DM	1961–1962 Ø
10	U. A. 1925	1958–1959 arthralgy 1968 Ø	1960–1961 SLE	1962 ?	1963 SLE	1964 ?	1965 Ø
11	F. T. K. 1938	1959 pleuritis	1960–1961 haematuria, hypertension	1962 epilepsy, th.: hydantoin	1963 SLE	1964 hypertension, subarachnoid haemorrhage	1965–1969 Ø
12	Sz. I. 1913	1963 SLE	1964 Ø	1966 Gr. D.	1967 ulcerative colitis	1968. IX.–1969. XII. Ø — SLE — RA — SLE	
13	B. J. 1897	1964 jaundice 1969. V.–VI. SLE, jaundice	1965 Ø –VII. Ø	1966 Ø	1967 LH	1968 SLE	1969 ?

* The treatment of SLE at the First Department of Medicine, University Medical School, Debrecen, has changed during the past two decades in the following way: 1st period, 1952–56, small doses of corticosteroids given only during acute exacerbations, occasionally supplemented by antimalarial drugs; 2nd period, 1957-61, vigorous corticosteroid treatment with large doses, then maintenance doses under careful supervision even during remissions; 3rd period, 1962–69, the above steroid treatment completed with 6-MP or cyclophosphamide in lupus nephritis, or occasionally with other cytostatic drugs. There is reason to believe that patients Nos 1, 2 and 3 observed in the first period would not have died with the treatment of the third period.

Abbreviations:

DLE = discoid lupus erythematosus
SLE = systemic lupus erythematosus
DM = dermatomyositis
RA = rheumatoid arthritis
A = arthritis without deformity
LH = lupoid hepatitis

Gr. D. = Graves' disease
? = uncertain symptoms and signs (e. g. arthralgy, occasional mild proteinuria) which are insufficient for a definite diagnosis
Ø = free of symptoms and signs

however, soon subside and the original symptoms of rheumatoid arthritis may return. According to the unitary concept of autoimmune diseases, the simultaneous occurrence or overlapping of various clinically monosystemic 'monoclonal' diseases and the presence of different autoantibodies confirm each other rather than causing difficulties in the differential diagnosis.

These views based on the author's clinical studies of more than 25 years differ in some respects from the views of the ARA Committee expressed in the seventh Primer on the Rheumatic Diseases [25]. The *Preliminary Criteria for the Classification of SLE* published by Cohen et al. [22], may be criticized because leaving out of consideration the differences in weight among the individual criteria, and the significance of antinuclear, viz. anti-DNA antibodies.

In many cases, vague complaints and uncertain symptoms such as subfebrility, elevated ESR, etc. may be observed for some time, even for many months, without any detectable involvement of any of the organs. In such cases, hyperimmunoglobulinaemia and increased titres of various autoantibodies may indicate SLE, or more precisely the aforementioned unspecified autoimmune syndrome, until the LE cell phenomenon, its histological equivalent (high anti-nuclear antibody titre) or skin-erythematodes appear and confirm the diagnosis.

As to the differential diagnosis, it is important to exclude all those diseases which may cause symptoms similar to those seen in SLE or in its different manifestations; such conditions are, e.g., microbial pneumonia, tuberculosis, chronic bacterial pyelonephritis, various haematological disorders (Hodgkin's disease, haemolytic anaemia, etc.). This is a particularly difficult task because these diseases may be present simultaneously. Difficulties may be encountered in distinguishing rheumatic fever since the anti-streptolysin O titre may be elevated in SLE, too. The LE cell phenomenon and high titres of anti-nuclear antibodies (particularly those reacting with native DNA) support the diagnosis of SLE, while in the absence of the classic criteria a follow-up of the patient should reveal the problem.

The most significant laboratory finding in SLE is the LE cell phenomenon, a method based on the supravital *in vitro* demonstration of anti-deoxyribonucleic acid antibody in the serum of the patient. Although there are sensitive techniques for the detection of anti-nuclear antibodies, e.g. immunofluorescence, complement fixation and passive haemagglutination, the diagnostic value and reliability of these methods have been debated [61]. Although anti-DNP and anti-DNA antibodies can be detected in almost all patients with active untreated SLE, they are often present (generally with lower titres) in other autoimmune diseases, and also in some chronic infections (e.g. in leprosy). Soluble nuclear antigens and anti-histon antibody are most frequently detected in patients with progressive systemic sclerosis. Anti-nuclear antibodies of SLE are usually found in the IgG class although they are often of the IgA, IgM and IgD type, while in patients with rheumatoid arthritis they are usually present in the IgM class. At present, determination of the immunoglobulin class to which the antibodies belong has no diagnostic significance [5].

The autoantibodies in SLE are non-tissue specific, they react with antigen present in more than one normal tissue or organ, e. g. nucleoprotein. Most of these autoantibodies often react more intensively with allogeneic and xenogeneic than with their isogeneic antigens. In clinical practice, allogeneic antigens obtained from surgically removed tissues or at necropsy are used for the detection of autoantibodies.

If the serum of a patient suspect of having SLE or some autoimmune disease is tested on an 'antigen panel' containing practically almost all autoantigens prepared from organs, cells or subcellular elements, it is often possible to detect antibodies in relatively high titres against antigens which are not involved in any pathological process *in vivo* [69*b*]. The more antibodies with possible pathogenetic roles are detected by refined techniques, the higher is the probability of the autoimmune or immune-derangement origin of the disease in question. The higher the titre of anti-DNP antibody, the more likely is the diagnosis of polysystemic autoimmune syndrome even if the cutaneous symptoms are missing and the LE cell phenomenon is also negative.

The reliability of the various diagnostic tests depends very much on the technique employed. Technical details, e.g. the preparation of antigens, etc., are beyond the scope of this review, although it is very important that antigens derived from various organs should be of sufficient purity, since if they contain high amounts of ribonucleoprotein and deoxyribonucleoprotein, biological false positive reactions may be obtained with anti-nuclear antibodies independently of organ specificity.

Methods for the detection of manifestations and depressed activity of cell-mediated immunity (delayed hypersensitivity), i.e. the cutaneous tests and *in vitro* methods so far evolved (lymphoid cell cultures, blast transformation to mitogens or autoantigens, lymphocyte migration test, T cell—B cell ratio, production of lymphokines, etc.) are mostly too laborious to be used for routine diagnostic purposes in SLE.

THE LE CELL PHENOMENON

Research work aimed at the clarification of the mechanism of the LE cell phenomenon has cast light on many theoretical problems and has also given rise to new approaches in several fields of clinical practice [40*a*]. The significance of the LE cell phenomenon is shown by the fact that the 20th anniversary of its discovery, or rather of its first description, was celebrated by a special symposium on SLE in 1968 [61]. Although numerous problems have been clarified recently, and considerable efforts have been made to elucidate the nature of anti-nuclear antibodies, most clinicians still believe the LE cell phenomenon to be the most specific of all the laboratory tests introduced to confirm the diagnosis of SLE.

The history of the discovery of the LE cell and LE factor is instructive [39]. Hargraves recognized that the LE cell was essentially an artifact formed *in vitro* in response to the LE factor present in the serum of patients with SLE. The LE factor gave also rise to this phenomenon if the SLE serum was incubated with white blood cell suspensions derived from healthy individuals [40].

The first method suitable for routine clinical work has been introduced by Zimmer and Hargraves and it is still widely employed [83]. Investigations have been directed at (*i*) technical perfection of the method, (*ii*) elucidation of the nature of the LE factor, and (*iii*) evaluation of the diagnostic significance of the phenomenon.

Technique of the LE cell test

The LE cell phenomenon is applied for the *in vitro* demonstration of the LE factor which is present in the blood plasma of SLE patients in certain active phases of the disease. Essentially, the method is based on the incubation of the patients' serum with a leukocyte suspension which contains both slightly damaged cells with easily accessible nuclei and surviving intact granulocytes capable of phagocytosis at 38 °C for periods varying between 30 min to 2 hours. During incubation, the LE factor is attached to the cell nuclei. These nuclei are soon surrounded by normal phagocytes, usually polymorphonuclear leukocytes (rosette formation). One or more of these cells take up the homogenized complex of LE factor

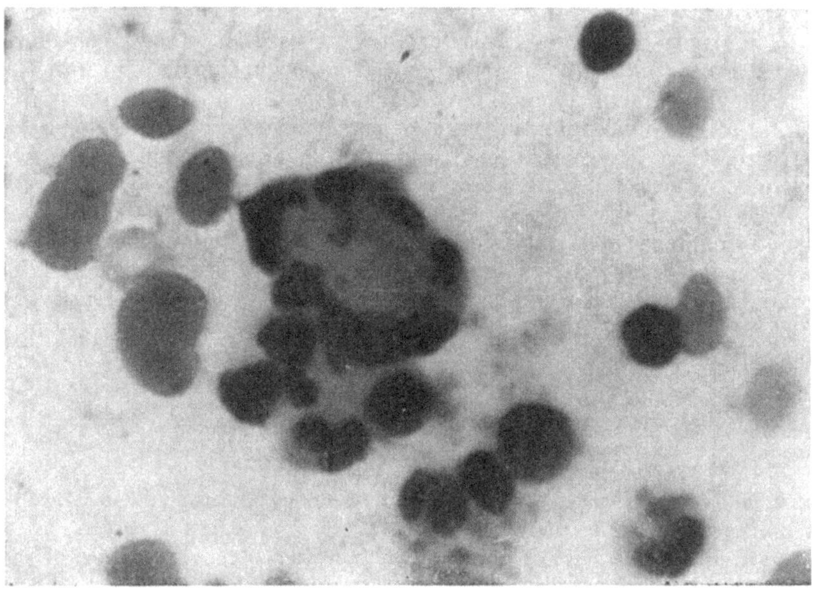

Fig. 35-1. LE cell phenomenon. Typical LE cell

and nucleoprotein, which then appears as a relatively large, rounded cytoplasmic inclusion and has a homogeneous salmon-pink colour with Giemsa staining. The inclusion body pushes the nucleus of the phagocyte to the side (Fig. 35-1). This is the LE cell which subsequently undergoes disintegration, the inclusions also appearing outside the cells as LE bodies. They are similar to the histologic haematoxyphil bodies (irregular aggregates of altered nuclear material found in the fibrinoid lesions) known to be characteristic of SLE. If the time of incubation is varied, the various phases of LE cell formation can be studied, however, for clinical diagnosis only the LE cell is conclusive. If there are many rosettes, or LE body formations, without characteristic LE cells, the examination has to be repeated with a somewhat longer or shorter incubation period before the film on a slide is made. The intensity of the reaction is commonly characterized by the number of LE cells per visual field or per 1,000 leukocytes.

Since the LE cell phenomenon involves, in addition to the serum of the patient, two further components (damaged cells with accessible nucleus or a suspension of nuclei, and surviving intact phagocytic leukocytes), the technique may vary depending on the source of these factors. The simplest way is to obtain all components from the patient with suspected SLE. Nevertheless, it is important that part of the leukocytes has to be damaged while intact cells capable of taking up the LE bodies must also be present. In the original '2-hour clot test' of Zimmer and Hargraves [83], 10 to 20 ml of blood is withdrawn from the patient and allowed to clot at room temperature. The material is then incubated for 1 hour. The clot is removed, and rubbed through a fine-meshed sieve; the cells released are centrifuged from the sediment and a smear is prepared and stained. This technique involves some damage of the leukocytes, however, it has proved superior in sensitivity to the method employing heparinized blood. The difference has been attributed to the process of clotting thought to render the reaction more sensitive; in fact, if coagulation is not inhibited with heparin, thrombocyte clumps are often seen in the centre of the rosette formed. Zimmer and Hargraves [83], however, demonstrated that the difference in sensitivity was due to damaging of the leukocytes in the course of clot formation; coagulation only provides a network along which the phagocytes migrate more readily, facilitating thereby the uptake of cell nuclei already attacked by antinuclear antibodies. This method, however, is laborious, and the smear contains many erythrocytes and disturbing debris. Bobory and Leövey [15] obtained the three factors by centrifuging at high speed the blood withdrawn with citrate, then pipetting off the plasma with part of the buffy coat (plasma with LE factor + intact leukocytes) into a separate tube, then allowing the remaining part of the buffy coat to haemolyse in distilled water, centrifuging, and adding the sediment to the tube containing the plasma and intact leukocytes. Zinkham and Conley [84] damaged leukocytes in a rotating ball mill. Traumatization with distilled water has the great advantage of simplicity, however, in both methods the time required for proper damaging of the cells prolongs the test procedure by about half an hour. Therefore, we have recommended traumatization of a part of the buffy coat by ultrasound [30]; this method has the advantage of being rapid and there being no loss and dilution of the serum or plasma which means that the required quantities are very small. The best smears are obtained when using defibrinated blood; defibrination can be mechanized, reducing thereby the amount of work significantly. There are also micromethods available [12, 67] when working with infants, or with mice, requiring only a drop of blood. If heparin is used as anticoagulant, the optimum concentration with the least effect on sensitivity has been found 0.1 mg per ml [13].

The LE cell phenomenon is a frequently used diagnostic tool which has become almost a routine test in clinical practice. It is, therefore, desirable to use a simple and quick technique which is, nevertheless reliable with regard to both pseudopositivity and pseudonegativity. The use of the patients' own leukocytes makes the test simpler, since no additional donor of the fresh phagocytes is required. On the other hand, it eliminates the possibility of ABO or H-LA incompatibility reducing the sensitivity of the method by increasing the number of pseudonegative cases. Therefore, homologous human leukocytes are no longer used in clinical practice.

The LE factor may be preserved for a considerable length of time if the serum is immediately frozen and stored at −20 °C. The LE cell phenomenon can be demonstrated subsequently by using fresh leukocytes separated from group O blood. Nevertheless, for reasons outlined above, it is more convenient to employ fresh leukocytes obtained from the same patient.

Since the LE cells are demonstrated by microscopic examination in a specially prepared blood film, evaluation will be quicker when the smear contains leukocytes in overwhelming numbers compared with the erythrocytes. If the titre of the LE factor in the serum is low, and there are relatively few leukocytes in the smear, many fields have to be examined under the microscope until a few LE cells are found. Therefore, it is essential to obtain a leukocyte preparation of maximum purity from the patient's blood. The preparation is first surveyed under low and medium magnification, then the areas containing the most leukocyte clumps and LE cells are examined and evaluated under high power using immersion oil.

The evaluation of the blood film under the microscope is the most laborious phase of the method, for which no automatic equipment is available. Care should be taken to avoid confusion of the LE cell with erythrocyte-containing and nucleophagocytosing cells. The latter have been denoted by Hargraves as 'tart cells' [39].

The nature of the LE factor

The LE factor is a 7S γ-globulin [43, 53] with the property of an IgG anti-nuclear antibody [29, 62*a*]. The LE factor has been shown to be neither organ- nor species-specific, giving a reaction with leukaemic leukocytes, with leukocytes of numerous mammalian species, with various spermatic nuclei and moreover with DNA and histones [48*a*, 66, 76]. The most specific antigen of the LE factor *in vitro* is the DNA-histone nucleoprotein [44]. There are several specific anti-nuclear antibodies directed against different nuclear components, e. g. against DNA-protein, nucleic acid, histone or RNA [36].

The LE cell phenomenon is the result of a complex biological reaction in which beside the anti-nuclear LE factor, other serum components also participate.

According to Bencze [7, 8*a*, *b*, 10], there are two types of the LE factor: a thermolabile one which is inactivated at 56 °C within 30 min and is more potent at room temperature, and a thermostable one which is not affected even by temperatures as high as 65 °C. The labile component could only be demonstrated by using the patient's own leukocytes. If the serum contained the thermostable factor, the LE cell phenomenon could be transferred by injecting a few ml of the LE-positive serum intravenously into healthy volunteers or dogs and withdrawing blood after a while from the acceptor; the thermolabile factor, on the other hand, could not be transferred in this way. Bencze has suggested that the stable transferable factor is present in only 4 per cent of SLE patients. Although there are also other possible explanations for these differences in transferability, e. g. binding of the anti-nuclear antibody [21], or the presence of activating and inhibitory factors, it is obvious that the LE cell phenomenon is the outcome of several biological reactions and thus can be affected by a variety of impacts.

Fresh serum contains a factor promoting LE phagocytosis, the activity of which is increased by magnesium ions [2]. Later on it became evident that this factor is identical with complement. The LE cell phenomenon has been successfully inhibited by sera containing specific antibodies against complement [34]. A serum LE factor belonging to the IgM class has also been described which, attached to the accessible cell nuclei, causes swelling and conversion of the nuclei into formations that are similar to the haematoxyphil bodies; however, this reaction is not followed by phagocytosis [25].

The LE cell phenomenon, like every biological test, has numerous sources of error. It is rather time-consuming and not really suitable for quantitative determination of the titre of the LE factor. It is, therefore, not surprising that there is an increasing demand for new, specific immunological methods for the determination of anti-nuclear antibodies. However, neither the antigen consumption test, nor the complement fixation reaction, nor the agar double diffusion technique has proved to be useful for this purpose. The passive haemagglutination method can be used for the routine detection of anti-nuclear antibody, however, opinions differ as regards the antigen to be attached to the erythrocytes. In our own studies involving more than 800 patients [69*b*], of whom more than 80 were SLE patients, anti-nuclear antibody levels were established by the passive haemagglutination method using nucleoprotein antigen prepared from thymus cell nuclei. It was found that the test was positive in patients showing the LE cell phenomenon, however, there was no close correlation between the titre of anti-nuclear antibody and the intensity of the LE cell reaction. While the LE cell phenomenon was positive only in patients suffering from SLE or some other autoimmune disease, anti-nuclear antibody could also be demonstrated in titres of 1:4–1:8 as compared with the normal serum pool also in patients with other diseases and occasionally in healthy subjects, too. There was, however, no appreciable correlation between the actual titre of anti-nuclear antibody and the severity of the autoimmune process.

The technique of immunofluorescence has proved to be of considerable value. Anti-nuclear antibody level in the serum can be established by this method [31]. It is also suitable for the demonstration of tissue-bound antibodies in biopsy specimens, giving typical fluorescent staining patterns. Three main types of immunofluorescence patterns may be encountered on the cell nuclei. These are the homogeneous pattern, the speckled and the nucleolar one, which all may be seen alone or in various combinations [3*a*, *b*]. A rim and an intranuclear fibrillary pattern have also been described [78]. The homogeneous pattern can most probably be resolved into a reticular and a nodular pattern, indicating that the homogeneous pattern is the product of at least two types of anti-nuclear antibodies [12]. Considering all these factors, there must be about 6 anti-nuclear antibodies of different specificities. It is, nevertheless, also possible that other factors present in the serum, e.g. enzymes or antibodies with an inhibitory action on enzymes, affect the tracer reaction. At present, it is not possible to establish a relationship between the various immunofluorescent patterns and the immunoglobulin classes [3*a*, *b*, 35]. Also, attempts to seek a relationship between LE factor and the patterns of immunofluorescence have so far been unsuccessful.

Significance of the LE cell phenomenon

It has already been pointed out that the LE cell phenomenon is not likely to have a significant role in the pathogenesis of SLE. The mechanism of the production of the LE serum factor and of the anti-nuclear antibodies is still unknown, similarly to the origin of other autoantibodies. Two mechanisms have been suggested. According to the first theory, autoimmune diseases are due to some pathologic alteration in the immune system: autoantibodies are produced by specific clones, the proliferation of which is essentially independent of an antigenic stimulus. The other concept is based on the assumption that the anti-DNA-protein antibody is raised against some abnormal DNA protein released into the circulation and the production of autoantibodies is induced by this pathologically altered antigen. In glomerular lesions of nephritic NZB and NZX mice, due to the deposition of circulating soluble antigen–antibody complexes, anti-DNA antibodies could be demonstrated, and in the blood of these mice an antigen containing DNA was found [50]. Administration of DNA caused deterioration of the nephritic lesion. The circulating DNA might have originated from cell nuclei of the organism, however, it might also have been of viral origin (see p. 5). A relationship between the positivity of the LE cell phenomenon and the titre of humoral anti-nuclear antibodies on one hand, and the appearance of the lupus nephritis on the other, could not be demonstrated in a material comprising 80 patients [71]. A much longer follow-up study would be, however, needed to prove or disprove definitely such a relationship.

If we regard the LE factor as *one* of the manifestations of autoimmune pathogenesis, the fact that the LE cell phenomenon may be positive in other monosystemic autoimmune diseases (e.g. rheumatoid arthritis and sicca syndrome) or, conversely, may be transiently absent in patients with SLE diagnosed by cutaneous manifestations, i. e. its specificity, will be readily understood. Although the diagnostic significance of the LE cell phenomenon was compared by Haserick [42] to that of the Wassermann reaction in the diagnosis of syphilis, there are substantial differences between the two tests. Positivity of the Wassermann reaction and the presence in the patient's serum of specific antibodies against the treponema antigens are permanent features, remaining positive for a long time. The LE cell phenomenon on the other hand furnishes no clue to the aetiology of SLE and its presence is also variable. Nevertheless, the presence in the serum of the LE factor is indicative of a pathological autoimmune process, irrespective of the severity and prognosis of the disease. Anti-nuclear antibodies should also be looked for since a high titre (over 1 : 16–32, depending on the method) will support the diagnosis of SLE, but their presence does not make the demonstration of the LE cell phenomenon superfluous.

CLINICAL FEATURES AND COURSE OF SLE

The various 'monosystemic' elements making up the clinical picture of SLE, which may occur in a great variety of combinations, can be most appropriately evaluated on the basis of their frequency in large patient materials (Table 35-I). Some of the components occur much more frequently than others and thus the polysystemic picture may show wide variations, particularly if one considers the time factor, i.e. the sequence of the different monosystemic constituents with their waxing and waning throughout the natural history of the disease (see Table 35-II).

In the first half of this century, SLE was considered to be a disease with fatal outcome to be expected within 1 to 2 years. This was due to the circumstance that the disease was usually recognized only in its full-blown grave form. Since the 1950's, however, significantly less dangerous atypical cases have also been recognized by means of the LE cell test changing the overall picture formed of the disease. At about the same time the introduction of corticosteroid treatment added to the possibility of a less grave prognosis even in cases where the outcome would earlier have been a rapid fatal course [27*b*, 28]. Since early diagnosis is now possible in the majority of cases, and the therapeutic means are of considerable efficiency, the general outlook of SLE has become considerably less severe.

The clinical picture may be judged mild if treatment results in a rapid complete remission lasting for years, occasionally for over 10 years, after treatment is discontinued, and autoimmune disease does not return even in a different form. In the early fifties when limited doses of cortisone were used many patients were lost due to acute general symptoms and the incidence of haemorrhagic exudative pleuritis and pericarditis requiring frequent aspiration was high. Such cases are no more seen if large doses of prednisolone are given in due time. However, there are patients who cannot be completely freed of the symptoms even with continuous high-dose steroid treatment.

Large-dose therapy may not only have dangerous side-effects, but may also be unable to arrest the progress of certain life threatening manifestations of the diseases, like myocarditis (coronaritis), or most often lupus nephropathy.

The frequency of the various elements of the clinical picture of SLE depends on the effectiveness of therapy during the follow-up of the patient. Considerable differences may be encountered when comparing earlier data characterized by striking predominance of acute exudative manifestations with more recent reports on the clinical features where chronic manifestations, at present still resisting therapy, are in the foreground. This change is apparent when studying the follow-up data of some patients of 20–30 years ago and nowadays (see Table 35-II).

The diagnosis of SLE is still based predominantly on the clinical picture, however, it should be recalled that SLE rarely commences with the characteristic polysystemic picture. Often months, years, or even decades may pass before the initial atypical symptoms are followed by the typical clinical appearance, and SLE with the characteristic combination of manifestations can be identified (Table 35-III). Examples listed in Table 35-II demonstrate this peculiarity of the disease. It is

TABLE 35-III

Frequency of the monosystemic manifestations as first signs of SLE in 250 patients (per cent)

Arthritis	38
Skin symptoms	23
Nephropathy	11
Pleurisy	9
Other	19

absolutely inappropriate to expect that all monosystemic lesions will appear simultaneously in the same patient, or even during the entire course of his life.

The monosystemic diseases (autoimmune nephropathies, chronic aggressive hepatitis, etc.) are discussed in detail in the appropriate chapters. It must be stressed, however, that we did not find any difference in the course and therapeutic susceptibility whether they occurred alone over the years or associated in the SLE syndrome.

EPIDEMIOLOGY

In our own material from 1952 to 1974 there was a constant increase in the number of freshly diagnosed SLE cases over the first 10 years (Fig. 35-2). Since then, the incidence remained fairly constant.

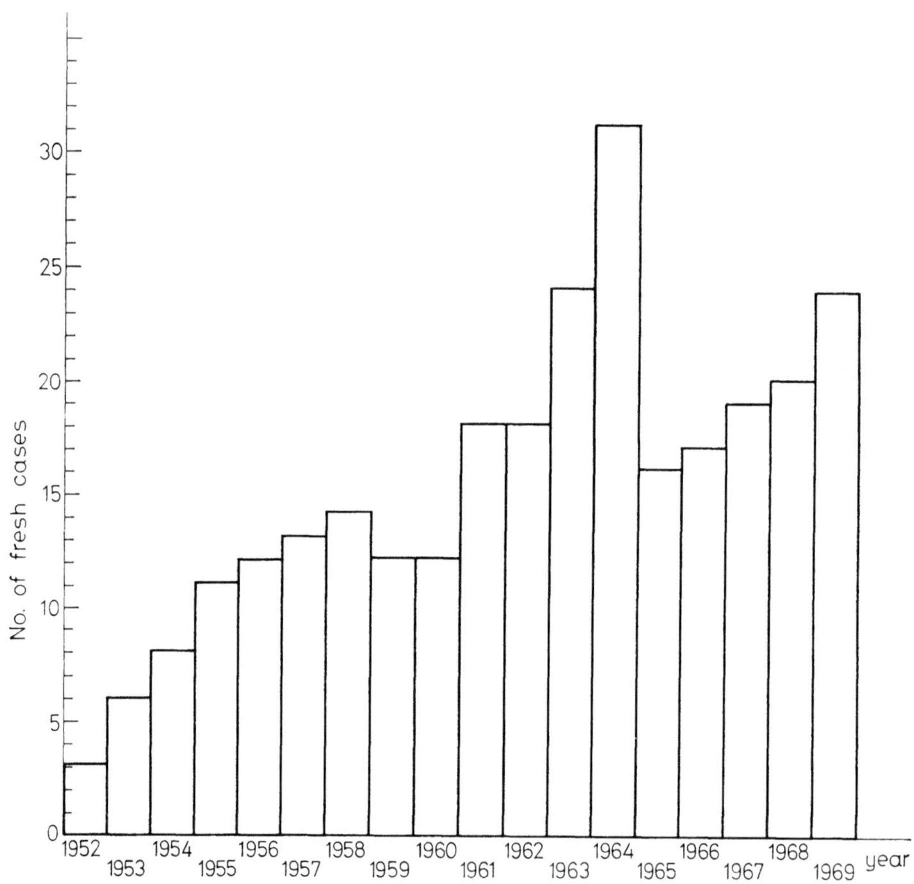

Fig. 35-2. Number of fresh SLE diagnoses made by the author between the years 1952 and 1969

This increase was only due to the more sensitive diagnostic methods and to a better understanding of the disease. Now the morbidity of SLE in our region (north-eastern part of Hungary with a genetically rather homogeneous population) varies around 25 cases per million inhabitants per year. This compares well with the incidence in white women in New York, whereas the incidence in black women (75.4) is considerably higher [25].

It is clear from Table 35-I that the distribution of the different manifestations of SLE in our own material comprising 250 patients did not significantly differ from the data published in the United States. No geographical or racial differences have been reported by other authors either.

THERAPY

The current therapy of SLE is mainly empirical. The consequences of pathogenetical theories including the introduction of anti-lymphocyte serum, have been discussed in the preceding chapter. The treatment of SLE is based on the use of corticosteroids, preferentially prednisolone (Δ-1-dehydro-hydrocortisone) or prednisone (Δ-1-dehydro-cortisone). The aim of the therapy is to free the patient from the symptoms within the shortest possible time and to maintain a possibly complete remission. We start with 40 to 60 mg (8–12 tablets) administered in the morning; if this fails to show an effect within 2 days, it should be increased by 20 mg every day (80, 100, 120 mg). The higher doses may be given in two parts ($2 \times$ 40–50–60 mg). If even this dosage fails to produce a marked effect, supplementary doses should be given intravenously.

During the numerous relapses observed in our 350 patients over a period of 22 years, we were forced to give doses in excess of this only on ten occasions. As soon as the patient feels better, and the fever declines, the corticosteroid dosage can be reduced, most conveniently by 20 mg every third day, until the 60 mg dose is reached; thereafter it is reduced by 10 mg every day down to 30–40 mg. This maintenance dosage is continued until all signs (including laboratory signs as elevated ESR) and reversible symptoms disappear. If the symptoms return, the steroid therapy is reinstituted, the dose is immediately raised to the level which has been found completely suppressive.

On corticosteroid treatment the acute general symptoms and exudations rapidly disappear. The maintenance dose necessary for a practically complete suppression might, after a time, become either insufficient or unnecessarily excessive. The actual suppressive dose should be determined individually and in accord with the requirements, to keep the patient possibly free of symptoms. Since the side-effects of corticosteroids depend largely on the maintenance dosage (size and duration), the dangers have to be considered in both respects. If the effect of corticosteroids is inadequate, antimalarial agent (e.g. chloroquine) may occasionally also be given as adjuvant, if it proves effective within 2–4 weeks and has no ocular or haematologic toxic side-effects. For maintenance the steroid may be given every other day, because the side-effects are better kept under control in this way.

Based on the autoimmune concept of SLE, cytostatic drugs have been employed since the 1950's in the treatment of this disease. Their value is still being debated. According to our own experience, the effect of cytostatic drugs on the various manifestations of SLE with different modes of immune pathogenesis is variable [69*d*]. Experience gained in connection with organ transplantations has suggested that long-term cytostatic treatment should be avoided in SLE. The best results so far have been obtained in the steroid-resistant nephrotic form of lupus nephritis with 6-mercaptopurine (6-MP), azathioprine or cyclophosphamide. We initiated the 6-MP treatment of autoimmune nephritis in 1962 as a routine. Cyclophosphamide may be given in 200 mg daily oral or 1–2 g weekly i.v. doses up to 4–6 g. The therapeutic efficacy of the cytostatics is dose-dependent, too, and an individual threshold must be passed, to get a good effect. This may not always be reached because of toxicity on the bone marrow. However, not infrequently, even daily doses as low as 50 to 100 mg of 6-MP given continuously for at least 5 to 8 weeks with regular control of haemopoiesis have produced complete remission [69*c*, *e*] without toxic side-effects or increased proneness to infections.

The regular and long-term use of corticosteroids in large doses has considerably reduced the frequency of lupus nephritis, while cytostatics may often completely cure severe nephrotic cases of lupus nephritis.

There is need to compare the efficacy of the therapeutic regime with the immune histological and electron-microscopic picture of repeated needle biopsy specimens. Until now the conclusions have been uncertain. Recently we use combinations of the effective drugs for two weeks followed by a fortnight's drug-free interval, to be able to lower the dose of each drug, potentiate their effect, and lessen the side-effects. This resembles the MOPP and VEPP, etc. schemes used in Hodgkin's disease. Preliminary results suggest that this method has some advantages. In non-reactive progressive cases of lupus nephritis the drug combination may be completed with antilymphocyte serum. This method is, however, still under investigation.

Heparin, in often repeated small doses, may give some help in acute exacerbations of lupus nephritis heralded by an early drop of the serum complement level. This may be explained either by its anti-complementary action, or by its anticoagulant action hindering the thrombotic obstruction of the small vessels and glomeruli. Its use is indicated by the finding of fibrin deposits in the biopsy specimen.

PROGNOSIS

Because of the extreme variability of the disease with regard to both manifestations and course, it is impossible to give an overall statement on prognosis. Obviously, there is no arithmetic mean of the two extremes, i.e. the seldom encountered acute cases with rapid course and relatively early lethal outcome, and the mild cases which escape recognition. Nowadays the immediate prognosis is good. The ultimate prognosis, however, must be judged individually, depending on the dose-response to the most adequate treatment. After a time, SLE tends to calm down, with increasingly less frequent relapses, and longer lasting remissions.

Prognosis is undoubtedly improved by regular supervision and adequate co-operation on the part of the patient.

Drug induced or provoked SLE (SLE-reaction) carries the best prognosis because it may completely disappear upon the immediate withdrawal of the provocative drugs or in response to a short course of prednisone.

REFERENCES

1. Aisenberg, A. C.: *J. clin. Invest.* **38,** 325 (1959).
2. Alarcon-Segovia, D., Worthington, J. W., Ward, L. and Wakim, G. K.: *New Engl. J. Med.* **272,** 462 (1965).

3*a*. Beck, J. S.: *Lancet* **i,** 1203 (1961).

3*b*. id., *Proc. Mayo Clin.* **44,** 600 (1969).

4. Baehr, G., Klemperer, P. and Schifrin, A.: *Trans. Ass. Amer. Phycns.* **50,** 139 (1935).
5. Barnett, E. V., Gondemi, J. J., Leddy, J. P. and Vaughan, J. H.: *J. clin. Invest.* **43,** 1104 (1964).
6. Bencze, Gy.: *Med. Mschr.* **23,** 494 (1969).
7. Bencze, Gy., Kovács, J. and Cserháti, I.: *Brit. med. J.* **ii,** 864 (1959).

8*a*. Bencze, Gy. and Lakatos, L.: *Brit. med. J.* **ii,** 1571 (1960).

8*b*. id., *Acta rheum. scand.* **8,** 52 (1962).

9. Bencze, G., Lakatos, L. and Hansági, G.: *Ann. rheum. Dis.* **21,** 76 (1964).
10. Bencze, Gy., Lakatos, L. and Ludmány, M.: *Brit. med. J.* **i,** 1707 (1960).
11. Bencze, G., Tiboldi, T. and Lakatos, L.: *Acta rheum. scand.* **9,** 209 (1963).
12. Bencze, Gy. and Watson, P.: *J. clin. Path.* **19,** 93 (1966).
13. Bidwell, E.: *Ann. Rev. Med.* **20,** 63 (1969).
14. Blondin, C. and McDuffie, G. C.: *Arthr. and Rheum.* **11,** 94 (1968).
15. Bobory, J. and Leövey, A.: *Acta med. Acad. Sci. hung.* **9,** 173 (1956).
16. Bobory, J. and Petrányi, Gy.: *Orv. Hetil.* **99,** 460 (1958).
17. Bridge, R. G. and Foley, F. E.: *Amer. J. med. Sci.* **227,** 1 (1954).
18. Burch, P. R. J. and Rowell, N. R.: *Amer. J. Med.* **38,** 793 (1966).
19. Cannat, A. and Seligman, M.: *Lancet* **i,** 185 (1966).
20. Cazenave, cited by 25.
21. Clark, R. F., Burkhart, C. R. and Bates, H. R., jr.: *Arthr. and Rheum.* **6,** 573 (1963).
22. Cohen A. S. et al.: *Bull. Rheum. Dis.* **21,** 643 (1971).
23. Comens, P.: *J. Lab. clin. Med.* **47,** 444 (1956).
24. Comens, P. and Schroeder, H. H.: *J. Amer. med. Ass.* **160,** 1134 (1956).
25. Committee of the ARA: *J. Amer. med. Ass.* **224,** 701 (1973).
26. Constantoulakis, M., Costen, N., Schwartz, R. S. and Dameshek, W.: *J. clin. Invest.* **42,** 1790 (1963).

27*a*. Dubois, E. L.: *Ann. intern. Med.* **38,** 1265 (1953).

27*b*. id., *Lupus Erythematosus.* Blakiston, New York 1966.

27*c*. Dubois, E. L. and Tuffanelli, D. L.: *J. Amer. med. Ass.* **190,** 104 (1964).

29. Fallet, G. H., Lospatullo, J. and Liff, M.: *Arthr. and Rheum.* **1,** 419 (1959).
30. Frick, P. G.: *Blood* **10,** 691 (1955).
31. Friou, S. J.: *Arthr. and Rheum.* **10,** 151 (1967).
32. Gardner, D. L.: *Brit. J. exp. Path.* **38,** 227 (1957).
33. Gennerich, W.: *Arch. Derm. Syph. (Chic.)* **138,** 403 (1922).
34. Golden, H. E. and McDuffie, F. C.: *Ann. intern. Med.* **67,** 780 (1967).
35. Gonzales, E. N. and Rothfield, N. F.: *New Engl. J. Med.* **274,** 1333 (1966).
36. Goodman, H. C., Fahey, J. L. and Malengren, R. A.: *J. clin. Invest.* **39,** 1595 (1960).
37. Gross, L.: *Amer. J. Path.* **16,** 375 (1940).
38. Hadley, W. K. and Roseman, W.: *Arch. Path.* **83,** 342 (1967).

39. Hargraves, M. M.: *Proc. Mayo Clin.* **44,** 579 (1969).
40*a*. Hargraves, M. M., Richmond, H. and Morton, R.: *Proc. Mayo Clin.* **23,** 25 (1948).
40*b*. ibid., **24,** 234 (1949).
40*c*. ibid., **27,** 419 (1952).
41. Harvey, A. M., Shulzman, L. E., Tumulty, A., Conley, C. L. and Schoenrich, E. H.: *Medicine (Baltimore)* **33,** 291 (1954).
42. Haserick, J. R.: *Arch. Derm. Syph. (Chic.)* **68,** 714 (1953).
43. Haserick, J. R., Lewis, L. A. and Bortz, D. W.: *Amer. J. Med.* **219,** 660 (1950).
44. Holman, H. R. and Deicher, H. R.: *J. clin. Invest.* **38,** 2059 (1959).
45. Kaposi, M.: In *Lehrbuch der Hautkrankheiten.* Vol. II. Ed. by Hebra, F. von and Kaposi, M. Enke, Stuttgart 1876, p. 298.
46. Klemperer, P.: *Amer. J. Path.* **26,** 505 (1950).
47. Koffler, D., Schur, P. H. and Kunkel, H. G.: *J. exp. Med.* **126,** 607 (1967).
48*a*. Lachmann, P. J.: *Immunology* **4,** 153 (1961).
48*b*. id., *Proc. roy. Soc. Med.* **60,** 464 (1967).
49. Ladd, A. T.: *New Engl. J. Med.* **267,** 1357 (1962).
50. Lambert, P. H. and Dixon, F. J.: *J. exp. Med.* **127,** 507 (1968).
51. Lange, K., Treser, G., Sagel, I., Ty, A. and Wasserman, E.: *Ann. intern. Med.* **64,** 25 (1966).
52. Larson, D. L.: *Systemic Lupus Erythematosus.* Little-Brown, Boston 1961.
53. Larson, D. L., Wilkens, R. F. and Dreschler, M.: *Arthr. and Rheum.* **2,** 364 (1959).
54. Leddy, J. P., Hiel, R. W., Swisher, S. N. and Vaughan, H. J.: In *Proc. 3rd Int. Symp. Immunopathology. La Jolla 1963.* Ed. by Miescher, P. A. and Grabar, P. Schwabe, Basel 1963, p. 318.
55. Lee, S. L., Rivero, I. and Siegel, M.: *Arch. intern. Med.* **117,** 620 (1966).
56. Leövey, A., Szegedi, Gy., Bobory, J. and Dévényi, I.: *Acta rheum. scand.* **13,** 119 (1967).
57. Libman, E. and Sacks, B.: *Arch. intern. Med.* **33,** 707 (1924).
58. Lindquist, T.: *Acta med. scand.* **158,** 131 (1957).
59. Marmont, A.: *Ann. N. Y. Acad. Sci.* **124,** 838 (1965).
60. McClusky, R. T., Vassali, O., Gallo, G. and Baldwin, D. S.: *New Engl. J. Med.* **274,** 695 (1966).
61. McDuffie, F. C.: *Ann. intern. Med.* **70,** 413 (1969).
62*a*. Miescher, P. A. and Fauconnet, M.: *Experientia (Basel)* **10,** 252 (1954).
62*b*. id., *Schweiz. med. Wschr.* **84,** 1036 (1954).
63. Miescher, P. A.: *Exp. Med. Surg. (Basel)* **11,** 173 (1953).
64. Miescher, P. A. and Paronetto, F.: In *The Textbook of Immunopathology.* Vol. 2. Ed. by Miescher, P. A. and Müller-Eberhard, H. J. Grune and Stratton, New York 1968, p. 675.
65. Morrow, J. D., Schroeder, H. A. and Perry, H. M.: *Circulation* **8,** 829 (1953).
66. Moyer, J. B. and Fischer, G. S.: *Amer. J. clin. Path.* **29,** 2022 (1950).
67. Mudrick, P., Lee, S. L. and Dividsohn, I.: *Amer. J. clin. Path.* **35,** 516 (1961).
68. Perry, H. M. and Schroeder, H. A.: *J. Amer. med. Ass.* **154,** 670 (1954).
69*a*. Petrányi, Gy.: *Acta med. Acad. Sci. hung.* **12,** 85 (1958).
69*b*. id., Unpublished data.
69*c*. id., *Acta med. Acad. Sci. hung.* **20,** 387 (1964).
69*d*. id., *V. Conf. Hung. Ther. Invest. Pharm. Budapest, 1968.*
69*e*. id., *Autoimmun betegségek* (Autoimmune diseases). Akadémiai Kiadó, Budapest 1974.
70. Petrányi, Gy. and Leövey, A.: *Orv. Hetil.* **94,** 1045 (1953).
71. Petrányi, Gy., Leövey, A., Szegedi, Gy., Kakuk, Gy. and Bobory, J.: *Acta med. Acad. Sci. hung.* **28,** 97 (1971).
72. Ruppli, H. and Vossen, R.: *Schweiz. med. Wschr.* **83,** 1555 (1957).
73. Shapiro, S. S.: *J. clin. Invest.* **46,** 147 (1967).
74. Shulman, L. E. and Harvey, A. M.: *Arthr. and Rheum.* **3,** 464 (1960).
75. Siegel, M., Lee, S. L. and Peress, N. S.: *Arthr. and Rheum.* **10,** 407 (1967).
76. Smith, J. B. and Prichard, R. W.: *Amer. J. clin. Path.* **44,** 487 (1965).
77. Talbott, J. H. and Ferrandis, R. M.: *Collagen Diseases.* Grune and Stratton, New York 1956, p. 27.
78. Tan, E. M.: *J. Lab. clin. Med.* **70,** 800 (1967).

79. Tan, E. M., Schur, P. H., Carr, R. I. and Kunkel, H. G.: *J. clin. Invest.* **45,** 1732 (1966).
80. Turk, J. L.: *Sci. Basis of Med. Ann. Rev.* 1969, p. 278.
81. Ullman, R.: *Klin. Wschr.* **41,** 1159 (1928).
82. Walsh, J. R. and Zimmermann, H. J.: *Blood* **8,** 65 (1953).
83. Zimmer, F. E. and Hargraves, M. M.: *Proc. Mayo Clin.* **27,** 424 (1952).
84. Zinkham, W. H. and Conley, C. L.: *Bull. Johns Hopk. Hosp.* **98,** 102 (1956).

CHAPTER 36

DERMATOMYOSITIS (DM), POLYMYOSITIS (PM)

by

S. KOROSSY

DEFINITION, SYMPTOMS AND PATHOLOGY

DM-syndrome is a severe, generalized inflammation of the skin and muscle tissue associated with degeneration and scar formation. Its aetiology is unknown. Not infrequently skin changes may be absent or insignificant in which case muscular weakness, myalgia, deformity, muscle atrophy dominate the picture. The term PM is applied to denote this condition. According to the generally accepted view [14, 54, 62, 79], the two conditions are the clinical variants of the same disease process.

DM is a relatively rare disease. It is two to three times less common than systemic lupus erythematosus (SLE) [54]. Females slightly outnumber males. The first onset occurs mainly in middle-aged individuals, though two peaks (1st and 5–6th decades) have been observed [34, 44, 61, 83]. The facial erythema (40 per cent) in the acute and subacute forms appears (Wagner–Hepp–Unverricht type) as oedema and a purplish red discolouration of the upper eyelids (Fig. 36-1), often described as 'heliotropic erythema' or 'alabaster facies', and is accompanied by a 'cape-like erythema' on the neck, shoulder girdle and arms. It may involve the nail matrix (Heuck–Gottron's sign) as a periungual telangiectasia, haemorrhagic necrosis or atrophy and keratosis. Furthermore, it may occur as a telangiectatic component with scaly, erythematous, maculopapular eruption over the knuckles and the wrists. In the chronic stage (Petges–Cléjat–Jacobi type) a poikiloderma-like picture (poikilodermatomyositis) develops with plaque-like areas of atrophy and hyper- or hypopigmentation with telangiectasia. Muscular changes (muscular soreness and weakness are the first symptoms) first involve the muscles of the neck and pharynx, later the weakness and tenderness are most apparent in the shoulder and pelvic girdles. With electromyography in two-third of the cases [9] the myogenic character of the process can be demonstrated, but it may be combined with signs of a neurogenic lesion [11]. The value of EMG is generally accepted [73]. The electrial patterns (spontaneous activity, morphology of the traces) permit not only the recognition of the myogenic impairment but also, to a certain degree, the evaluation of the potential development and prognosis of the disease.

Frequently, the histological picture of the skin is non-specific [38, 59]. Many biopsies of the skin show only slight telangiectasia and oedema of the papillary dermis. In the early stage it may resemble SLE (vacuolar pathologic change of the dermoepidermal interface), while later the collagen bundles are homogenized in the

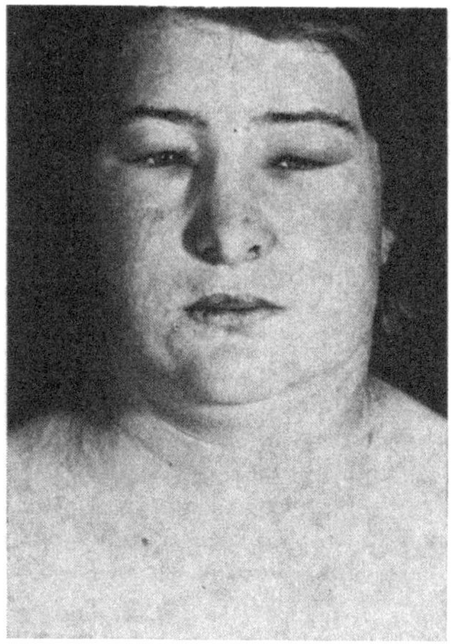

Fig. 36-1. Dermatomyositis. Characteristic binoculars: the eyelid is purplish red, hyperaemic, and oedematous

dermis, and the cutaneous arterioles display a thickening and homogenization of their wall, accumulation of large amounts of PAS-positive substance and fibrinoid necrosis [70]. The muscle biopsy [9, 78, 79] should preferably always be obtained from a muscle which is tender. Myositis is focal. In the acute phase the degeneration of the muscle fibres (loss of cross-striations and a waxy or coagulative type of eosinophilic necrosis) [17] (Fig. 36-2) accompanied by interstitial inflammation is characteristic, where the muscular parenchymal alterations are the primary. There may be a considerable variation in fibre size, some being swollen above the normal diameter and others reduced to collapsed sarcolemmal membranes. The number of sarcolemmal nuclei may appear to be increased (Fig. 36-3). The severely degenerated muscle fibres are surrounded by intact fibres, which is a characteristic feature. The inflammatory cellular infiltrate may vary in composition and intensity consisting first of histiocytes and macrophages and later of lymphocytes and plasma cells (Fig. 36-4). If the process becomes chronic, sclerosis and atrophy of the muscle fibres develop with fibrotic replacement. Interpretation of the electron-microscopic findings is not easy. Damage of muscle fibres in DM is analogous with that found in other autoimmune diseases where the involvement of the muscular system is secondary, merely the degree of the changes exceeds the former [36.] The changes in the mitochondria and endoplasmic reticulum, as well as the presence of numerous lysosomes, are probably secondary, depending on the impairment of the cell functions and on destructive processes.

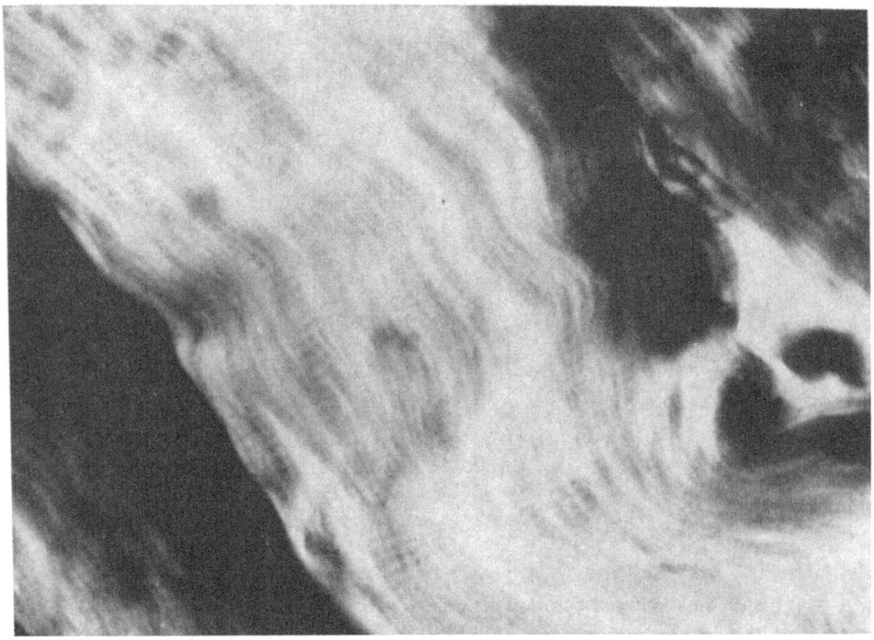

Fig. 36-2. Muscle biopsy specimen from a patient with dermatomyositis. Note the loss of cross-striation at many sites. Iron haematoxylin; ×240 (Courtesy of Professor L. Szodoray, Department of Dermatology, Debrecen University Medical School)

The most striking pathologic changes on capillaries are the following [41]: frequent thickening of the basement membrane and an increased number of cytoplasmic micropinocytotic vesicles in the endothelial cells, which may be due to an inhibition of the transendothelial passage (cytopempsis). The changes of the blood vessels obviously appear earlier than the muscular parenchymal changes. The findings on the sarcomeres strongly support the assumption that the mitochondria and the sarcoplasmic reticulum completely disappear before the glycogen granules are discharged. After that the myofibrils appear altered or show a granular degeneration of part of the myofilaments.

The leading symptom of PM is the weakness of the striated muscles (myogenic paresis) which may be preceded by swelling (subcutaneous oedema). Muscular

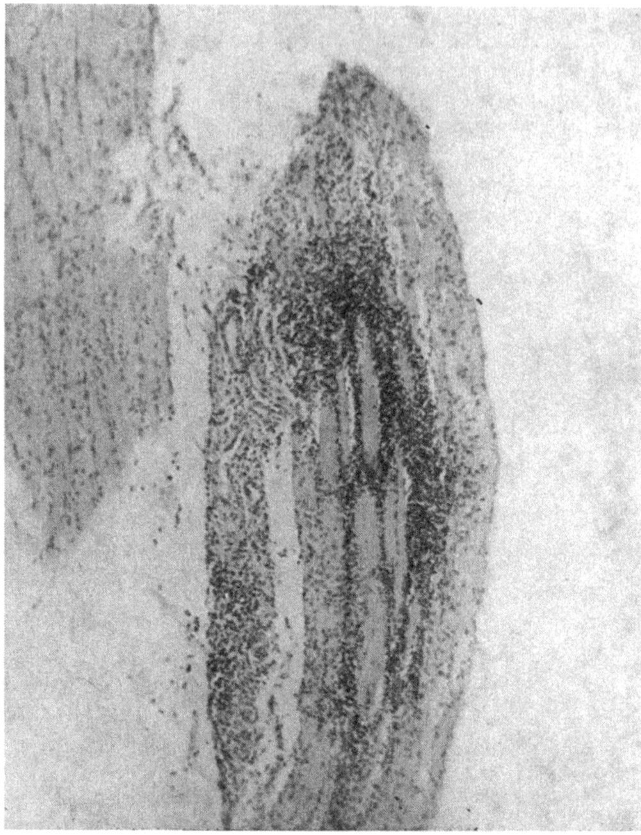

Fig. 36-3. Muscle biopsy specimen from a patient with dermatomyositis: among the bundles of muscle fibres there is massive inflammatory cell infiltration. Note the high number of sarcolemmal nuclei on the left. Some muscle fibres have undergone hyalinization. Haematoxylin-eosin; ×12 (Courtesy of Professor M. Simon, Department of Dermatology, Szeged University Medical School)

pain comes in the foreground when the inflammation reaches also the peri- and endomysium, then follow induration, extensive necrosis of the muscle fibres and weakening of the reflexes; finally myatrophy develops.

Walton and Adams [79] called PM without skin symptoms 'α-type DM', the condition characterized by PM, or DM and combined with other connective tissue diseases 'β-type DM', whereas in cases when PM is associated with neoplasm, they applied the term 'γ-type DM'.

A condition, possibly related to PM but usually considered a separate entity, is paroxysmal myoglobinuria [54]. It is characterized by acute febrile attacks of muscular pain and cramping with myoglobinuria, as a consequence of which tubular renal insufficiency may manifest itself.

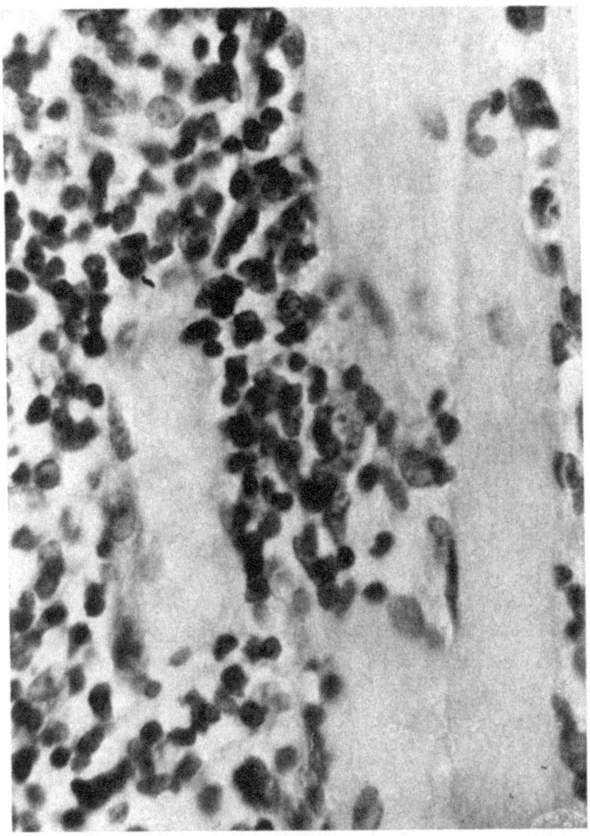

Fig. 36-4. Muscle biopsy specimen showing characteristic dermatomyositic alterations. In the inflammatory infiltration lymphocytes predominate. Haematoxylin-eosin; × 160 (Courtesy of Professor M. Simon, Szeged)

Other organs (heart, lungs, brain, joints, gastrointestinal tract, etc.) may also become involved in the DM syndrome [43]. The myocardium participates in the process in 25–33 per cent [45]. Simultaneously, lesion of the peripheral nerves may develop, though the nervous system may also become secondarily affected, as e. g. in the secondary neuromyositis syndrome. Fatigue, weakness and atrophy appear in succession. Paresis appears relatively late. The pain is not constant, and the contractures are late [8, 77]. (The peripheral neurones are mostly involved, therefore the term distal neuronitis is used [73].) PM may involve the mucous membranes of the mouth and of the genitalia, and the conjuctiva in 10–20 per cent in the form of papules and shallow ulcers. This condition is called dermatomucomyositis (Oppenheim). In contrast to SLE, inflammatory renal disease does not occur in DM, also serositis and leukopenia are rare. Since the clinical and pathological features are particular to DM in children, some authors [7] regard DM of childhood as a clinical-pathological entity ('systemic angiopathy').

Laboratory findings of the syndrome are not characteristic. Erythrocyte sedimentation is slightly increased, total serum protein content is low. Hypergammaglobulinaemia, albumin reduction and α_2-globulin accumulation are not so regular and not so extensive as in SLE. CSF electrophoresis shows a massive α_1-globulin accumulation and a slight initial albumin decrease [29]. Serum enzyme levels (aldolase, myokinase, glutamic oxalacetic transaminase, creatine phosphokinase, lactic dehydrogenase, etc.) are elevated, indicating enzyme activity. Late in the disease when severe muscle atrophy has occurred, enzyme levels may return to normal. Creatine clearance in the urine is augmented while creatinine clearance is reduced, indicating reduction of the active, functioning mass of muscles. Establishment of the correct diagnosis of DM still relies upon the clinical picture, skin and muscle biopsy. Enzyme determinations and other laboratory data are merely complementary.

AETIOLOGY AND PATHOGENESIS

No final standpoint has so far been reached in this respect [14, 34, 39, 40, 49, 54, 61, 62, 79, 83].

Earlier, as aetiological factors, chronic inflammatory processes with poor symptomatology or of latent infectious disease origin (chronic appendicitis, tuberculosis, toxoplasmosis, endogenous infective streptogenic focus) had been mentioned [74]. There are several reports [46, 58, 80] concerning its manifestatiton after viral infections of the upper respiratory tract, chronic hepatitis, enterocolitis, rubella.

Search for a possible viral origin has come into the fore in recent years. Namely, viral antigens, or muscle antigen leaking from muscle fibres damaged by a virus, could trigger off a self-perpetuating delayed hypersensitivity reaction. Viewed against a background of genetically determined immunological hyperreactivity to nucleoprotein antigens, infection with a persistent 'slow' virus or with a defective virus may result in excessive antibody production to these agents or to cell-complexed antigens of these agents with a consequent 'autoimmune' disease [31]. Several electron-microscopic studies have been published reporting the occurrence of endothelial inclusions [58] and paramyxo- or related virus-like structures [18, 31, 41, 42] in the cytoplasm of the endothelial cells of vessels, in the nuclei of muscle cells, and in the fibroblast of skin lesions; further picorna-virus-like inclusions [12, 63], tubular cytoplasmic inclusions and tubuloreticular structures have been found in the skin and lymph nodes [46]. Occasionally, inclusions corresponding to ribonucleic acid-ribonucleproteins are detected in the myositic cells, which are believed to be the closest to a Coxsackie virus variant [22]. Antibody against picorna- and myxovirus can be demonstrated in the serum of patients [39]. Coxsackie B6 and measles virus as eliciting factors are hoped to be excluded by age-specific titre [39]. Presumably, the structures appear as short helical microfilaments within the cell nuclei [31]; others [64] believe that the tubular inclusion types appear like a common denominator to autoimmune disease in man. Nevertheless, since the viral nature of the inclusions is not a decided fact yet, attempts to isolate the virus by tissue culture from such tissue remained unsuccessful, and the use of helper virus did not reveal the presence of incomplete or deficient virus material [32], the possibility remained that these inclusion bodies are merely the side products of myolysis and are not the pathogens of DM-syndrome.

Beside the infectious aetiology it has also been suggested [1, 74, 83] that DM may occur following the injection of foreign proteins such as vaccines or drugs.

As to the pathogenesis of DM, several hypotheses have been put forward (allergy, autonomic nervous dystrophy, endocrine imbalance, altered immune response) [49] indicating a possible multiple pathogenesis of DM.

Primary importance should be attributed in the human pathogenesis to predisposition determined by heredity, the genetic factors of the individual and above all to the entire immune system. Indirect evidence yielded by recent research has suggested that immunopathological mechanisms are involved in the DM syndrome [67]. This theory has been refuted by several authors. It may be classified into the group of the so-called 'diffuse connective tissue diseases' or 'collagen diseases' characterized by the primary disturbance of connective tissue or ground substance, or both, accompanied by fibrinoid alteration and by varying degrees of vasculitis [38, 70], upon the effect of eliciting and deteriorating factors, such as certain physical impacts (mechanical or cold) [83]. However, these signs only define a morphological concept and do not necessarily mean an immune pathogenesis. The individual diseases of the group only differ in their responses to the fundamental lesion [47]. The dysgammaglobulinaemia suspected by Ehrich [26] as a primary pathogenetic factor, is not present in every case. An increase in the level of α_2-lipoproteins in the sera of both tumorous and tumour-free patients occurs, but this is not found exclusively in diseases with an autoimmune origin [66]. In part of the cases proneness to hypergammaglobulinaemia may be found [27], occasionally with increased IgA levels [39], but this is not characteristic of DM, for there are cases even with hypo- or agammaglobulinaemia [69]. It has been described in conditions in which deficiency of humoral or cell-mediated immunity existed. In other cases absence of immunoglobulin or β_1C-globulin in skin or muscle specimens, or failure of the peripheral blood lymphocytes to respond to specific antigens were found [28]. In a patient with DM with agammaglobulinaemia an adenovirus was isolated from several organs; the patient had humoral antibody deficiency and a relative impairment of cell-mediated immunity as well (involving only some environmental antigens) [28].

AUTOIMMUNE THEORY

There are several, mainly indirect data indicating autoimmune origin, though the pathogenetic correlation is unclear [25]. Association of DM with other so-called autoimmune diseases [54, 57, 62], mainly with SLE and PSS has been reported. The muscular tissue may be involved in the pathological process in several autoimmune diseases. In rheumatoid arthritis there may be a myositic focus but without the necrosis of muscle tissue. In polyarteritis nodosa the focal necrosis of muscle tissue is frequent; oedema, pain and the swelling of the muscles being the characteristic signs. In SLE the musculature is affected less and in a well circumscribed manner, but sometimes muscular weakness may be so far advanced that it reminds of PM. In Sjögren's syndrome characteristic muscular changes may sometimes be observed. In progressive systemic sclerosis the muscular weakness may occasionally be stronger than the degree of sclerosis.

The appearance of DM as a paraneoplastic syndrome is worthy of consideration [65]. Namely, association of DM with malignant tumours is fivefold (15.3 per cent) of what could be expected on the basis of probability calculations. Over 40 years of age, malignant tumour has been demonstrated in one-fourth to half of the DM cases [6, 54]. DM is not tumour specific. It occurs mainly in carcinoma, more seldom in lymphoblastoma, sarcoma, thymoma and even in myelomatosis [10]. In 81 per cent of the cases the appearance of DM preceded the clinical recognition or post-mortem diagnosis of the tumour. Since DM may transiently improve or may even disappear in response to the surgical or X-ray therapy of the tumour, while in other cases DM reappears simultaneously with tumour recurrence, an antigenic role has been attributed to the myotoxic metabolic products of the tumour [21]. According to the other hypothesis, muscle and tumour tissue might share some common antigenic components toward which a cross-reacting antibody response is induced. The possibility that the tumour would interfere with the mechanism suppressing, under normal conditions, the 'prohibited clones' has also been suggested. In theory it is not excluded that DM and tumour would be the result of a common pathogenic agent (virus?). In intracutaneous tests carried out with homogenized tumour filtrate [30] or with tumour tissue extract (tumour protein?) [21], an immediate-type reaction was obtained [30]. No antigen could be detected in intact tissue parts. The skin sensitizing humoral antibody could be passively transferred. Naturally, a positive skin test with autologous tumour cell homogenate cannot in itself be regarded as clinical diagnostic evidence of DM. By means of immunoelectrophoresis, an increase in the α_1-lipoprotein fraction was found mainly in the tumorous cases of DM [75]. It is, therefore, important to screen all DM patients for tumours most thoroughly, especially if massive corticosteroid therapy remains ineffective.

The therapeutic benefit derived from anti-lymphocyte serum and immunosuppresive drugs is a further indirect sign pointing to autoimmune origin [67], though the anti-inflammatory effect of these substances must not be forgotten either. The occasional hyperplasia of the entire immune apparatus is noteworthy (generalized lymph node swelling, hepatosplenomegaly). Deterioration in response to physical exertion and UV irradiation may be signs of a self-perpetuating autoimmune mechanism.

Several methods are currently in use for the demonstration of antibodies. With the gel diffusion test [53] positive results have been obtained with striated muscle protein, thus the possibility of humoral anti-myogenic or anti-myoprotein antibody has been raised [62, 68]. In a case of juvenile DM, beside the usual muscle and skin lesions there was frizzy hair and circulating antibodies to hair follicles and striated muscles were demonstrated [3]. According to the authors, the damaged hair follicle would initiate in certain cases of DM the production of anti-hair-follicle antibodies. The indirect immunofluorescent studies did not in general prove to be a principal diagnostic method for DM [82]. Using striated muscle antigen for the test [39], in the acute phase of DM, in the degenerative or inflammatory alterations anti-sarcolemma antibody could be demonstrated, but the sarcolemma fluorescence is not specific for DM because it is positive also in other disease (SLE, amyotrophic lateral sclerosis). With the direct immunofluorescent method, antibody deposition could be demonstrated in certain cases in the basement membrane zone of the epidermis [2, 17]. Positive staining mainly occurred with anti-IgA- and anti-IgM-conjugated globulin, more seldom with anti-β_1C/β_1A-globulin and anti-IgG [82]. In contrast to the shaggy fluorescence pattern characteristic of SLE, the pattern found in DM is less specific and rather homogeneous [15]. The weak nuclear fluorescence is usually associated with anti-nuclear factor eluted from the dermis and allowed to react with epidermal nuclei of skin lesions during the staining process. The cytoid-like bodies are not disease-specific and are of little, if any, diagnostic use [82]. The accumulation of tissue-bound IgG at the site of connective tissue lesion corresponds to the situation of fibrinoid [38]. In the muscle the immune reaction takes place at the site of antibody deposition in the sarcolemma or in the subsarcolemmal plasma [2], where the immunoglobulins are bound to the damaged muscle fibres (tissue antigen) [39]. The location of the immunoglobulin granules along the capillary wall may correspond to the site of the lipoprotein granules originating from myolyis [39]. It must also be borne in mind that globulin deposition along the dermo-epidermal junction may be the consequence of telangiectasis instead of an immunological event [35]. No significant difference has been found between the immunofluorescent behaviour of the intact and affected muscles by some authors [66]. The anti-myosin antibody binding [16] demonstrated in about half of the DM patients is not considered characteristic for this condition because it may also occur in muscular dystrophy, neurogenic muscle atrophy, myasthenia gravis, and even in healthy individuals. Based on these facts it can be stated that the immunofluorescent staining of the basement membrane zone is a useful diagnostic tool in the recognition of DM, though the phenomenon is not disease specific and the evidence is not striking enough to argue DM as an autoimmune disease [66].

With passive haemagglutination and immunoconglutination anti-myosin antibodies can be demonstrated more frequently in the serum of patients with PM than in healthy controls, but not more frequently than in some other diseases (neurogenic atrophy, muscle dystrophy) [16]. The result of passive haemagglutination carried out with striated muscle extract is independent of the degree of inflammation [46]. Therefore, the humoral anti-myosin antibody reaction is more likely to be the consequence than the cause of the disease. The serum of PM patients as well as immunoglobulins [46] may have a toxic effect upon the muscle cell culture, but the toxic effect of the serum on myo- and fibroblast cultures has not been confirmed [39]. In autologous, homologous, and heterologous tissues, a humoral serum factor reacting with DNA proteins has been demonstrated in about one-third of the cases [16, 71]. LE factor may be found occasionally. Tests for rheumatoid factor are positive in about 10 per cent of the cases [9]. The autoantibodies mentioned could be detected only in part of the patients, and also the titres are lower than in other autoimmune diseases. Thus, it is presumable that they are not pathogenic, their function being rather the removal of breakdown products.

CONNECTION BETWEEN DM SYNDROME AND VASCULITIS

This can be best studied in cases of DM of childhood which is predominantly a vasculitis involving connective tissue structures as well as the skin and skeletal muscle [7]. It is found in small arterioles that show intimal hypertrophy and the deposition of fibrin and platelet material in the lumen, which may lead to occlusion. Inflammatory infiltration of the vascular wall or vascular deposits of immunoglobulin and C [81] may be seen (Fig. 36-5). Nevertheless, non-immune aggregation of IgG in DM patients also occurs [33]. Necrosis does not occur, a feature which distinguishes these lesions from those of other forms of vasculitis. Acute muscular weakness may rarely be the presenting manifestations of systemic vasculitis. In contrast to DM, this is almost always associated with a polyneuropathy. Evidence

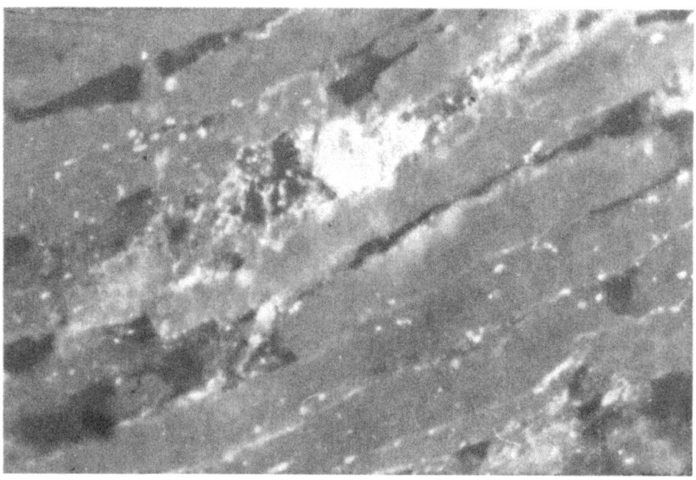

Fig. 36-5. Dermatomyositis. Immunofluorescent technique. Blood vessels between the fibres contain immunoglobulin in great quantities; staining of the muscles is of no diagnostic value. RAHu (IgA)FTC. Leitz Ortholux (Courtesy of Professor M. Simon, Szeged)

of vasculitis in parenchymatous organs other than the gastrointestinal tract is not found in DM. Perivascular infiltration of cerebral vessels has been reported at autopsy in DM [56]. One case of DM with agammaglobulinaemia was associated with central nervous system vasculitis [28].

CELL-MEDIATED IMMUNITY IN DM

In vitro lymphocyte studies have revealed evidence of a cell-mediated immunity against skeletal muscle [23*a*]. The round cell infiltration seen in histological specimens suggests lymphocyte activation [39, 50], reminescent of that found in muscle grafts undergoing rejection [51]. Increased lymphocyte transformation with a muscle homogenate [20, 72] is a rare finding and is mostly only positive in neurogenic muscle atrophy [39]. On the contrary, migration inhibition factor production can be elicited in the effector lymphocytes using muscle extract as antigen [55]. Direct evaluation of the cell-mediated hypothesis would be possible with a cytotoxicity assay that measured the muscle-specific injury induced by patients' lymphocytes *in vitro*. Lymphocytes from patients with α-type DM either destroy human and rat foetal muscle cultures (or fibroblast and epithelial cell cultures in the case of β-type DM) [19, 20, 23*b*] or only exert a toxic effect on mixed myo- and fibroblast cultures [39]. By means of a ^{51}Cr isotope method lymphocyte mediated myotoxicity was shown to be elevated in patients with active disease [25]. There was no evidence of antibody-mediated cytotoxicity. Immunosuppressive therapy (prednisone, azathioprine) exerts its clinical effect by decreasing lymphocyte myotoxicity [25]. Positive intracutaneous test elicited by the autologous thrombocytes of a patient with PM has also been reported [5]. According to recent studies [36*a*], production of lymphotoxins could be demonstrated incubating muscle pieces with autologous lymphocytes and using human foetal muscle monolayer as the target cell. Further, muscle fibre destruction and creatine phosphokinase release from muscle occurred in Maximow chambers challanged with lymphocytes from patients with PM [31*a*].

It is still not known [67] whether the role of cell-mediated immunity is also important in causing DM or whether it is a secondary phenomenon and the mechanism of the initial sensitization remains obscure.

EXPERIMENTAL AUTOALLERGIC MYOSITIS

If heterologous (rabbit) muscle suspension is given to guinea-pig together with complete Freund's adjuvant, a diffuse inflammation, histologically similar to human PM, arises [24]. In some animals the muscle extract elicits a delayed-type skin reaction [23*a*, 37]. This reactivity can be transmitted with lymphocyte suspension to non-immunized animals [76]. The lymphocytes originating from the immunized animals are toxic to the foetal muscle cells, but show no such effect on some other (e.g. renal) tissue cultures [63]. Anti-muscle antibody has been demonstrated [37] in such animals by indirect immunofluorescence technique reacting with the I band and H zone. Other authors [60] using epifluorescence and phase-contrast microscopy on preparation of relaxed glycerinated myofibrils have found that the antibodies are present principally in the A band and Z line regions of the sarcomere. Because A band staining can be absorbed with actin-free myosin, it seems that at least one antibody present is directed against a myosin-associated antigen. Further, experiments by the same authors [60] have shown that the 'myofibrillar' fraction of homogenized muscle produces both a severe myositis and a high and persistent antibody response in injected animals.

In conclusion, Pearson's [62] opinion may be quoted who maintains that clinically and pathologically there is a possibility that some, if not all, cases result from a hypersensitivity reaction. The animal models and the tissue culture results strongly suggest that at least delayed hypersensitivity and possibly circulating antibody are somehow involved in human DM syndrome.

THERAPY

Spontaneous remission may occur, but there are also refractory cases [74]. Treatment may consist of two phases [13]. First only prednisolone is given (occasionally combined with antibiotics, daily 60–100 mg prednisone or its equivalent) because it may suppress the inflammatory mechanisms. After sufficient subjective and objective improvement a logarithmic (first rapid, later slow) decreasing of doses is recommended. Muscular weakness concomitant with the disease may be aggravated by hypokalaemia. Because corticosteroid analogues, such as triamcinolone and dexamethasone, may themselves produce considerable myopathy, prednisone is the drug of choice. Immunosuppressive therapy is then initiated (100–150 mg azathioprine daily, but it may also be amethopterine or 6-mercaptopurine). The beneficial effect of combined corticosteroid and immunosuppressive treatment is noticeable after 3–4 weeks, and thus the corticosteroid dose can be maintained sufficiently low to avoid producing Cushing's disease [13] or, in favourable cases, corticosteroids can completely be abandoned. If remission follows, they should be started again [48]. Anabolic steroids of the testosterone group have been used in an effort to overcome the catabolic effects of corticosteroid and to stimulate muscle hypertrophy. In the treatment of DM the use of antilymphocyte serum has recently been introduced [4, 41]. If the patient is refractory to corticosteroid therapy and shows only temporary improvement to immunosuppressive drugs, thymectomy and azathioprine combined with actinomycin C may be attempted [48]. This combination has been found only just to arrest the progress of the disease and brief exacerbations followed after stopping actinomycin C (which has been given to suppress the activity of T lymphocytes left in the organism after thymectomy). Physiotherapy might be applied to prevent muscle contracture. However, as massage of the striated muscles may raise the serum enzyme level, it should not be applied until enzyme levels are normalized.

PROGNOSIS

While earlier 50–60 per cent of the patients died, by now mortality has dropped to about 15 per cent [68]. The prognosis is favourable in cases not complicated by tumour, but sequelae are frequent (defective state). Muscular wasting is irreversible, therefore the strength of the muscles returns only gradually.

REFERENCES

1. Adams, R. D., Denny-Brown, D. and Pearson, C. M.: *Diseases of Muscle: A Study in Pathology.* Kimpton, London 1967, p. 345.
2. Alexander, S. and Forman, L.: *Brit. J. Derm.* **80,** 86 (1968).
3. Alexander, S. and Stimmler, L.: *Arch. Dis. Childh.* **46,** 363 (1971).
4. Amiel, J. L.: *Münch. med. Wschr.* **112,** 497 (1970).
5. Argenziano, G. and Rossi, A. G.: *Italia derm.* **110,** 517 (1969).
6. Arundell, F. D., Wilkinson, R. D. and Haserick, J. R.: *Arch. Derm.* **82,** 772 (1960).
7. Banker, B. Q. and Victor, M.: *Medicine (Baltimore)* **45,** 261 (1966).
8. Barron, K. D. and Fine, D. I. M.: *J. nerv. ment. Dis.* **128,** 497 (1959).
9. Barwick, D. D. and Walton, J. N.: *Amer. J. Med.* **35,** 646 (1963).

10. Beck, P.: *Brit. med. J.* **i**, 747 (1968).
11. Bekény, Gy.: *Ideggyógy. Szle.* **18**, 65 (1965).
12. Ben Bassat, M. and Machtey, I.: *Amer. J. clin. Path.* **58**, 245 (1972).
13. Braun-Falco, O. and Burg, G.: *Hautarzt* **21**, 391 (1970).
14. Bugár-Mészáros, K. and Korossy, S.: In *Allergie und allergische Erkrankungen.* Vol. II. Ed. by Rajka, E. Akadémiai Kiadó, Budapest 1959, p. 723.
15. Burnham, T. K., Fine, G. and Neblett, T. R.: *Ann. intern. Med.* **65**, 9 (1966).
16. Caspary, E. A., Gubbay, S. S. and Stern, G. M.: *Lancet* **ii**, 941 (1964).
17. Chorzelski, T., Jabłońska, S. and Blaszczyk, M.: *Arch. klin. exp. Derm.* **233**, 219 (1968).
18. Chou, S. M.: *Science* **158**, 1453 (1967).
19. Currie, S.: *Acta neuropath. (Berl.)* **15**, 11 (1970).
20. Currie, S., Saunders, M., Knowles, M. and Brown, A. F.: *Quart. J. Med.* **40**, 63 (1971).
21. Curtis, A. C., Hackenan, J. H. and Wheeles, A. H.: *J. Amer. med. Ass.* **178**, 571 (1961).
22. Daróczy, J. and Walter, E.: *Morphol. Ig. Orv. Szle. (Budapest)* **12**, 81 (1972).
23*a*. Dawkins, R. L.: *J. Path. Bact.* **90**, 619 (1965).
23*b*. id., In *Myology*. Ed. by Kakulas, B. A. Excerpta Medica Foundation, Amsterdam 1973.
24. Dawkins, R. L., Eghtedari, A. and Holborow, E. J.: *Clin. exp. Immunol.* **9**, 329 (1971).
25. Dawkins, R. L. and Mastaglia, F. L.: *New Engl. J. Med.* **288**, 434 (1973).
26. Ehrich, W. E.: *Amer. Heart J.* **43**, 121 (1952).
27. Gertler, W., Helldorf, E. von, Sönnichsen, N. and Thormann, Th.: *Derm. Wschr.* **150**, 227 (1964).
28. Gotoff, S. P., Smith, R. D. and Sugar, O.: *Amer. J. Dis. Child.* **123**, 53 (1972).
29. Göpel, W. and Linke, E.: *Dtsch. Gesundh.-Wes.* **28**, 1272 (1973).
30. Grace, J. T. and Dao, T.: *Cancer* **12**, 648 (1959).
31. Györkey, J., Sinkovics, J. G., Min, K. W. and Györkey, Ph.: *Amer. J. Med.* **53**, 148 (1972).
31*a*. Haas, D. C. and Arnason, B. G. W.: *Arch. neurol.* **31**, 192 (1974).
32. Hashimoto, K., Robinson, L., Velayos, E. and Niizuma, K.: *Arch. Derm.* **103**, 120 (1971).
33. Heimer, R., Martinez, J. and Abruzzo, J.: *J. Immunol.* **104**, 738 (1970).
34. Holborow, E. J.: In *Clinical Aspects of Immunology*. Ed. by Gell, P. G. H. and Coombs, R. R. A. Blackwell, Oxford 1968, p. 871.
35. Jabłońska, S., Chorzelski, T. and Maciejowska, E.: *Brit. J. Derm.* **83**, 242 (1970).
36. Jabłońska, S., Jakubowicz, K., Biczysko, W. and Dabrowski, J.: *Acta med. pol.* **12**, 187 (1971).
36*a*. Johnson, R. L., Fink, Ch. W. and Ziff, M.: *J. clin. invest.* **51**, 2435 (1972).
37. Kakulas, B. A.: *J. Path. Bact.* **91**, 495 (1966).
38. Kierland, R. R.: In *Dermatologic Allergy*. Ed. by Criep, L. H., Saunders, Philadelphia 1967, p. 481.
39. Király, K., Horváth, A., Daróczy, J. and Nagy, É.: *Allergie Immunologie* **18**, 141 (1972).
40. Klemm, D.: *Med. Klin.* **64**, 1065 (1969).
41. Klug, H. and Jost, W.: *Derm. Mschr.* **160**, 81 (1974).
42. Klug, H. and Sönnichsen, N.: *Derm. Mschr.* **159**, 97 (1973).
43. Korossy, S.: *Bőrgyógy. vener. Szle.* **23**, 201 (1947).
44. Korossy, S. and Fehér, E.: *Derm.-vener. Halad.* **6**, 261 (1957).
45. Krosch, H., Schäbitz, J. and Rikirsch, P.: *Z. ges. inn. Med.* **25**, 424 (1970).
46. Landry, M. and Winkelmann, R. K.: *Proc. Mayo Clin.* **47**, 479 (1972).
47. Lever, W. F.: *Histopathology of the Skin.* Lippincott, Philadelphia 1961, p. 382.
48. Lurati, M. and Mertens, H. G.: *Dtsch. med. Wschr.* **99**, 697 (1974).
49. Mankovsky, N. B., Vainshtok, I. B. and Kazakevich, R. L.: *Sovetsk. Med.* **32**/9, 18 (1969).
50. Mastaglia, F. L. and Currie, S.: *Acta neuropath. (Berl.)* **18**, 1 (1971).
51. Mastaglia, F. L., Dawkins, R. L. and Papadimitriou, J. M.: In *Myology*. Ed. by Kakulas, B. A. Excerpta Medica Foundation, Amsterdam 1973.

52. Melly, G. and Mazzei, D.: *Münch. med. Wschr.* **112,** 523 (1970).
53. Midana, A. and Martina, G.: *Dermatologica (Basel)* **135,** 375 (1967).
54. Mills, J. A.: In *Dermatology in General Medicine.* Ed. by Fitzpatrick, Th. B., Arndt, K. A., Clark, W. H., jr., Eisen, A. Z., Van Scott, E. J. and Vaughan, J. H. McGraw-Hill, New York 1971, p. 1518.
55. Moulins, R., Goust, J. M., Deville Chabrolle, Mlle A., Buffet, Mlle C. and Muller-Berat, Mme C. N.: *Presse méd.* **78,** 2315 (1970).
56. Mozai, T.: *Jap. Circulat. J.* **30,** 1292 (1966).
57. Nagy, E., Szodoray, L. and Pongrácz, E.: *Z. Haut-Geschl. Kr.* **33,** 26 (1962).
58. Norton, W. L., Velayos, E. and Robinson, L.: *Ann. rheum. Dis.* **29,** 67 (1970).
59. O'Leary, P. A. and Waisman, M.: *Arch. Derm. Syph. (Berl.)* **41,** 1001 (1940).
60. Partridge, T. A., Mangani, D. and Sloper, J. C.: *Lancet* **i,** 676 (1973).
61. Pascher, F.: In *J. Jadassohn's Handbuch der Haut- und Geschlechtskrankheiten.* Erg.-Werk. Vol. II/2. Ed. by Miescher, G. and Storck, H. Springer, Berlin 1965, p. 523.
62. Pearson, C. M.: In *Immunological Diseases.* 2nd ed. Vol. II. Ed. by Samter, M. Little-Brown, Boston 1971, p. 1039.
63. Prunieras, M., Grupper, Ch., Durepaire, R., Bourgeois-Spinasse, J. and Edelson, Y.: *Presse méd.* **79,** 1463 (1971).
64. Prunieras, M., Grupper, Ch., Durepaire, R., Eisenmann, D. and Regnier, M.: *Nouv. Presse méd.* **1,** 1133 (1972).
65. Reinert-Dietkey, J.: *Z. Haut-Geschl. Kr.* **45,** 241 (1970).
66. Remy, W. and Bockendahl, H.: *Allergie Immunologie* **18,** 183 (1972).
67. Ridley, A.: *Clin. Allergy* **1,** 311 (1971).
68. Rose, A. L. and Walton, J. N.: *Brain* **89,** 747 (1966).
69. Rosen, F. S. and Janeway, C. A.: *New Engl. J. Med.* **275,** 709 (1966).
70. Roszkiewicz, A. and Niedzwiecka Kotowicz, A.: *Pat. Pol.* **23,** 433 (1972).
71. Rowell, N. R. and Swanson Beck, J.: *Arch. Derm.* **96,** 290 (1967).
72. Saunders, M., Knowles, M. and Currie, S.: *J. Neurol. Neurosurg. Psychiat.* **32,** 569 (1973).
73. Schneider, Cl.: *Schweiz. med. Wschr.* **103,** 1145 (1973).
74. Schuermann, H. and Hornstein, O.: In *Dermatologie und Venerologie.* Vol. II/1. Ed. by Gottron, H. A. and Schönfeld, W. Thieme, Stuttgart 1958, p. 543.
75. Stachów, A. and Jabłońska, S.: *Arch. klin. exp. Derm.* **222,** 138 (1965).
76. Takayanagi, T.: *Folia psychiat. neurol. jap.* **21,** 117 (1967).
77. Thiébaut, F., Gruner, J. E., Isch, F. and Isch-Tressard, C.: *Rev. neurol.* **108,** 575 (1963).
78. Vignos, P. J., Bowling, G. E. and Watkins, M. P.: *Arch. intern. Med.* **114,** 263 (1964).
79. Walton, J. N. and Adams, R. D.: *Polymyositis.* Livingstone, London 1958.
80. Westerman, M. P., Martinez, R. C., Medzger, V. A., jr., Tosten, R. S. and Rodnan, G. P.: *Arch. intern. Med.* **122,** 39 (1968).
81. Whitaker, J. N. and Engel, W. K.: *New Engl. J. Med.* **286,** 333 (1972).
82. Winkelmann, R. K., Jordon, R. E. and Moragas, J. M. de: *Dermatologica (Basel)* **145,** 42 (1972).
83. Winkelmann, R. K., Mulder, D. W., Lambert, E. H., Howard, F. M. and Diessner, G. R.: *Proc. Mayo Clin.* **43,** 545 (1968).

CHAPTER 37

PROGRESSIVE SYSTEMIC SCLEROSIS (PSS)

by

S. KOROSSY

PSS (synonyms: diffuse generalized scleroderma, systemic sclerosis, diffuse sclerosis, scleropathy) is a generalized disorder of the connective tissue characterized by inflammatory, fibrotic and degenerative changes, accompanied by vascular lesions in the skin, synovium and certain internal organs. The clinical picture is variable. There occur 4.5–12 fresh cases per 1 million inhabitants per year. Females are affected two to three times more often than males. Onset of the disease is rare before puberty, starting most of the time between the 4th and 6th decades of life.

CLINICAL FEATURES AND PATHOLOGY

In the clinical course two phases can be distinguished: (*i*) a non-characteristic prodrome (oedematous phase); (*ii*) the phase of fully developed true symptoms (indurative phase).

The first oedematous signs appear principally on the acrae. Hypotonic perfusion defect followed by vascular spasms occurs on the fingers or toes, and angiopathy or Raynaud's syndrome is found in 90 per cent of the patients [55*b*]. Then soft tissue atrophy of the fingertips develops. Capillary microscopy, though of secondary importance in the diagnosis [65], is suitable for the separation of PSS from Raynaud's disease on the basis of the deformed, frequently fragmented capillary loops observed in PSS. Plethysmography cannot be used for this purpose [65]. Histologically, at the beginning intima proliferation, hypertrophy of the media then hyalinization, furthermore, sclerosis (without obliteration) and atrophy can be seen in the arterioles and minor arteries. As the disease progresses, elec-

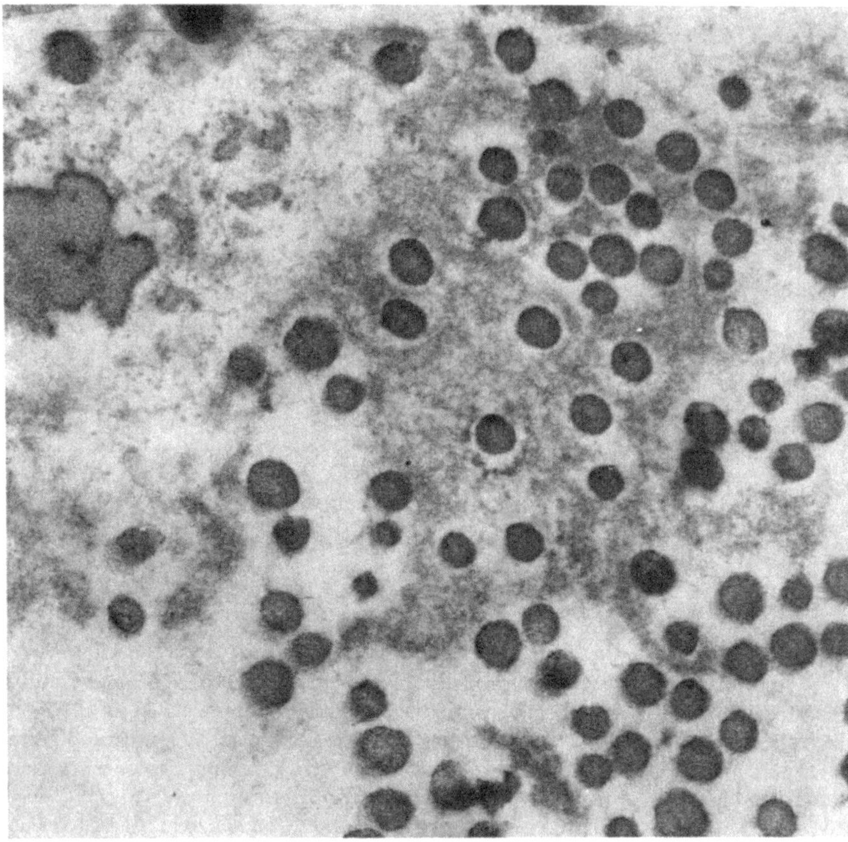

Fig. 37-1. Collagen bundles seen in transection are ensheathed by a granulofilamentous ground substance. Accumulation of this material is primary; it determines the further fate of the collagen bundles and the clinical course of the disease. (Courtesy of Professor K. Király, Department of Dermatology, Semmelweis University Medical School, Budapest)

tron microscopy of the skin [17, 38, 39*b*, 53*b*, 54, 75, 115, 122] reveals, besides mature collagen fibrils arranged in bundles, 700 to 800 Å in diameter, with normal periodicity and surrounded by clear ground substance, more and more fine, immature collagen fibrils, arranged in random fashion; these are 200 to 400 Å in diameter and show an incomplete cross-banding pattern. Abnormal fibroblasts, furthermore, an amorphous mass in the ground substance represented by granular or structureless material that is proportional to the degree of the swelling may also be seen. Homogenization of the dermis appears as well. The protofibrils (the so-called pearl necklace filaments) are reminiscent of the immature collagen fibres of embryonic tissue. The fine parallel filaments with repeated dense bands represent increased fibrinogenesis (Figs 37-1 and 37-2).

Between the collagen fibrils and altered elastic fibres (degenerated and containing granular glycoprotein material) considerable amounts of threads with knobs

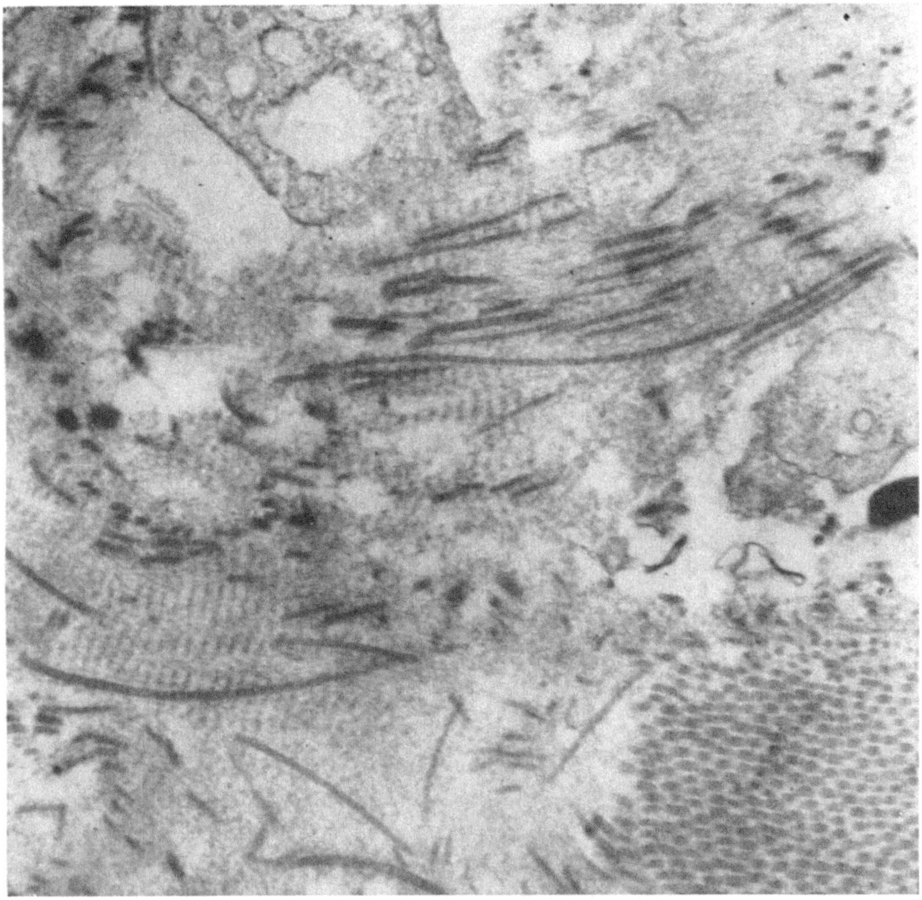

Fig. 37-2. Under pathological intercellular conditions polymerization of the collagen precursors is also pathological. Along with the collagen bundles with normal periodicity, a crossbanding pattern between the bundles is noticeable, due to the altered ground substance eliciting the formation of the so-called fibrous long spacing collagen. The collagen precursors are arranged into 1,800 Å long periods and have a very high acid and neutral mucopolysaccharide content. (Courtesy of Professor K. Király, Budapest)

and lattice-like filaments are located; they represent avid glycosaminoglycans. Using techniques of polarization microscopy [86], the skin compliance, an intrinsic property of the normal dermal architecture, was seen markedly reduced.

PSS is preceded in 4–15 per cent by isolated circumscribed scleroderma (the plaque consists of yellow-brown sclerotic zones that extend continuously), by sclerodactylia or anasclerosis [26, 148]. The opposite may also occur: PSS without scleroderma (dysphagia, oesophagopathy, pulmonary lesion, dental lesion, calcification of the fingertips) [107]. The chest X-ray shows initial diffuse interstitial fibrosis reminiscent of pulmonary tuberculosis or Boeck's disease. Dysphagia only occurs in 10–20 per cent.

The oedematous phase is followed by an indurative, sclerotic condition and, later on, by atrophy (Fig. 37-3). Decreased motility of the fingers, sclerodactylia (33–80 per cent), acroosteolysis, dilated capillary loops with haemorrhage on the fingertips, occlusion of the digital artery, microinfarcts, then scars resembling

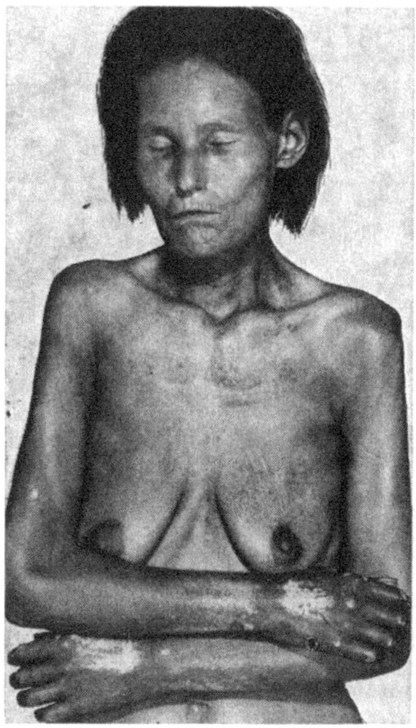

Fig. 37-3. The skin of the melanodermic asthenic female patient is compact all over her body, displaying marked atrophy at sites. (Courtesy of Professor L. Szodoray, Department of Dermatology, Debrecen University Medical School)

rat bites, are the presenting signs (Fig. 37-4). Histologically, the skin [39*a*, 89, 136] is characterized by: (*i*) atrophy of the epidermis and its appendages; (*ii*) thickening of the dermis by fibrosis, closely packed thick collagen bundles but with normal staining properties; (*iii*) homogenization or hyalinization of the connective tissue; (*iv*) vascular changes; (*v*) atrophy of the subcutaneous tissue, replacement of fat by hyalinized connective tissue (Figs 37-5, 37-6 and 37-7). Though the prominent change is often an abnormality and coarseness of the collagen fibres in the dermis, the total collagen may not be increased [14]. Early changes can be

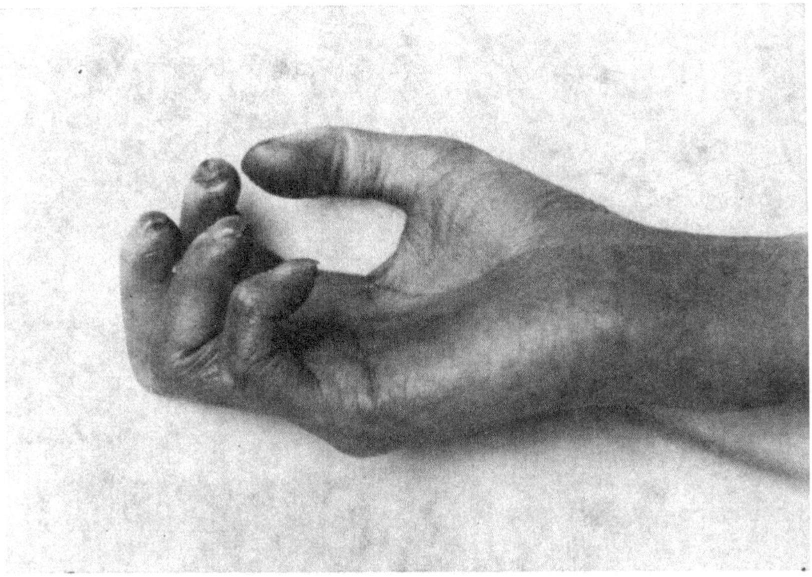

Fig. 37-4. Sclerodactylia, acroosteolysis on the hand, microinfarcts on the fingertips, retracted scars. (Courtesy of Professor L. Szodoray, Debrecen)

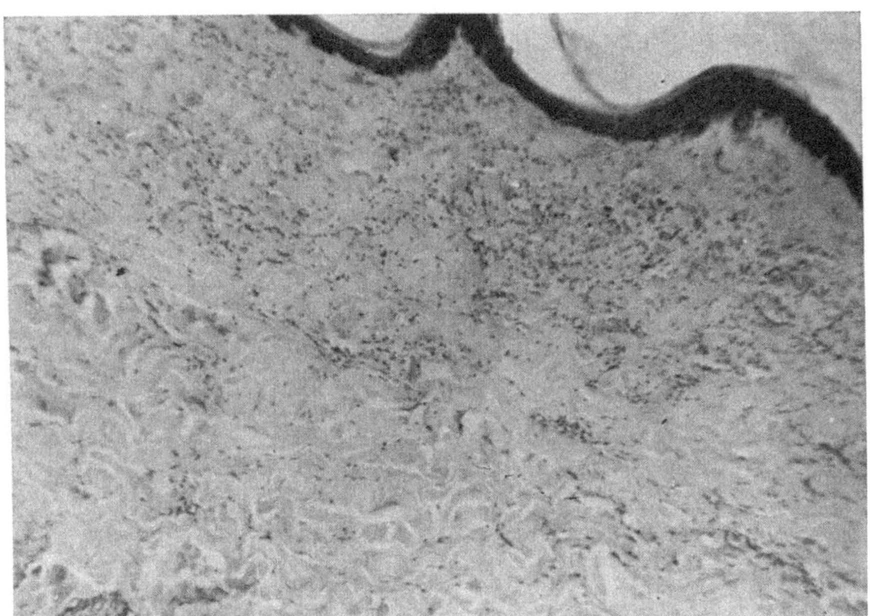

Fig. 37-5. Histological picture of the skin. Note the homogenized collagen bundles and some inflammatory traces under the thin epidermis. HE; ×20 (Courtesy of Professor L. Szodoray, Debrecen)

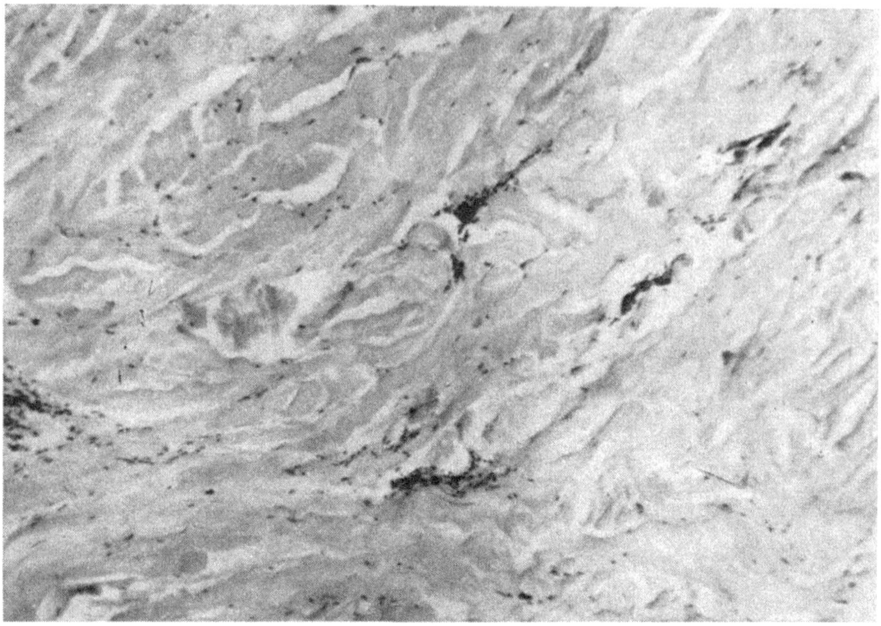

Fig. 37-6. The same specimen as in Fig. 37-5, at higher magnification. HE; ×60

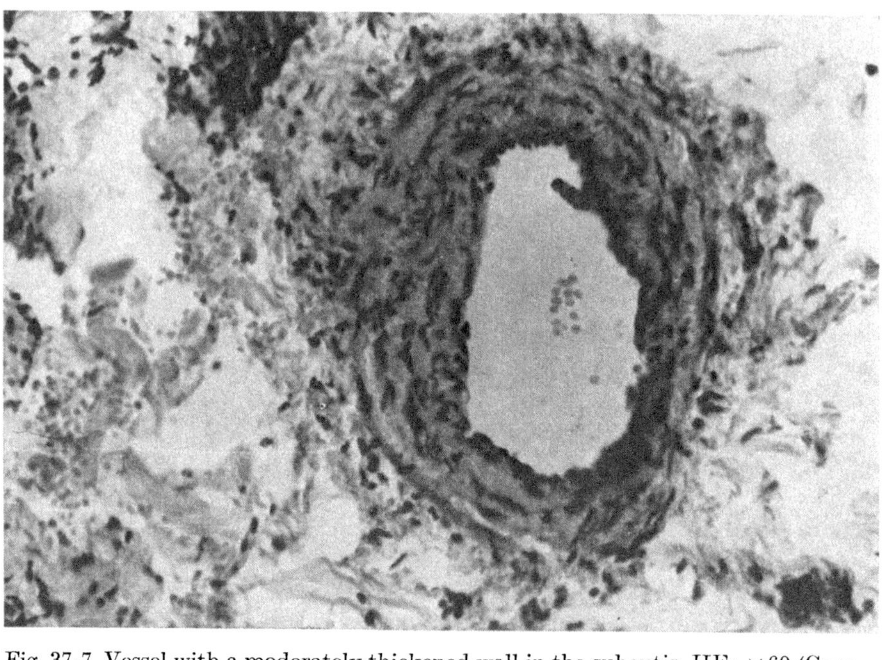

Fig. 37-7. Vessel with a moderately thickened wall in the subcutis. HE; ×60 (Courtesy of Professor L. Szodoray, Debrecen)

found in the subcutaneous tissue [40] and the sclerosis may be partly due to an abnormal architecture of the collagen with a tethering of the underlying tissues or to abnormal forces binding the individual fibres together [94]. As a consequence of the increased Ca content of the skin, circumscribed calcification in the subcutis may arise (Thibièrge–Weissenbach syndrome; 12 per cent). The syndrome in which calcinosis, Raynaud's phenomenon, scleroderma and telangiectasia can be observed simultaneously is called CRST syndrome.

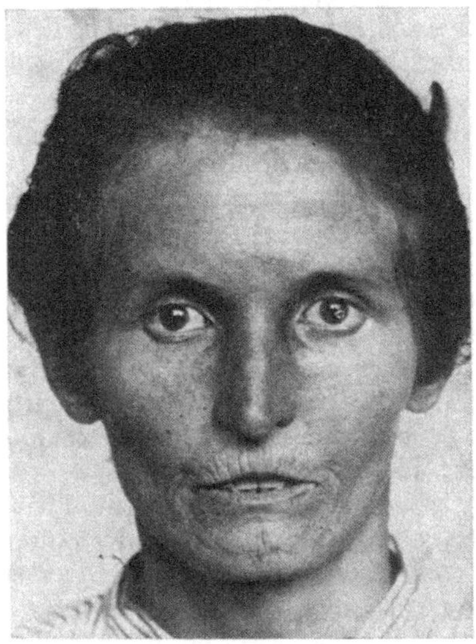

Fig. 37-8. Characteristically tight facial skin (mask-like expression), microstomia, radial wrinkles, loss of the lower teeth. (Courtesy of Professor L. Szodoray, Debrecen)

The symptoms of the indurative phase include tight facial skin, sharp nose, microstomia, radial wrinkles, dry, retracted tongue (microglossia) and loss of the teeth (Fig. 37-8). The involvement of the oral tissues is shown by the widening of the periodontal ligament, the induration and atrophy of the musculature of the tongue, lips and soft palate, resorption of alveolar bone, pseudoankylosis of the temporomandibular joint and sclerodermatous patches in the gingival tissues [43].

INVOLVEMENT OF DIFFERENT ORGANS IN THE SYSTEMIC PROCESS

In the lungs progressive, diffuse interstitial fibrosis (74 per cent; [11, 87]), then bronchiectasis may arise. This is followed by pulmonary sclerosis. At autopsy diffuse interstitial pulmonary fibrosis (23–82 per cent) or compact cystic pulmonary fibrosis ('honeycomb lung') (55–74 per cent), pulmonary vascular changes (18–82 per cent), and seldom pleuritis are found [116*a*]. Pulmonary function test generally shows diminution in lung volumes [60, 91, 116*a*]. The bronchograms show dilatation and distortion of the airways as might be seen in cylindrical bronchiectasis but without the characteristic clinical signs [116*a*]. Body plethysmographic findings show dilated airways, values for conductance may exceed predicted normal values, often diminished lung compliance, i.e. an increase in lung stiffness [116*a*]. The pulmonary findings are not specific for PSS, they are found in all conditions producing pulmonary fibrosis. Sackner [116*a*] described a unique entity characterized by clusters of 'fibrinoid nodules' in the lung and a serum γ-globulin level of 5.78 g per 100 ml. Fibrinoid alterations occur on the pleura.

Sclerodermic heart disease is much more a pathological than a clinical entity. It is characterized by widespread proliferation of connective tissue and degeneration of myocardial fibres [116*b*], pericarditis (fibrinous 18–35 per cent, fibrous 24–30 per cent), pericardial effusion (12–35 per cent), myocardial fibrosis, valvular complication or endocarditis [92]. In the ECG non-specific ST-T complex change and signs of right ventricular hypertrophy are seen [116*b*]. The kinetocardiogram has a greater diagnostic and probably also a greater prognostic value than ECG in PSS [91]. Pulmonary hypertension is an almost ubiquitous finding at cardiac catheterization [116*b*]. The cardiac involvement is evidently rather a secondary phenomenon, the consequence of pulmonary hypertension or systemic hypertension with renal involvement [11, 106*b*, 116*b*].

Sclerodermic kidney is observed in 8–58 per cent of the cases [71, 74]. In contrast to SLE and dermatomyositis, where diminished glomerular function is the outstanding finding, this condition is characterized by vascular changes. The focal alterations consist of intimal hyperplasia of the interlobar and smaller arteries marked by the deposition of a material rich in mucopolysaccharides, furthermore, by 'fibrinoid alteration' of the small arteries, afferent arterioles and glomerular tufts [37*a*, 135]. These changes appear to be indistinguishable from those in malignant nephrosclerosis. In both conditions a preferential concentration of fibrinogen has been reported in the walls of the small arteries. In PSS the renal involvement generally appears in the 5th year of the disease as a severe arterial hypertension associated with rapidly progressive and irreversible renal insufficiency. Terminally, there is oliguria and uraemia, and usually from a few to many small infarcts [19, 106*b*]. The angiogram may show striking constriction of the interlobar arteries and afferent arterioles with a sharp decrease in glomerular filling [82, 110, 145]. This is, however, not disease-specific, because it is also present in arterial hypertension. Some of the renal vascular changes may be the result of spasm. In normotensive patients, effective renal plasma flow was found to be reduced in the majority of cases, while glomerular filtration was normal in all but a few [78, 146], which indicates efferent arteriolar constriction. Normotensive patients displayed a hyperreactivity to angiotensin and cold pressor responses, which suggests the existence of an intrinsic alveolar abnormality [109]. The increased intravascular coagulation may play a role in the precipitation or aggravation of the renal changes, however, the underlying mechanism still awaits clarification. It is also undecided [106*b*] whether corticosteroids have a provoking or precipitating role (inducing or accelerating the progression of pre-existing lesions) because intimal thickening of interlobar vessels in the kidney occurs also in normotensive patients.

Hypotonia and atonia of the oesophagus (54 per cent), dysphagia (55 per cent), gastro-oesophageal reflux, finally *Glasröhren* oesophagus concomitant with muscle atrophy (80 per cent) are the prominent gastrointestinal changes [23, 32, 45, 113, 121]. Involvement of the stomach is less frequent (10 per cent); the incidence of hypochlorhydria is 87 per cent, others failed to find histamine-refractory achlorhydria [15]. In the intestines X-ray examination reveals alterations (sclerodermic enteropathy) in 20–44 per cent, which include duodenal stasis with the sign of the 'mesenteric clamp', delayed evacuation, distension with crumpling of the mucosa as well as pulsion diverticula of the colon [59]. Histological findings in the intestines occur in 48 per cent in the form of circular smooth muscle fibrosis, degeneration and atrophy. Their consequences in the majority of the patients (some years after the first presenting symptoms on the skin) are abdominal pain, vomiting, diarrhoea, increased small intestinal calibre, hypomotility of the small intestine, often atonic and dilated duodenum (loop sign), which may lead to ileus. Steatorrhoea and malabsorption are due to oesophageal dyskinesia. Large colonic diverticula, vasculitis with mucosal microinfarcts, lymphatic obstruction by fibrosis, deconjugation of bile salts and jejunal bacterial overgrowth have also been described. Hepatic involvement may occur, but primary biliary cirrhosis is rare [58]. Attention has been called to disturbances of hepatic kynureninase activity (tryptophan → nicaine-pathway) [13].

Sclerodermic polyarthralgia or arthritis [27, 49, 52, 73, 87, 106c] is characterized corresponding to the lymphoplasmocytic inflammation of the synovial membrane, by swelling, tenderness, redness and warmth with morning stiffness, and decrease in motion of the interphalangeal joints. Later the fingers tend to become fixed by fibrosis and contracture. The radiogram shows absorption of the tufts of the terminal phalanges of the fingers (akroosteolysis) which is often accompanied by subcutaneous calcinosis. Erosion of the bones (80 per cent) first occurs on the palmar aspects of the fingertips. Destruction of the muscle parenchyma may be primary. The electromyogram mainly exhibits myositis-type tracings [7], which are not specific for the disease as they can be observed in other autoimmune diseases as well [65].

Lesions of the central nervous system and the ganglia are rare findings [133]. The sensitive chronaxy is also delayed on seemingly intact skin areas [65].

PROGNOSIS

The outcome of the disease is not always fatal. Remissions may occur at any time. The 5-year survival rate of 727 patients from the Mayo Clinic was 70.3 per cent; after 10 years 58.9 per cent were still alive [142]. In two-thirds of the cases the full course of the disease takes years. The cause of death of those who die within 5 years is visceral involvement and rapid progress. With the onset of renal sclerosis the outlook becomes graver. Death is due in general to renal insufficiency (severe hypertension and eyeground symptoms, increasing oliguria, then anuria and finally uraemia) or to right heart failure (e.g. in connection with intercurrent or aspiration pneumonia) [74].

LABORATORY FINDINGS

Erythrocyte sedimentation rate is moderately increased in one-third of the cases, while in another one-third it is markedly increased [28]. Anaemia occurs (29 per cent) mainly on an Fe-deficient or on an autoimmune haemolytic basis [25, 150]. In the serum the α_1-seromucoid, α_1-glycoprotein, hydroxyproline and glycine levels are elevated [77, 128], while the β-glycoprotein titre may be diminished [24]. The rise in coeruloplasmin oxidase activity is proportional to the extent and intensity of the process [100]. Serum creatine phosphokinase activity is increased [33]. Mucoprotein (protein-bound hexosamine) and glucoprotein tolerance tests are positive [93]. Glucidogram may be used as means of orientation. The values of plasma hyproprotein (collagen-like plasma protein) are significantly greater than those observed in unaffected relatives and healthy young subjects [81, 106*d*]. Urinary hydroxyproline is derived from the breakdown of soluble collagen and more from the degradation of insoluble collagen. In the early stage of the disease 34 per cent of the patients with PSS, while in the late stage only 26 per cent of the cases were hyperexcretors, which is in keeping with the extent and speed of progress of the disease. Urinary glycosaminoglycans is not necessarily an index of collagen metabolism, but may furnish useful information about the connective tissue ground substance and cellular function.

AETIOPATHOGENESIS

PSS is a complex clinical disorder of unknown aetiology and pathogenesis. In the study of the postulated causal factors particular attention is being paid to infectious agents. The occasional streptococcal origin was suggested on the basis of preceding streptococcal angina, increased anti-streptolysin-O titre and positive intracutaneous test. Acid fast Gram-positive bacteria [21], mycobacteria [20] and toxoplasma [31] have also been mentioned. It is of great interest that cytoplasmic filamentous structures, resembling unenveloped nucleocapsid of paramyxo- or related viruses were found in vascular endothelial cells of the kidney and skin and in circulating leukocytes from patients with PSS [48, 70, 96, 141*a*]. Nevertheless, the pathogenic role of the inclusions is not satisfactorily supported. Susceptibility to slow virus infection may be genetically determined.

BIOCHEMISTRY

The skin thickening and fibrosis of internal organs in PSS is the result of an increase in the quantity of collagen [106*a*] although reports on normal or even decreased collagen content of sclerodermatous skin are also known. In the ground substance there is a network of fibrous collagen in all stages of maturation, ranging from the microfibrils secreted by fibroblasts to the tri-helical fibrils with 640 Å periodicity. Microfibrils are released into the ground substance in solution (tropocollagen) and can only be seen by electron microscopy. The tri-helical fibrils are insoluble and undergo progressive cross-linking until they grow into adult collagen fibres [10].

The stability of the collagen fibre depends on the formation of specific lysine-derived intermolecular cross-links between the tropocollagen molecules making up the fibre [138, 139]. The cross-links formed in the newly synthesized collagen are labile aldimine bonds [3]. Analysis of skin collagen from patients with active scleroderma revealed the presence of a high proportion of reducible aldimine bond cross-links. These cross-links are replaced by more stabile, non-reducible ones during maturation. The absence of reducible cross-links in the centre of older plaques and in inactive disease suggests that the diseased skin matures more rapidly than normal skin.

Electron-microscopic studies of sclerodermatous skin have revealed the presence of numerous collagen fibres of narrow diameter and immature banding pattern and of double-stranded periodic beaded filaments identical with those found in embryonic skin. The ultrastructural appearance of dermal fibroblasts also points to the resumption of active fibrillogenesis [53*a*]. A series of drugs, hormones, amino acids and chelating agents were shown to interfere with collagen synthesis [16]. The total collagen content of the dermis is measurable by its content of amino acid hydroxyproline [14, 143], but the evaluation is rendered difficult by the fact that it rises with age, varies with sex and different sites [125] and falls in response to corticosteroid therapy [126]. Increased transformation of radioactive proline into hydroxyproline and also the protocollagen-proline hydroxylase activity increase responsible for it have been demonstrated *in vitro* [69, 143]. The latter findings are, however, not specific for PSS, they are merely the signs of a non-specific generalized reparatory process. The salt-soluble collagen content of the dermis has been found elevated in PSS [144]. The observation of collagenase in the dermis of patients with PSS drew attention to the possible role of collagen metabolism in the disease [151].

The collagen in the dermis is shown qualitatively normal by physical and chemical measurements. The occasional evidence for its altered synthesis or catabolism in PSS is fragmentary whether studied by amino acid quantity, turnover, or metabolism in the skin, blood or urine. The reported changes are probably related to the severity of the disease and may indicate a number of metabolic, toxic or nutritional alterations rather than a primary collagen change causing the disease. The most frequently mentioned qualitative abnormalities of skin collagen in PSS are an increase in the stability of the collagen fibres, an increase in tensile strength and elevated levels of dermal collagen-bound hexose and hexosamine [151]; also the collagen is less soluble in acid buffers and the soluble fraction has a lower ratio of α to β chains than normal collagen [46]. In PSS the collagen fibres do not contain glycosaminoglycans; 1–2 per cent of the fibres have been found to contain neutral carbohydrate components, but the role of these has not yet been clarified.

Several investigators have emphasized the presence in PSS of abnormalities of the ground substance and of its metabolism [17, 46, 47, 58, 151]. The ground substance contains glycosaminoglycans and proteoglycans in considerable amounts. The two major glycosaminoglycans of vertebrate and human skin are hyaluronic acid and dermatan sulphate. Heparin presumably is found in mast cells and not in the ground substance [42]. The hyaluronidase content is normal in the majority of the cases [41]. The specific radioactivity of sulphate ester groups, radioactive hexosamine and proline increase in patients with PSS as compared to the controls [12]. Radiobiochemical and infrared analysis of the *in vitro* synthesized product of skin cells of patients with PSS was found to exhibit a relative increase in C_6-esterified sulphate groups [79]. An increased deposition of chondroitin-4,6-sulphate and total (acid and sulphated) glycosaminoglycans was demonstrated with histochemical methods in the skin [79, 143]. The levels of glycosaminoglycans in the dermis are not routinely altered, but in severe disease, the urinary values are elevated as expressed by the ratio of uronic acid to creatine [50]. The content of uronic acid grows to 4.4-fold in the skin of patients with PSS [79].

A binding to collagen of chondroitin-4-sulphates, dermatan sulphates, heparan sulphates, heparin and proteoglycans of chondroitin sulphate and dermatan sulphate was observed [41, 98]. The complex formation was electrostatic in nature and was abolished with increasing ionic strength. Keratan sulphate did not bind to collagen. The interaction seemed to be increased with increasing chain length of the polysaccharide and increasing charge density. The properties of the polysaccharide chains *per se* are of importance for the mode of reaction between the proteoglycans and collagen. Hyaluronic acid was not to any significant extent bound to collagen [98].

The importance of biochemical findings is doubted by some investigators on the ground that these findings are in a great number of cases the consequences of the activated non-specific repair and do not indicate primary alterations. These biochemical examinations, nevertheless, do have some bearing, because the final form and arrangement of collagen fibres in any area are the result of the interplay between the tropocollagen molecules in solution and the protein–polysaccharide complexes also present. It seems probable that the sclerotic nature of the lesions in PSS is the result of a disturbance in the interaction of these two major connective tissue constituents [46]. The disturbed function, the acid mucopolysaccharides (proteoglycans) having a matrix-like function, may increase the rate of biosynthesis of fibrillar collagen which is normally in balance with the former [72]. It has been suggested that the imbalance between production and reabsorption of the fibrils may lead to collagen excess and to overstabilization of the fibrils by excessive cross-linkage either within the fibrils or between the tropocollagen molecules [46]. The qualitative and quantitative deviation of the ground substance from the normal can be imagined in various ways; it may be due to the genuine damage of fibrocytes, i.e. pathological production of intercellular substance and fibrous precursor, but it may also be due to a vascular process.

VASCULAR INJURY

Vascular changes in PSS can be distinguished from other types of vasculitis by the mucoid proliferation of the intima.

Although the cause of vascular injury is unknown, it has been postulated [97] that systemic vasculature may be the primary target organ of the disease process. Large-artery disease is extremely rare; lesions of minor arteries and arterioles are common, while capillary lesions are virtually universal [97]. The most characteristic feature is a concentric thickening of the intima through deposition of a mucoid substance which stains with PAS and Alcian blue. The thickening may considerably narrow the lumen of the vessels, but without thrombus formation. The mucoid substance deposition may gradually give way to hyalinization. The fibrinoid alteration of the vessel wall, the infiltration by fibrin of the muscle tissue of the media and its necrosis resemble allergic necrotizing arteritis [58]. It appears that after the primary involvement of the vessels, mucopolysaccharides pass from the blood into the connective tissue ground substance in the form of exudation towards the tissues. The vascular changes, especially in the more active form of PSS, can be found in all organs involved, but their presence in the kidney has been most closely documented. In the kidney the fibrinoid alteration of the afferent glomerular arterioles is indistinguishable from the lesions in malignant hypertension. The larger vessels, such as the interlobar arteries, show a more specific lesion in the form of pronounced luminal restriction by considerable intimal and subintimal deposition of some mucoprotein.

Small foci of lymphocytes may be observed about the blood vessels [151]. The mast cell population is normal. A major feature of PSS is the minimal cellular inflammation [151]. Inflammation reaction, best seen in the involved synovial membrane of the joints [27], is almost exclusively of a mononuclear character, implying an immunological association [46]. Polymorphonuclear cells are not seen, and their absence helps to exclude not only the presence of pyogenic microbial agents but perhaps those examples of antigen–antibody complexes which fix complement and hence attract neutrophil cells [46].

THE ROLE OF DIFFERENT FACTORS IN THE PATHOGENESIS

A genetical background is suggested by immunological abnormalities which may be found in the family of PSS patients (hypergammaglobulinaemia, hypocomplementaemia, the presence of rheumatoid and anti-nuclear factors, biological false positive syphilis seroreaction), and by the sporadically occurring scleroderma [63, 77]. Chromosomal breakage has also been described in PSS [35, 57], which implies some toxic change and perhaps genetic susceptibility to toxic substances [151].

Endocrine disorders may be involved as suggested by the therapeutic benefit derived from sex hormones [76, 77] and by the role of progestogens in delaying the cross-linking of collagen. Participation of the adrenals has also been suggested on the basis of generalized melanodermia, asthenia profunda and hypotension occurring in severe PSS [58]. The hypothesis that excess of endogenous catecholamines (norepinephrine and/or epinephrine) in the plasma, which is due to the inability of the tissues of these patients to destroy them oxidatively, may play a role in the pathogenesis of PSS [118] has failed to find support.

Attempts have been made to clarify the role of the nervous system. Apparently, it plays some part in scleroderma of all types [62]. Reference has been made to the zoniform appearance of certain types of localized scleroderma (*en coup de sabre*, or facial atrophy variants) [59], to the disturbed functional balance of the autonomic nervous system in PSS, which can be noted in the terminal part of the vessels [22, 58, 74], to the impaired motility of the oesophagus [58], though the latter may also be of a myogenic nature, to a variety of autonomic and somatic nervous symptoms and disturbances observed at neurological examination [22].

A certain degree of syntropy with malignant diseases, mainly lung cancer (bronchoalveolar carcinoma in half of the cases) can be established, and females are affected in the majority [8, 90, 116*a*]. Although the correlation did not prove to be significant, a rising tendency has been evident for the last 20 years.

The role of environmental factors has been suggested by the frequency of the disease in coal miners, where silicosis perhaps may serve as a predisposing factor [108]. The possible triggering role of external stimuli has also been investigated [141*a*].

IMMUNOLOGY

Of the postulated pathogenetic conceptions the immunopathological mechanisms have been the most thoroughly studied in recent years. Classification of PSS into the group of autoimmune diseases has been raised; nevertheless, almost all the criteria can be refuted by so many counterarguments. Thus (*i*) the systemic 'fibrinoid alteration' of the connective tissue of the intercellular ground substance is not a disease-specific morphological feature and does not in itself prove an autoimmune origin. (*ii*) Laboratory findings occurring in several autoimmune diseases, e. g. autoantibodies (principally anti-nuclear factor) have been demonstrated in PSS, which may have a significance in the pathogenesis. Nevertheless, it is important to distinguish between cause and effect. (*iii*) The viscerocutaneous phenomena in PSS show the same distribution as in autoimmune diseases. Nevertheless, this analogy may be attributed to the occurrence of a mixed connective tissue disease or overlap syndrome, and does not necessarily imply a common pathogenesis. (*iv*) The simultaneous occurrence of PSS with, or its transition into, other autoimmune diseases like SLE, dermatomyosis, rheumatoid arthritis, Sjögren's syndrome, or autoimmune thyroiditis has also been reported [123]. Positivity of the LE cell phenomenon varies between 2.5 and 5 per cent in PSS. In case of positivity its association with SLE must be excluded [34]. It is hard to decide in some cases whether the organic changes are due to PSS or some previous disease. Thymic hyperplasia is an isolated autopsy finding [12]. (*v*) The self-perpetuating character of the disease is a common feature of autoimmune diseases. The antibody titre response if e. g., PSS has been preceded by some infectious disease, may remain in the background, or may even be absent. In other cases immune reactions come into the fore both clinically and serologically.

It has also been proposed that the constituents of the body's own tissues, e.g. the cellular components or ground substance of the connective tissue might have an autoantigenic role. The shift of pH to acidity in the inflamed area, the rise in temperature and enzyme activation may be jointly responsible for the release of the soluble tropocollagen, partly denatured collagen, or gel-precursor (self-antigens) giving rise to autoimmunization. The antibodies produced would enter into reaction not only with the determinants of the altered collagen substance ('anti-hapten') but also with the non-altered collagen ('anti-conjugate'), and even with the carrier substance ('anti-carrier protein') because of the possibility of cross-reaction. The antigen–antibody reaction, taking place primarily in the fibrocytes, would start the production of immune cells (lymphocytes and plasma cells committed against collagen). There is, however, no explanation for the beginning and initial phase of the process.

The possible role of collagen as an antigen has intrigued several investigators, for though collagen is metabolically inert, it is possible that it does have an antigenic potential. Animal experiments carried out with certain collagen fractions and immunological studies [88, 99, 105, 111, 132, 137, 147] have demonstrated that the antigenic activity of collagen does not depend on the genuine conformation of the molecule. This is compatible with the localization of the major antigenic determinants in N-terminal and C-terminal non-helical sequences for which no function in information and maintenance of the triple-helical structure is assumed. Conformation-independent antigenic determinants have also been recognized in the central regions of the unfolded polypeptide chains, having a helical conformation in the native molecule.

Several antigenic determinants (e.g. with general collagen specificity, with species specificity, etc.) mediating humoral antibody production are known [88, 117, 130]. Antiserum prepared against serum-free medium from human fibroblast cultures reacted specifically with protropocollagen, the soluble precursor of tropocollagen [124]. Amino acid sequences corresponding to the telopeptides and helical α chains of tropocollagen were not recognized by the antiserum. Antigenic effect of foetal and denatured acid soluble dermal collagen was shown by immunofluorescence in autoimmune diseases (SLE, dermatomyositis), but also in hypertrophic scars and chronic pyoderma [117]. Precipitating anti-collagen antibodies were also demonstrated in the serum of healthy individuals [29]. These results do not, in themselves, indicate the pathogenetic effect of antibodies produced to such antigens [120]. In human serum 'anti-elastin', most probably autoantibody, could be demonstrated [104]. It is presumed that cathepsin-like enzymes decompose the elastin as a result of which soluble peptides enter circulation. The antigen–antibody complex would then participate in the local tissue reaction.

Publications concerning the problem of delayed-type reactions to collagen are much less abundant. Collagen from different species exhibited various degrees of cross-reactivities in the skin reaction. Calf and rat skin collagen in the native, triple helical conformation [2] but also in its denatured state in which the constituent α chains are present as random coils [1] is active as sensitizer as well as elicitor in cutaneous delayed hypersensitivity reactions in guinea pigs. α_1 chains as well as α_2 chains are capable of sensitizing guinea pigs for the delayed reaction [83]. This is in contrast to humoral antibody production, where the major collagen antigen determinant of the skin of rats and guinea pigs is localized at the amino terminal part of the α_2 chain which does not have a helical conformation [88]. The saline-soluble collagen, the gelatin and acid mucopolysaccharides yield in intracutaneous test both immediate and delayed reactions [117]. With slightly denatured collagen and gelatin precursor mainly the delayed type skin reaction can be elicited. The rabbit antiserum against the acid-soluble collagen of the human skin was found to have a cytoxic effect on human embryonic fibroblasts. Patients with PSS showed significantly increased degree of migration inhibition using autologous lymphocytes, liver microsomes and mitochondria, and the myelin basic protein [57*a*].

The presence of anti-muscle antibodies in PSS cases in which the electromyogram was of a pathologic type was shown by haemagglutination and haemagglutination inhibition using antigenic muscle component [7]. Crude muscle homogenate used as mitogen in lymphocyte transformation test appeared to stimulate the lymphocytes of the patients with PSS in whom there was evidence of myopathy (possibly the collagen was antigenic) [30].

According to the other hypothesis, the responsible autoantigen is the ground substance (the structural glycoproteins of the connective tissue), more particularly one or more of its protein-polysaccharide complexes [29]. These consist of a core of protein to which a series of polysaccharide side chains are attached. These may vary from molecule to molecule of protein and more than one type of polysaccharide side chain is usually attached to a single protein core [46]. Thus, in the cartilage, e. g., the side chains may include both chondroitin sulphate and keratan sulphate. The immunological specificity resides, at least in part, in the polysaccharide side chains, since their partial removal, e. g. by hyaluronidase, significantly affects the specificity and enhances the cross-reactivity with homologous material in the immunized animal itself [34].

There is no immunopathological alteration that would be specific to PSS. Dysproteinaemia is not characteristic. The complement level is normal. In about one-fourth of the cases [28, 112, 127] there is hypalbuminaemia or hypergammaglobulinaemia; α_1-, α_2- and β-globulin studies have failed to demonstrate changes specific for PSS, or disease-specific protein. Speckles of fluorescence have been found confined to scleroderma and Raynaud's disease, while nuclear fluorescence is mainly found in scleroderma. The data are, however, not of predictive or diagnostic value, nor do they indicate immunological activity [127].

Anti-nuclear factor has been demonstrated in 21–91 per cent of the cases using different methods [9, 49, 55*b*, 74, 85, 101*a*, 112]; the factor belonged to the IgG class in 75–100 per cent, to IgM in 4–18 per cent, to IgA in 0–11 per cent; but occasionally it was present only in a single Ig class. A tendency of the IgM-type antibodies occurring first and the IgG-type later but in a higher concentration [6] has been observed. The anti-nuclear factor content in the serum may change considerably but there is no parallelism with either the duration or the severity of the disease; it does not seem to affect the clinical picture or course either [65, 67]. Positivity of the anti-nuclear factor is more frequent in PSS than in rheumatoid arthritis or dermatomyositis, but more infrequent than is SLE [67, 112]. At the same time the anti-ADN antibody is more common in PSS (25 per cent) than in SLE (4 per cent) [58]. Rounal haematoxylin body in PSS is found in 2 per cent [9]. With immunofluorescence anti-nuclear factors have been demonstrated in 36–80 per cent [6, 65, 67, 85, 101*a*, *b*, 114, 122], in the majority of cases in low or medium titre. The anti-nuclear factors are heterogeneous [101*b*]: ADN, nucleoproteins, histones, soluble nuclear components; with the various dilutions of the serum these can be separated by immunofluorescent technique. Fine speckles in a reticular network were found more frequent than large speckles or homogeneous staining. However, the inhomogeneous fluorescence of the 'non-DNA-nucleoprotein' is the most frequent finding. Anti-nucleolar staining has been observed in 10–20 per cent [85, 112]. Presumably, the serum anti-nuclear factors react with the non-chromatin components of the nucleus [101*a*]. From the anti-nuclear factors found by means of the indirect immunofluorescent method some workers have inferred to the genuine autoantibody origin of the process [95]. In 50 per cent of the cases the anti-nuclear factors, mainly IgG of slow (γ_2) electrophoretic motility, bind complement [63, 101*a*, *b*]. This is important because thus they are able to form soluble complexes [101*b*]. The nuclear antigen + anti-nuclear factor + complement complex may have a pathogenic role through deposition in the tissues, principally in the renal glomeruli. But since the anti-nuclear factor titre is low in PSS, the possibility for complex formation is slight [101*b*]. No relationship has been found between the complement fixing ability of the anti-nuclear factor and the renal involvement in PSS [63]. The presence of 7S γ-globulin and complement components was verified in the necrotic areas of renal vessels of two patients, but this can also be found in malignant hypertension [119]. Fibrinogen deposition has been reported in renal lesion as well. Results of intracutaneous tests with DNA have shown no abnormality in patients with PSS in contrast to patients with SLE [36]. It can be regarded as generally accepted today [46] that the anti-nuclear factors in themselves do not lead to PSS; their demonstration does not alone strengthen the diagnosis, neither are they decisive in the prognosis of PSS [65]. But if the anti-nuclear factor level exceeds 1/64 and the multisystemic symptoms are obvious, it is certain that we are facing either SLE or PSS. If on examination the clinical symptoms are missing or uncertain, then we might expect the symptoms of SLE or PSS to manifest themselves later. In clinically symptom-free neonates anti-nuclear factor is demonstrable; later it disappears gradually. The occurrence of rheumatoid factor ranges between 17–41 per cent [28, 55*b*, 85, 112] but after the inactivation of the serum it is positive only in 12 per cent [85]. Biologically false positive syphilis seroreaction is obtained in about 5 per cent [28]. Occasionally, cold agglutinin and kryoglobulin have also been detected.

Tissue-specific antibodies against collagen, thymus nucleus and vascular homogenate have been determined with the antiglobulin consumption test [131]. The anti-thyroid-cytoplasm factor was found in about 9 per cent, and the anti-gastric-parietal-cell factor in 6 per cent [85]. Autoimmune haemolytic anaemia, which may reach 40 per cent in SLE, is very rare in PSS. Immunofluorescent techniques have not pointed to a preferential localization of γ-globulin and other proteins within cutaneous lesions [37*b*].

Presuming an enhanced sensitivity of the immune apparatus in PSS patients who, therefore, respond even to antigenic stimuli which leave a normal individual indifferent, immunization with blood group substance has been attempted [134]. The production of isohaemagglutinin, Rhesus antibody, anti-nuclear factor and anti-coagulant factor have been studied but only a minor disturbance of the immune system of PSS patients could be found. Apparently, the hyperreactivity is not the main cause of PSS. On the other hand, a search for antibodies to human collagen in the serum of subjects with a relative IgA deficiency disclosed antibodies in 44 per cent as compared to the 2.5 per cent found in the normal controls [149]. Investigating the ability of patients to manifest a cutaneous delayed-type reaction (using bacterial, fungal and viral antigens intracutaneously) and the *in vitro* lymphoproliferative response to the nonspecific mitogen PHA, it has been demonstrated [153] that both *in vivo* and *in vitro* criteria of the mechanism of cell-mediated immunity are intact in patients with PSS. Since their history does not contain hints to undue susceptibility to viral, fungal, protozoal or other intracellular infections, the integrity of cell-mediated immune defence mechanisms can be taken for granted [106*a*, 153]. Lymphocytes from patients have destroyed fibroblasts from human embryos in tissue culture [140]. With the use of cultures of skin fibroblasts, an increase in the synthesis of soluble collagen and glycoprotein has been demonstrated in the skin of patients with PSS [80]. Lymphocyte cytotoxicity of muscle, fibroblast and epithelial cells in PSS suggests that cell-mediated sensitivity may underlie the multisystemic involvement in these disorders [30, 102]. Stastny et al. [129] found that a form of runt disease induced in adult rats by the administration of allogeneic lymphocytes to which the recipients had previously been made tolerant was characterized by skin lesions remarkably similar to those of human scleroderma.

Sclerogenic action has been attributed by some workers to serotonin when released from malignant carcinoid tumours. It is, therefore, quite possible that some substances released during immunological reactions could affect the interfibrillar ground substance, especially if the antigen itself was intimately associated with them [46]. The presence of complement potentiates, i.e. locally increases the concentration of vasoactive amines and in this way vascular disturbance, or tissue destruction may arise.

The question arises whether there is a principal difference between the localized (focal as morphoea or linear) scleroderma and PSS. There is a counterargument [64], viz. that with electromyography [7] and electron optic studies phenomena identical in type though less intensive can also be demonstrated in the former. The light-microscropic and electron-microscopic changes of PSS and morphoea are essentially similar apart from slight differences, e.g. in the lesions of small blood vessels [61]. Also the immunological evidence speaks in favour of a transition [49, 114]. In the opposite way, on the basis of reciprocal full-thickness skin grafts (exchange between involved and uninvolved skin) the skin involvement in PSS appeared to be generalized or irreversible (if sclerodermatous skin is placed in a normal bed, it remains sclerodermatous; clinically normal skin in sclerodermatous bed becomes sclerodermatous), in contrast to the findings in morphoea, where the disorder has been found to be localized and reversible [44]. These suggest the importance of extracutaneous factors in PSS determining the localization and severity of cutaneous involvement [106*d*].

Surveying the pathogenetic theories and the presently available experimental and clinical evidence, we can only say that PSS occupies a particular position among the diseases of the connective tissue [74] and with respect to autoimmune activity it does not belong to the same class as SLE [55*b*].

THERAPY

No single drug or combination of agents has proved to be of value or is generally accepted as useful [108, 141*b*, 152]. The situation is rendered more difficult inasmuch as the parameters (skin temperature, pulmonary function, oesophageal motility, laboratory data) suitable for measuring the efficacy of the various drugs do not appear to relate well with clinical activity [141*b*]. To promote perfusion of the peripheral vessels, vasodilators (phenoxybenzamine, Tolazoline, α-methyldopa, reserpine, nicotinic acid, procaine) are given [152], whereas to reduce blood viscosity and intravascular cell aggregation plasma volume expanders in drip infusion are used together with sympatholytics (procaine) [55*a*, 56]. They are effective in the early stage before organic changes have appeared. Glycocorticosteroids decrease collagen neogenesis, but accelerate the maturation of collagen [4], therefore, in indebilitating arthritis, extensive cutaneous oedema, and acute toxic phases of the disease they are used in low doses (10 mg prednisolone per day [77, 141*b*]. They have done more harm than good in cases with hypertension and renal changes [4, 56]. In females progestogens delay the cross-connection of collagen [76], therefore norethisterone acetate, ethinylnortestosterone acetate, in males progesterone, 17-α-hydroxyprogesterone caproate treatment for several months may be considered [56, 77, 103]. Effects like softening of the skin, improved reflex plethysmogram, appearance of a collagen-like protein in the serum as a consequence of intensification of collagen metabolism, rise in urinary hydroxyproline excretion, normalization of the increased mucopolysaccharide excretion have been described, but no definite changes in the function of the internal organs have been noted [56, 103]. The use of immunosuppressive agents (azathioprin, amethopterin, 6-mercaptopurine) and of cytostatics (cyclophosphamide) have aroused general interest, though it is still too early to make a statement about their value. Chloroquine inhibits collagen synthesis and increases the catabolism of neocollagen only in toxic doses [4]. ε-aminocaproic acid, the chelate-producing EDTA, and hyaluronidase treatments have not fullfilled hopes [4]. Recently, D-penicillamine has been increasingly used. This is an agent known to interfere with the intermolecular cross-linking of collagen and to increase the acid solubility [51] and solubility in 0.14 M sodium chloride of dermal collagen [84]. If it is given in sufficiently large doses and for a long time (5–15 months), the starting value of the increased collagen solubility is reduced by half and the elasticity of the skin increases [15]. However, the biochemical improvement is not followed by simultaneous clinical and functional amelioration (e.g. cardiac passage). Its wider application is greatly hindered by its side-effects, i.e. fever, conjunctivitis, rhinitis, otititis media and drug exanthem appearing on the 8–11th day of treatment [4]. Since often the drug proves to be toxic (leukopenia, thrombocytopenia, loss of taste perception, renal damage) it must be administered with extreme caution [66]. Attempts have been made to employ hyperbaric oxygen therapy [5]. Results of thoracic and cervical sympathectomy are usually transient [141*b*]. Amputation of chronically infected, ulcerated digits is indicated. Of the other systemic agents, as penicillin, griseofulvin, vitamin E, relaxin with oestrogen, potassium para-aminobenzoate, ethylenediamine tetraacetic acid, none have proved effective in carefully controlled clinical studies [141*b*]. Due to excessive toxicity (exfoliative dermatitis, haemolytic anaemia, lathyric bone changes) the use of β-amino propionitrile cannot be recommended [141*b*], though it augments the urinary hydroxyproline excretion [68]. If the gastrointestinal tract is involved, broad-spectrum antibiotics, multivitamins, antidiarrhoeal agents, antiulcer diet [32] can be tried. With renal lesions (hypertension, renal sclerosis) antihypertensive medication becomes necessary. Corticosteroids are contraindicated [141*b*]. In the presence of cardiopulmonary symptoms the basic therapy must be complemented with cardiotonic drugs and broad-spectrum antibiotics. Local medications (heparinoid + hyaluronidase ointment, dimethylsulphoxide) are only partially effective. Certain general measures [141*b*] like the avoidance of stimuli which precipitate vasospasm (cold, nicotine, fatigue, stress, etc.), adequate rest (in the polyarthralgic or arthritic form), physiotherapy (warm, whirlpool baths, infrared irradiation, passive and graduated muscle exercise), changes in life style and occupation may prevent complications [152].

REFERENCES

1. Adelmann, B. C., Glynn, L. E. and Kirrane, J.: *Fed. Proc.* **27,** 263 (1968).
2. Adelmann, B. C., Kirrane, J. and Glynn, L. E.: *Immunology* **23,** 723 (1972).
3. Bailey, A. J. and Robins, S. P.: In *Frontiers in Matrix Biology*. Ed. by Robert, L. Vol. I. Basle 1973, p. 130.
4. Balda, B.-R.: *Dtsch. med. Wschr.* **97,** 1876 (1972).
5. Barr, P.-O., Enfors, W. and Eriksson, G.: *Brit. J. Derm.* **86,** 631 (1972).
6. Barthelmes, H.: *Derm. Mschr.* **158,** 702 (1972).
7. Bădănoiu, Al. and Bucur, G.: *Derm.-Vener. (Buc.)* **17,** 17 (1972).
8. Belisario, J. C.: *Hautarzt* **22,** 185 (1971).
9. Bencze, Gy.: *Rheum. Balneol. Allerg. (Budap.)* **14,** 151 (1973).
10. Berger, H.: *Hautarzt* **20,** 225 (1969).
11. Bessler, W. and Meyer, C.: *Radiol. clin. biol.* **39,** 230 (1970).
12. Biggard, J. D. and Nevin, N. C.: *J. Path. Bact.* **93,** 334 (1967).
13. Binazzi, M. and Calandra, P.: *Arch. derm. Forsch.* **246,** 142 (1973).
14. Black, M. M., Bottoms, E. and Shuster, S.: *Brit. J. Derm.* **83,** 552 (1970).
15. Bluestone, R., Grahame, R., Holloway, V. and Holt, P. J. L.: *Ann. rheum. Dis.* **29,** 153 (1970).
16. Blumenkrantz, N. and Asboe-Hansen, G.: In *Abstr. 14th Int. Congr. Derm., Padua–Venice 1972*. Ed. by Flarer, F., Paton, P. M., Rabito, C., Serri, F. and Kleinman, R. L. Excerpta Medica Int. Congr. Ser. No. 248. Amsterdam 1972, p. 34.
17. Braun-Falco, O.: In *Scleroderma*. Ed. by Delbarre, F. and Saporta, L. Masson, Paris 1972, p. 21.
18. Burnham, Th. K.: Meeting Dermat. Section of Amer. Med. Assoc., New York 1973, cited by *Derm. News* **6**/7, 7 (1973).
19. Calvert, R. J. and Owen, T. K.: *Lancet* **ii,** 19 (1956).
20. Cantwell, A. R., Craggs, E. and Wilson, J. W.: *Dermatologica (Basel)* **136,** 141 (1968).
21. Cantwell, A. R., jr. and Kelso, D. W.: *Arch. Derm.* **104,** 21 (1971).
22. Čapuşan, I., Stern, A. and Maier, N.: *Derm.-Vener. (Buc.)* **14,** 407 (1969).
23. Čapuşan, I., Stern, A., Maier, N., Dimitrescu, I. and Neumann, E.: *Derm.-Vener. (Buc.)* **14,** 105 (1969).
24. Carniol, M., Popescu, E. and Pirojinski, M.: *Derm.-Vener. (Buc.)* **16,** 405 (1971).
25. Chaves, F. C., Rodrigo, F., Franco, M. L. and Esteves, J.: *Brit. J. Derm.* **82,** 298 (1970).
26. Christianson, H. B., Dorsey, C. S. and O'Leary, P.: *Arch. Derm.* **74,** 629 (1956).
27. Clark, J. A., Winkelmann, R. K., McDuffie, F. C. and Ward, L. E.: *Proc. Mayo Clin.* **46,** 97 (1971).
28. Clark, J. A., Winkelmann, R. K. and Ward, L. E.: *Proc. Mayo Clin.* **46,** 104 (1971).
29. Crouzet, J., Camus, J.-P. and Robert, L.: *Presse méd.* **78,** 1185 (1970).
30. Currie, S., Saunders, M. and Knowles, M.: *Brit. J. Derm.* **84,** 400 (1971).
31. David, R. J.: In *Immunopathology*. IV. Symposium. Ed. by Miescher, P. A. and Grabar, P. Schwabe, Basel 1966, p. 253.
32. Debray, Ch. and Leymarios, J.: In *Scleroderma*. Ed. by Delbarre, F. and Saporta, L. Masson, Paris 1972, p. 99.
33. Debreczeni, M. and Ladányi, É.: *Hautarzt* **21,** 81 (1970).
34. Dubois, E. L., Chandor, S., Friou, G. J. and Bischel, M.: *Medicine* **50,** 199 (1971).
35. Emerit, I., Housset, E., de Grouchy, E. and Camus, J. P.: *Rev. europ. Ét. clin. biol.* **16,** 684 (1971).

36. Fardal, R. W. and Winkelmann, R. K.: *Arch. Derm.* **91,** 503 (1965).
37*a*. Fisher, E. R. and Rodman, G. P.: *Arch. Path.* **65,** 29 (1958).
37*b*. id., *Arthr. and Rheum.* **3,** 536 (1960).
38. Fleischmajer, R. and Damiano, V.: *J. invest. Derm.* **56,** 414 (1971).
39*a*. Fleischmajer, R., Damiano, V. and Nedwich, A.: *Science* **171,** 1019 (1971).
39*b*. id., *Arch. Derm.* **105,** 59 (1972).
40. Fleischmajer, R. and Nedwich, A.: *Arch. Derm.* **106,** 509 (1972).
41. Fleischmajer, R. and Perlish, J. S.: *J. invest. Derm.* **58,** 129 (1972).
42. Fleischmajer, R., Perlish, J. S. and Gaisin, A.: *J. invest. Derm.* **61,** 1 (1973).
43. Foster, T. D. and Fairburn, E. A.: *Brit. dental J.* **124,** 353 (1968).
44. Fries, J. F., Hoopes, J. E. and Shulman, L. E.: *Arthr. and Rheum.* **14,** 571 (1971).
45. Garrett, J. M., Winkelmann, R. K., Schlegel, J. F. and Code, Ch. F.: *Proc. Mayo Clin.* **46,** 92 (1971).
46. Glynn, L. E.: In *Scleroderma*. Ed. by Delbarre, F. and Saporta, L. Masson, Paris 1972, p. 279.
47. Guiraudon, C., Saporta, L. and Delbarre, F.: In *Scleroderma*. Ed. by Delbarre, F. and Saporta, L. Masson, Paris 1972, p. 263.
48. Györkey, J., Sinkovics, J. G., Min, K. W. and Györkey, Ph.: *Amer. J. Med.* **53,** 148 (1972).
49. Hanson, V., Drexler, E. and Kornreich, H.: *Arthr. and Rheum.* **13,** 798 (1970).
50. Hardy, K. H., Rosevear, J. W., Sams, W. M., jr. and Winkelmann, R. K.: *Proc. Mayo Clin.* **46,** 119 (1971).
51. Harris, E. D., jr. and Sjoerdsma, A.: *Lancet* **ii,** 996 (1966).
52. Hartmann, F. and Deicher, H.: In *Klinische Pathophysiologie*. Ed. by Siegenthaler, W. Thieme, Stuttgart 1970, p. 806.
53*a*. Hayes, R. L. and Rodnan, G. P.: *Anat. Rec.* **163,** 197 (1969).
53*b*. id., *Amer. J. Path.* **63,** 433 (1971).
54. Hernández-Richter, H. J. and Struck, H.: *Die Wundheilung. Theoretische und praktische Grundlagen.* Thieme, Stuttgart 1970.
55*a*. Holti, G.: *Brit. J. Derm.* **77,** 560 (1965).
55*b*. id., *Practitioner* **204,** 644 (1970).
56. Holzmann, H., Korting, G. W. and Morsches, B.: *Act. dermo-sifilogr. (Madr.)* **62,** 1 (1971).
57. Housset, E., Emerit, I., Baulon, A. and De Groucky, J.: In *Scleroderma*. Ed. by Delbarre, F. and Saporta, L. Masson, Paris 1972, p. 283.
57*a*. Hughes, P., Holt, Sh. and Rowell, N. R.: *Brit. J. Derm.* **91,** 1 (1974).
58. Huriez, Cl.: *Lille méd.* **16,** Sér. 3, No. 10, 1 (1971).
59. Huriez, Cl., Bergoend, H., L'Hermine, C., Thomas, P., Piette, F. and Brouet, J.-F.: *Ann. Derm. Syph.* **100,** 481 (1973).
60. Hutás, I., Urai, L., Böszörményi-Nagy, G. and Grosz, A.: *Respiration* **30,** 141 (1973).
61. Ishikawa, H. and Mori, S.: *Hautarzt* **23,** 440 (1972).
62. Jabłońska, S.: *Scleroderma and Pseudo-scleroderma.* Polish Medical Publ., Warsaw 1965.
63. Jabłońska, S. and Chorzelski, T.: *Allergie Immunologie* **18,** 187 (1972).
64. Jabłońska, S., Jakubowicz, K., Biczysko, W. and Dabrowski, J.: *Derm. Mschr.* **156,** 162 (1970).
65. Jabłońska, S. and Szczepanski, A.: In *Scleroderma*. Ed. by Delbarre, F. and Saporta, L. Masson, Paris 1972, p. 253.
66. Jaffe, I. A., Treser, G., Sazuki, Y., Ehrenreich, T.: *Ann. intern. Med.* **69,** 549 (1968).
67. Jordon, R. E., Deheer, D., Schroeter, A. and Winkelmann, R. K.: *Proc. Mayo Clin.* **46,** 111 (1971).
68. Keiser, H. R. and Sjoerdsma, A.: *Clin. Pharmacol. Ther.* **8,** 593 (1967).
69. Keiser, H. R., Stein, H. D. and Sjoerdsma, A.: *Arch. Derm.* **104,** 57 (1971).
70. Kerl, H. and Auböck, L.: *Hautarzt* **24,** 95 (1973).
71. Kierland, R. R.: In *Dermatologic Allergy*. Ed. by Criep, L. H. Saunders, Philadelphia 1967, p. 481.
72. Kimmig, J. and Kreysel, H. W.: *Klin. Wschr.* **51,** 207 (1973).
73. Klein, G. and Schneider, G.: *Wien. klin. Wschr.* **84,** 27 (1972).

74. Klemm, D.: *Med. Klin.* **64,** 1065 (1969).
75. Kobayashi, T. and Asboe-Hansen, G.: *Acta derm.-venereol.* **52,** 81 (1972).
76. Korting, G. W.: In *Dermatologie und Venerologie.* Vol. II/2. Ed. by Gottron, H. A. and Schönfeld, W. Thieme, Stuttgart 1958, p. 886.
77. Korting, G. W. and Holzmann, H.: *Die Sklerodermie und ihr nahestehende Bindegewebeprobleme.* Thieme, Stuttgart 1967.
78. Kreysel, H. W.: *Z. Haut- u. Geschl.-Kr.* **40,** 173 (1966).
79. Kreysel, H. W., Köhler, A. and Kleine, T. O.: *Klin. Wschr.* **51,** 214 (1973).
80. LeRoy, E. C.: *J. exp. Med.* **135,** 1351 (1972).
81. LeRoy, E. C., Kaplan, A., Udenfriend, S. and Sjoerdsma, A.: *J. biol. Chem.* **239,** 3350 (1964).
82. Lester, P. D. and Koehler, P. R.: *Radiology* **99,** 517 (1971).
83. Lindsley, H., Mannik, M. and Bornstein, P.: *J. exp. Med.* **133,** 1309 (1971).
84. Lorenzen, I., Uitto, J. and Ohlenschlaeger, K.: *Scand. J. Rheumatol.* **1,** 121 (1972).
85. McGiven, A. R., de Boer, W. G. R. M., Batnett, A. R. and Coventry, D. A.: *Med. J. Austr.* **2,** 533 (1968).
86. McNeal, J. E.: *Arch. Derm.* **107,** 699 (1973).
87. Meszaros, W. T.: *Radiology* **70,** 313 (1958).
88. Michaeli, D., Martin, G. R., Kettman, J., Benjamini, E., Leung, D. Y. K. and Blatt, B. A.: *Science* **166,** 1522 (1969).
89. Montgomery, H.: *Dermatopathology.* Hoeber, New York 1967.
90. Monti, M.: *Schweiz. med. Wschr.* **102,** 1023 (1973).
91. Morpurgo, M., Rampulla, C., Beulcke, G., Casaccia, M., Finardi, G. and Venco, A.: *Schweiz. med. Wschr.* **102,** 605 (1972).
92. Nasser, W. K., Mishkin, M. E., Rosenbaum, D. and Genovese, P.-D.: *Amer. J. Cardiol.* **22,** 538 (1968).
93. Năstase, Gh., Carniol, M., Popescu, E. and Pirojinski, M.: *Derm.-Vener. (Buc.)* **14,** 11 (1969).
94. Neal, J. E.: *Arch. Derm.* **107,** 699 (1973).
95. Nebe, H. and Blume, N.: *Derm. Mschr.* **157,** 27 (1971).
96. Norton, W. L.: *J. Lab. clin. Med.* **74,** 369 (1969).
97. Norton, W. L. and Nardo, J. M.: *Ann. intern. Med.* **73,** 317 (1970).
98. Obrink, B.: *Eur. J. Biochem.* **33,** 387 (1973).
99. O'Dell, D. S.: In *Treatise on Collagen.* Vol. II. Ed. by Gould, B. S. Academic Press, New York 1968, p. 311.
100. Olszewska, Z. and Dudek, H.: *Przegl. Derm.* **58,** 537 (1971).
101*a*. Peltier, A.-P.: *Presse méd.* **78,** 1969 (1970).
101*b*. id., In *Scleroderma.* Ed. by Delbarre, F. and Saporta, L. Masson, Paris 1972, p. 235.
102. Perlmann, P. and Holm, G.: *Advanc. Immunol.* **11,** 117 (1970).
103. Raul, R., Randurovic, L. and Böni, A.: *Dtsch. med. Wschr.* **97,** 1283 (1972).
104. Robert, M., Stein, F., Pezess, M.-P. and Poullain, N.: *Arch. Mal. Coeur* Suppl. **1,** 233 (1967).
105. Rodermund, O. E.: *Arch. klin. exp. Derm.* **234,** 315 (1969).
106*a*. Rodnan, G. P.: In *Immunological Diseases.* 2nd ed. Vol. II. Ed. by Samter, M. Little-Brown, Boston 1971, p. 1052.
106*b*. id., In *Scleroderma.* Ed. by Delbarre, F. and Saporta, L. Masson, Paris 1972, p. 135.
106*c*. ibid., p. 157.
106*d*. ibid., p. 271.
107. Rodnan, G. P. and Fennell, R. H.: *J. Amer. med. Ass.* **180,** 665 (1962).
108. Rodnan, G. P., McEwen, C. and Wallace, St. L.: *J. Amer. med. Ass.* **224,** Suppl. to No. 5, 711 (1973).
109. Rodnan, G. P., Shapiro, A. P. and Krifcher, E.: *Ann. intern. Med.* **60,** 737 (1964).
110. Rodnan, G. P., Shapiro, A. P., Moutsos, S. E. and Bron, K. M.: *Arthr. rheum. Dis.* **8,** 464 (1965).
111. Rothbard, S. and Watson, R. F.: *J. exp. Med.* **129,** 1145 (1969).
112. Rothfield, N. F. and Rodnan, G. P.: *Arthr. and Rheum.* **11,** 607 (1968).
113. Rowell, N.: *Brit. med. J.* **i,** 514 (1968).

114. Rowell, N. R. and Swanson Beck, J.: *Arch. Derm.* **96,** 290 (1967).
115. Rupec, M. and Braun-Falco, O.: *Arch. klin. exp. Derm.* **218,** 543 (1964).
116*a*. Sackner, M. A.: In *Scleroderma*. Ed. by Delbarre, F. and Saporta, L. Masson, Paris 1972, p. 29.
116*b*. ibid., p. 71.
117. Sano, Sh.: *Jap. J. Derm. Ser. B.* **79,** 292 (1969); cited by *Z. Haut- u. Geschl. Kr.* **128,** 5 (1971).
118. Sapira, J. D., Rodnan, G. P., Scheib, E. T., Klaniecki, Th. and Rizk, M.: *Amer. J. Med.* **52,** 330 (1972).
119. Schäfer, H. E. and Schäfer, A.: *Arch. klin. Med.* **214,** 187 (1968).
120. Scott, D. G.: *Ann. rheum. Dis.* **18,** 207 (1959).
121. Scudamore, H. H., Green, P. A., Hoffman, H. N., Rosevear, J. W. and Tauxe, W. N.: *Amer. J. Gastroent.* **49,** 193 (1968).
122. Seville, R. H.: *Brit. J. Derm.* **64,** 467 (1952).
123. Sharp, G. C., Irvin, W. S., Tan, E. M., Gould, R. G. and Holman, H. R.: *Amer. J. Med.* **52,** 148 (1972).
124. Sherr, C. J. and Goldberg, B.: *Science* **180,** 1190 (1973).
125. Shuster, S. and Bottoms, E.: *Clin. Sci.* **25,** 487 (1963).
126. Shuster, S., Raffle, E. J. and Bottoms, E.: *Lancet* **i,** 525 (1967).
127. Spencer, St. K. and Winkelmann, R. K.: *Proc. Mayo Clin.* **46,** 108 (1971).
128. Stachów, A. and Jabłońska, S.: *Arch. klin. exp. Derm.* **222,** 127 (1965).
129. Stastny, P., Stembridge, V. A. and Ziff, M.: *J. exp. Med.* **118,** 635 (1963).
130. Steffen, C., Dichtl, M. and Brunner, H.: *Z. Immun.-Forsch. allerg. klin. Immun.* **140,** 408 (1970).
131. Steffen, C., Schuster, F., Tausch, G., Timpl, R. and Pecker, I.: *Klin. Wschr.* **46,** 976 (1968).
132. Steffen, C., Timple, R. and Wolff, I.: *Immunology* **15,** 135 (1968).
133. Stork, J.: *Schweiz. Arch. Neurol. Neurochir. Psychiat.* **110,** 83 (1972).
134. Stringa, S. G., Sanchez Avalos, J. C., Andrada, J. A., Casala, A. and Bianchi, G.: *Arch. Derm.* **103,** 394 (1971).
135. Szinnay, Gy.: Data to the Morphology of Collagen Diseases. Thesis. Budapest 1968.
136. Szodoray, L.: In *Autoimmun betegségek (Autoimmune diseases)*. Ed. by Petrányi, Gy. Akadémiai Kiadó, Budapest 1974, p. 95.
137. Timpl, R., Wolff, I., Furtmayer, H. and Steffen, C.: *Immunology* **15,** 145 (1968).
138. Traub, W. and Piez, K. A.: *Advanc. Protein Chem.* **25,** 243 (1971).
139. Traub, W., Yonath, A. and Segal, D. M.: *Nature* **221,** 941 (1969).
140. Trayanova, T. G., Sura, V. V. and Svet-Moldavsky, G. J.: *Lancet* **i,** 452 (1966).
141*a*. Tuffanelli, D. L.: *Dermatologica (Basel)* **138,** 93 (1969).
141*b*. id., in *Scleroderma*. Ed. by Delbarre, F. and Saporta, L. Masson, Paris 1972, p. 291.
142. Tuffanelli, D. L. and Winkelmann, R. K.: *Arch. Derm.* **84,** 359 (1961).
143. Uitto, J., Helin, G., Helin, P. and Lorenzen, I.: *Acta derm.-venereol.* **51,** 401 (1971).
144. Uitto, J., Laitinen, O., Hannuksela, M. and Mustakallio, K. K.: *Scand. J. Lab. Invest.* **19,** Suppl. 95, 41 (1967).
145. Urai, L., Munkácsi, I. and Szinnay, Gy.: *Brit. med. J.* **i,** 713 (1961).
146. Urai, L., Nagy, Z., Szinnay, Gy. and Wiltner, W.: *Brit. med. J.* **ii,** 1264 (1958).
147. Watson, R. F., Rothbard, S. and Vanamee, P.: *J. exp. Med.* **99,** 535 (1954).
148. Weidner, F. and Braun-Falco, O.: *Hautarzt* **19,** 345 (1968).
149. Wells, J. V., Michaeli, D. and Fudenberg, H. H.: *Clin. exp. Immunol.* **13,** 203 (1973).
150. Westerman, M. P., Martinez, R. C., Medzger, V. A., jr., Tosten, R. S. and Rodnan, G. P.: *Arch. intern. Med.* **122,** 39 (1968).
151. Winkelmann, R. K.: *Proc. Mayo Clin.* **46,** 83 (1971).
152. Winkelmann, R. K., Kierland, R. R., Perry, H.-O., Muller, S. A. and Sams, W. M., jr.: *Proc. Mayo Clin.* **46,** 128 (1971).
153. Winkelstein, A., Rodnan, G. and Heilman, J. D.: *Ann. rheum. Dis.* **31,** 126 (1972).

CHAPTER 38

RHEUMATOID ARTHRITIS

by

L. BAKOS and S. BOZSÓKY

CRITERIA OF DIAGNOSIS

In 1958 the American Rheumatism Association set up criteria for the easier diagnosis of this disease [12, 68]. The criteria are widely known, and they have also been adopted by the International League against Rheumatism. At the same time it also listed those diseases and laboratory results in the presence of which rheumatoid arthritis could be excluded.

The question may arise whether the work done so far in this field is correct and sufficient, or whether there is a need for revision of some current standpoints. There is no doubt, however, that this widespread disease of unknown aetiology and with many clinical presentations requires an exact delineation.

The criteria of rheumatoid arthritis are:

1. Morning stiffness.
2. Pain on motion or tenderness in at least one joint.
3. Swelling (soft tissue thickening or fluid—not bony overgrowth alone) in at least one joint continuously for not less than six weeks.
4. Swelling of at least one other joint (any interval free of joint symptoms between the two joint involvements may not be more than three months).
5. Symmetrical joint swelling with simultaneous involvement of the same joint on both sides of the body (bilateral involvement of proximal interphalangeal, metacarpophalangeal or metatarsophalangeal joints is acceptable without absolute symmetry). Distal interphalangeal joint involvement will not satisfy this criterion.
6. Subcutaneous nodules over bony prominences, on extensor surfaces or in juxta-articular regions.
7. X-ray changes typical of rheumatoid arthritis (which must include at least bony decalcification localized to, or greatest around, the involved joints and not just degenerative changes). However, degenerative changes do not exclude the diagnosis of rheumatoid arthritis.

8. Positive sheep cell agglutination test. (Any modification will suffice that does not give more than 5 per cent of positive results in non-rheumatoid control subjects.)

9. Poor mucin precipitate from synovial fluid (with shreds and cloudy solution).

10. Characteristic histologic changes in synovial membrane with three or more of the following: marked villous hypertrophy; proliferation of superficial synovial cells often with palisading; marked infiltration of chronic inflammatory cells (lymphocytes or plasma cells predominating) with tendency to form 'lymphoid nodules', deposition of compact fibrin, either on the surface or interstitially; foci of cell necrosis.

11. Characteristic histologic changes in nodules showing granulomatous fcci with central zones of cell necrosis, surrounded by peripheral fibrosis and chronic inflammatory cell infiltration, predominantly perivascular.

'Classical rheumatoid arthritis' is the diagnosis if at least seven of the criteria may be found, and if the joint symptoms including swelling last for at least six weeks. 'Definite rheumatoid arthritis' is the diagnosis if five criteria may be found, and the signs and swelling in the joints last for six weeks. If three criteria are found and the joint changes last for four weeks, 'probable rheumatoid arthritis' is the diagnosis. In the presence of two of the following criteria—1, 2, 3, and 6—accompanied by an elevated ESR or an iritis, the diagnosis is one of 'possible rheumatoid arthritis'.

Factors excluding rheumatoid arthritis are:

1. The typical rash of systemic lupus erythematosus.

2. High concentration of lupus erythematosus (LE) cells (four or more in two smears). However, because of the frequent finding of LE cells in patients with clinically typical rheumatoid arthritis, the Committee suggests that such patients be listed separately.

3. Histologic evidence of polyarteritis nodosa with segmented necrosis of arteries associated with nodular leukocytic infiltration extending perivascularly and tending to include many eosinophils.

4. Weakness of neck, trunk and pharyngeal muscles or persistent muscle swelling of dermatomyositis.

5. Definite scleroderma (not limited to the fingers).

6. A clinical picture characteristic of rheumatic fever with migratory joint involvement and evidence of endocarditis, especially if accompanied by subcutaneous nodules of erythema marginatum or chorea. (An elevated anti-streptolysin-O titre will not rule out the diagnosis of rheumatoid arthritis.)

7. A clinical picture characteristic of gouty arthritis with acute attacks of swelling, redness and pain in one or more joints, especially if relieved by colchicine.

8. Tophi.

9. A clinical picture characteristic of acute infectious arthritis of bacterial or viral origin with: an acute focus of infection or in close association with a disease of known infectious origin; chills; fever; and an acute joint involvement, usually migratory initially (especially if there are organisms in the joint fluid or response to antibiotic therapy).

10. Tubercle bacilli in joints or histological evidence of joint tuberculosis.

11. A clinical picture characteristic of Reiter's syndrome with urethritis and conjunctivitis associated with acute joint involvement, usually migratory initially.

12. A clinical picture characteristic of the shoulder-hand syndrome with unilateral involvement of shoulder and hand, with diffuse swelling of the hand followed by atrophy and contractures.

13. A clinical picture characteristic of hypertrophic osteoarthropathy with clubbing of fingers and/or hypertrophic periostitis along the shafts of the long bones especially if an intrapulmonary lesion is present.

14. A clinical picture characteristic of neuroarthropathy with condensation and destruction of bones of involved joints and with associated neurological findings.

15. Homogentisic acid in the urine detectable grossly with alkalinization.

16. Histological evidence of sarcoid or positive Kveim test.

17. Multiple myeloma as evidenced by marked increase in plasma cells in the bone marrow, or Bence–Jones protein in the urine.

18. Characteristic skin lesions of erythema nodosum.

19. Leukaemia or lymphoma with characteristic cells in peripheral blood, bone marrow or tissues.

Ad criteria 1–5. The first criterion in the diagnosis of rheumatoid arthritis is morning stiffness in the joints. It is a prodromal, early symptom. In the prodromal stage, the following other symptoms and signs may be observed: fever, anorexia, paraesthesia in the hands and feet, a tendency to perspiration, mild joint pains, small degree of muscle atrophy, anaemia. In fact a number of these signs may also be the early features of quite a number of diseases. They may be present for weeks or months, and only after this period does there appear swelling of the joints, with marked pain and in the majority of cases, symmetrically. It may happen that the swelling in one joint with spontaneous pain or pain on pressure or movement lasts for years in the form of a monarthritis or only periarticularly with a picture of tendinitis or tenovaginitis, before progression starts.

In a large part of the cases symmetrical pain, swelling, and restriction of movement in the joints of the hand and the wrist are the signs of the disease in the first half year. It is not infrequent to find a slight erythema over the interphalangeal joints. If these clinical signs are evident, the disease may be regarded on the presence of five criteria as 'definite rheumatoid arthritis'. Thus the diagnosis may be based purely on the clinical picture disregarding any radiological, serological or histological features. An early diagnosis is quite important from the patient's point of view, as hope for a definite improvement rests on treatment at this stage. In a smaller proportion of cases the prodromal phase is followed by high fever, tachycardia, swelling of joints, intense pain, limitation of movement, fatigue and loss of weight these being also accompanied by the involvement of internal organs. This is the malignant or septic form of rheumatoid arthritis, which is important to be differentiated from rheumatic fever and systemic lupus erythematosus.

Irrespective of how the disease commences, its process continues relentlessly throughout the years, as a rule, with periods of remissions and exacerbations. The most dangerous event is contracture formation, which most frequently affects the elbows and knees, generally symmetrically, but on occasions it may also affect the shoulders, ankles, feet, and hands. The later alterations in the hands are characteristic of rheumatoid arthritis. Atrophy of the interosseous muscles and ulnar deviation of the fingers are already noticeable if the patient is inspected from a distance.

The variable commencement and clinical progress of the disease gave an opportunity for Schulhof to classify it into types [73*b*]. Type I includes those cases which commence without any fever, insidiously in the joints of the hand, progressing with symmetrical subacute exacerbations. The highest percentage of positive agglutination reactions is found in this type. Type II commences without fever and progresses asymmetrically. Type III commences with fever and progresses symmetrically. Type IV commences without fever with the involvement of large joints asymmetrically, these remaining affected through the whole course of the disease.

Tichy classifies rheumatoid arthritis into three types, based on serological data: agglutination, anti-streptolysin-O and a mixed type [81]. It is still useful to take into account the presence of the rheumatoid factor. On this basis, seropositive and seronegative rheumatoid arthritis can be differentiated.

Classification into types may have some significance if conclusions can be drawn from them as to the progression of the disease. However, a prognosis is very difficult to predict. Irrespective of the disease type, an unexpected, transient or lasting remission, and a more or less severe relapse may occur at any time. With a view to estimation of the current status of the patients, Steinbrocker arranged a staging based partly on clinical and radiological data, and partly on functional ability [78]. Namely, the clinical and radiological status are not in strict correlation with the functional ability. Despite serious anatomical alterations or deformities, the patient may still have good functional ability, and on the other hand, with minimal anatomical alterations the patient may be incapacitated due to severe pain. Up to now no classification has taken into account the degree of activity of the disease (ESR, CRP values), although this should determine to a large extent the actual way of treatment.

Ad criterion 6. The most characteristic site for the Meynet nodules is on the elbow above the olecranon. However, they may be distributed all over the body, mainly over bony prominences, bursae, and around tendon sheaths. It occurs in barely 10 per cent of patients with rheumatoid arthritis, characteristically in the more severe forms. They are painless, as a rule. Quite identical nodules to the subcutaneous rheumatic nodules may be found infrequently in the pericardium, in the annulus fibrosus, in the lung parenchyma, and also in the sclera.

Ad criterion 7. The radiological and clinical picture generally develops in parallel. Osteoporosis is typical of the early stage, developing in the adjacent bone to the affected joint, and is particularly significant if radiograms of two symmetrical joints show a greater degree of porosis on the side more severely affected clinically. With progression of the disease the radiological signs are delayed, but later a similar parallel state of affairs will arise. With the appearance of cartilaginous destruction, there is evidence of narrowing of the joint space. In later stages the cartilaginous defects caused by pannus formation will become obvious.

Several causes may explain the osteoporosis in rheumatoid arthritis (toxic factors, inactivity). The toxic form is characterized by an increased osteoclast activity, which can only be distinguished from an osteoblast porosis by histological means, and which has been classified by Nordin amongst the local osteoporoses [60]. In the pathological events synovitis in the early stage may be followed by the accumulation of fluid, capsular thickening, and radiological evidence of changes in soft tissue contours. As a result of the necrosis of cartilage, the joint surfaces come closer to each other, and as a result of the deeply extending inflammation, bony erosions, caries, and cysts occur which already indicate an osteolytic process.

Arthritis mutilans is a severe form of rheumatoid arthritis; clinically the fingers become shortened, and appear shrunken. Radiologically a picture of bone necrosis is seen where the bony structure of the finger bones is to a large extent reabsorbed. Bone necrosis on such a large scale, either complete or incomplete, occurs not only in the fingers, but in other bone ends involved in joints (femur, knee, elbow). From a functional point of view, however, these joints remain more mobile than those tending towards ankylosis.

Ad criterion 8. When in the 1940's it became known that most rheumatoid arthritis sera agglutinate haemolysin sensitized sheep red cells, the Waaler–Rose test soon gained recognition in the serological diagnosis of the disease. The serum component responsible for the reaction, named rheumatoid factor, is only infrequently found in other musculoskeletal disorders [2, 15*b*, *c*, *e*, 44, 53].

Rheumatoid factor reacts with IgG globulin of different species, this property being used for its demonstration. In the Wealer–Rose reaction, haemolysin produced in rabbits, i.e. rabbit IgG is involved. However, for the demonstration of rheumatoid factor human or, e.g. bovine γ-globulin may also be used, and for the carrier, instead of red blood cells, synthetic particles (polystyrol-latex) [15*a*, 75*a*, *b*,], bentonite [11, 66], quartz, etc. The rheumatoid factor–γ-globulin reaction can also be demonstrated by direct precipitation, both in a fluid or semisolid medium, but this method is not sensitive enough for clinical practice. The differential diagnostic significance of the demonstration of rheumatoid factors of varying specificity, e.g. reacting only with human IgG, or reacting both with animal and human IgG, will be referred to later on.

The nature, origin, and significance of rheumatoid factor, or rather, of the varying rheumatoid factors, have not been clarified. They belong to the IgM globulin class, although IgG and IgA rheumatoid factors have also been reported [10, 19, 36]. Based on its reactivity with human IgG, rheumatoid factor is considered as an antibody against human γ-globulin, cross-reacting also with γ-globulins of different animal species. The rheumatoid factors, just as the antibodies, are produced by plasma cells. However, this fact in itself would be little proof for the antibody nature of rheumatoid factor, since plasma cells may produce not only antibodies but paraproteins as well. The production of rheumatoid factor cannot be inhibited with steroid treatment. Serum with high titres of rheumatoid factor can be injected without any consequences into human beings, or into experimental animals [35]. These observations are at variance with the antibody or autoantibody nature of rheumatoid factor.

The question also arises that if rheumatoid factor is an antibody against human IgG, why does it not also react with the circulating IgG globulins? Ultracentrifugation of serum of patients with rheumatoid arthritis, in occasional cases, showed the presence of soluble complexes with a 22S sedimentation constant. These complexes could be dissociated into 7S and 19S components; the former corresponded to IgG, the latter to IgM-rheumatoid factor [31, 72]. According to this, rheumatoid factor can react also *in vivo* with IgG molecules, but presumably without any serious consequences. If to rheumatoid factor, or even to the 22S complex, denatured, e.g. lightly heat-treated γ-globulin is added, a precipitate is formed. It appears, therefore, that rheumatoid factor exhibits a more definite reactivity towards denatured human γ-globulin. Hence was born the proposition that rheumatoid factor is an antibody to human denatured IgG. The free surface antigenic determinants of the native IgG molecules are recognized by the organism as 'self', and no antibody is produced against them. Various events, e.g. enzymatic digestion, heat treatment, or binding of the molecule with its specific antigen, lead to structural alteration of the IgG molecule. This may be accompanied by the exposition of new, previously hidden antigenic determinants from the interior of the molecule, evoking rheumatoid factor production [38, 39, 61, 71]. This view is supported by the fact that in experimental animals, after the injection of their own γ-globulin which had been slightly heat- or alkali-denatured rheumatoid factor-like substances are produced [57, 87]. Rheumatoid factor production can also be elicited if the animals are immunized over long periods with various bacteria, e.g. with *E. coli* [20, 29, 64]. What could in this case the explanation be for rheumatoid factor production? Antibodies form antigen–antibody complexes with the regularly introduced bacterial antigens. The antibody in this complex, i.e. the IgG molecule, undergoes certain structural alterations as a result of the linkage, which are similar to denaturation. This *in vivo* denatured γ-globulin would initiate the formation of rheumatoid factor. Perhaps this may be an explanation for the frequent, but transient, rheumatoid factor positivity in subacute bacterial endocarditis.

If the antigenic determinants of the IgG molecule are altered by iodination, desamination, acetylation or other treatments, the reactivity of these γ-globulin samples will be reduced or suspended both against rheumatoid factors, and Coombs' serum. Thus, the specificity of the rheumatoid factor–γ-globulin reaction closely resembles the specificity of the true antigen–antibody reaction, this being a further proof for the antibody nature of rheumatoid factor [17].

It is still not clear which factors or conditions can initiate denaturation of some IgG molecules (?by linking with antigen, ?by disordered metabolism). It may also be possible that rheumatoid factor production is not an answer at all to antigenic stimulation by denatured IgG antigen, but that an alteration of the immunologically competent cells is the primary event. As a result of the disturbed protein synthesis of these cells, such proteins are produced which, 'by chance', give antibody-like specific reactions with the denatured human or animal γ-globulins [63*a*, *b*]. An example of such 'accidental' specificity is that some plant extracts (lectins) agglutinate quite specifically certain types of red blood cells, although in this case antigenic stimulation is obviously out of question. Possibly, the various anti-γ-globulin factors are not produced by identical mechanisms. In some instances an alteration of the immune system is more likely while in other instances it may be an autoantigenic change of γ-globulin.

After the addition of various antigens to *in vitro* cultures of lymphocytes, the immunologically competent cells 'recognize' those antigens with which the organism has already been in contact and, as a result, transform into blast cells [15*d*]. In rheumatoid arthritis lymphocyte cultures, when treated with autologous or homologous joint fluid or synovial extracts, or even with γ-globulin prepared from serum of patients with rheumatoid arthritis, in a proportion of the cases blast transformation can be induced. However, blast transformation does not occur after stimulation with normal human γ-globulin, or heat denatured human γ-globulin [16, 43, 69]. According to these data, the serum and synovial fluid of rheumatoid arthritis patients may contain antigenic substances, but their exact nature has not yet been clarified. The rheumatoid factor, on a cellular basis, can be demonstrated by rosette formation (human erythrocytes coated with rabbit immunoglobulin form rosettes around lymphocytes of rheumatoid patients). The reaction is species-specific and is positive in 69 per cent of seronegative cases of rheumatoid arthritis [3, 44*a*].

The diagnostic significance of the demonstration of rheumatoid factor is limited because in the early stage of rheumatoid arthritis, in the first half to one year of the disease, the rheumatoid factor generally cannot be demonstrated either in the serum or the joint fluid [6, 15*c*, 32, 73*a*]. It is interesting, however, and demands an explanation, that patients with clinically verified rheumatoid arthritis are negative for rheumatoid factor in 10–20 per cent of the cases.

Rheumatoid factor tests frequently give positive results in systemic lupus erythematosus and other autoimmune diseases. This observation, just as much as the varying LE cell positivity in rheumatoid arthritis, reaffirm the close connection between rheumatoid arthritis and other autoimmune diseases [7, 8, 9, 24, 63*a*]. Patients suffering from psoriatic arthritis, or ankylosing spondylitis, however, do not, as a rule, have rheumatoid factor in their sera [15*c*, 49, 80]. Transient or sometimes long-lasting latex or even Waaler–Rose positivity is a frequent finding in acute and chronic hepatitis, in hepatic cirrhosis, subacute bacterial endocarditis, sarcoidosis, and several other chronic disease processes accompanied by hypergammaglobulinaemia [2, 14, 15*c*, 58, 67, 70]. According to general experience, in rheumatoid arthritis, rheumatoid factors reacting with both human and rabbit IgG can be demonstrated, and the serum is therefore latex and Rose positive. Rheumatoid factor positivity occurring occasionally in other diseases is, however, primarily directed against human IgG. Thus, the Waaler–Rose test would be comparatively more specific for rheumatoid arthritis.

This view, however, requires revision in the light of recent evidence. The production and demonstration of rheumatoid factors with differing specificity is largely influenced by the time factor, or more correctly by the time interval from the commencement of the disease. In early cases of rheumatoid arthritis the latex test becomes positive first, as a rule, and positivity of the Rose test is only a later feature. At the same time, however, not infrequently we obtain both a positive latex and Rose test in diseases other than rheumatoid arthritis, in cases where the disease process has been established for a longer time. If the antigen initiating rheumatoid factor production is, indeed, denatured autologous human γ-globulin, it is understandable that during the first period of the disease, rheumatoid factor reacts only with human γ-globulin, i.e. the serum is latex positive but Rose negative. The specificity of antibodies produced in the first phase of immunization is usually rather well expressed. During the course of the disease the specificity of the antibodies diminishes, and cross-reactions will appear. The rheumatoid factor will now react not only with human IgG, but also with the γ-globulins of other species, and the serum therefore gives a positive Rose reaction also in addition to the positive latex test. Such types of change in specificity equally relate to rheumatoid arthritis and other disease processes. Thus in the evaluation of rheumatoid factor tests, the significance of the time factor must be taken into consideration. One must also note, however, that in certain viral, and parasitic infections, a positive Waaler–Rose reaction may be found, accompanied by a negative latex test. No definitive explanation is yet available for this phenomenon.

Rheumatoid factor can be demonstrated in clinically healthy individuals, too; according to wide population surveys, it occurs in 3–5 per cent of the normal population. The extent of positivity is increased with age; in the age group above 80 years positivity may even reach 30–50 per cent, especially with the latex fixation test. At times rheumatoid factor can be shown in the serum of healthy blood relatives of patients suffering from rheumatoid arthritis, although on the basis of results of recently completed extensive analyses, the familial aggregation of positive rheumatoid factor tests is thrown into doubt. The observed positive Rose or latex tests in clinically symptom-free cases cannot simply be regarded as biological 'mistakes'. It has been observed that rheumatoid factor-positive healthy individuals will develop manifest rheumatoid arthritis in the later years in a higher frequency than the general occurrence of this disease. A persisting positive Rose or latex test — if it cannot be correlated with the clinical picture — may indicate an inclination towards rheumatoid arthritis [18, 21*a*, 23, 46*a*, 51, 52, 56].

The leukocytes in rheumatoid arthritis synovial fluid contain inclusion bodies measuring 0.5–1.5 μ in diameter. With phase-contrast microscopy these inclusion bodies show a dark ring-like appearance [40, 41, 42]. Immunofluorescence studies have verified that a part of the inclusion bodies contain IgG and IgM molecules [65, 83, 84]. From these white blood cells, rheumatoid factor was successfully extracted. Therefore it would appear that these so-called 'RA cells', or rhagocytes, developed as a result of the phagocytosis of rheumatoid factor–γ-globulin complexes.

Subsequent analyses also verify that lysosomal enzymes are released from those white blood cells which incorporate the complexes during phagocytosis [1, 13]. As is known, the various enzymes in the cytoplasm (acid hydrolase, desoxyribonuclease, ribonuclease, etc.) do not exist in the free state, but are situated in the lysosomes surrounded by a lipoprotein membrane [50, 59]. The permeability of the lysosome membrane determines the quantity of lysosomal enzyme which can come into contact with other substances in the cell, and with the environment. If the membrane becomes excessively permeable, the cell itself will be destroyed, and the enzyme causes tissue damage in the surrounding tissues. The granules of the neutrophil granulocytes are in fact lysosomes.

The infiltrating plasma cells of the rheumatoid synovial tissue produce in part γ-globulin, and also rheumatoid factor [89]. These can react with each other, especially if the γ-globulin becomes partly denatured for some reason. This complex is then phagocytosed by white blood cells which then develop into RA cells, while some of their enzyme content is released into the joint cavity. Rheumatoid synovial fluids are in fact quite rich in lysosomal enzymes [33, 34, 48, 76]. On the other hand, most drugs used in the treatment of rheumatoid arthritis possess a lysosomal membrane stabilizing effect [27, 62]. The role of lysosomes in the pathomechanism of rheumatoid arthritis appears to be likely [26, 85, 86*a*, *b*, 88*a*].

Electron-microscopically and histochemically it was possible to demonstrate in RA cells not only IgG–IgM complexes, but also numerous other types of inclusions such as fibrin, nuclear particles and DNA–protein complexes. RA cells can be demonstrated not only in rheumatoid arthritis, but also in other joint inflammatory diseases, although generally in a considerably smaller number. In these cases the inclusion bodies do not contain γ-globulin–rheumatoid factor complexes, but other phagocytosed substances [4, 37, 55, 77, 88]. Thus the RA cell phenomenon is not specific for rheumatoid arthritis, and so in fact the term is misleading. Similarly, the justification for the term rheumatoid factor is also debatable; however the more correct term 'anti-γ-globulin factor' has still not been able to replace the former one in usage. The fact that RA cells can be demonstrated in numerous joint conditions refers to the probable role played by lysosomes in the perpetuation of different types of joint inflammations. The pathogenesis of rheumatoid arthritis, however, has not received support from the recognition of the RA cell phenomenon.

Ad criterion 9. Apart from the slight mucin content of the synovial fluid, the cellular elements of the joint fluid also have a certain diagnostic significance [25]. In the early stage polynuclear cells, clasmatocytes, can be found, the rheumatoid factor may be negative; in more advanced cases the rheumatoid factor is positive, and rhagocytes are present in larger numbers. In cases of seronegative rheumatoid arthritis the number of rhagocytes is less.

Ad criteria 10 and 11. Just like the clinical, radiological, and serological data, the histological picture is not characteristic either. The synovial inflammation, at the beginning, affects the synovial membrane only slightly; later the synovial membrane surrounds the edge of the surface cartilage, it becomes thicker, the synovial cells proliferate and destroy the joint surface by pannus formation.

HISTOLOGY

The pathohistological picture appears in several phases, but a typical tissue structure, like the Aschoff body in rheumatic fever, cannot be found. There is no characteristic tissue destruction, but a particular type of tissue reaction is characteristic [30*a*, *b*]. The noxious process affects the whole organism, and even the ground substance of the connective tissue and the fibrous tissue are involved. The overactivity of the synovial membrane, its change to a shaggy appearance, an increase of capillarization, the deposition of connective tissue cells around vessels, and infiltration with round cells and plasma cells are characteristic. This is accompanied by an oedematous swelling and deposition of fibrin. Fibrinoid change and necrosis complete the picture. Fibrinoid change must be regarded as one of the most characteristic processes. One may find in the fibrinoid not only connective tissue elements, but also proteins and globulins. Granulation tissue and scar tissue appear in the last stages of the process.

In adults the different organs are less often involved in the disease process than in juvenile arthritic inflammations, but it cannot be disregarded, as in some individuals it may have serious consequences.

Heart. The endocardium, myocardium, and pericardium may become involved; thus all those constituents of the heart which may also be affected in rheumatic fever. It is striking how large the discrepancy between the clinically detected alterations and the post-mortem findings is. At autopsy higher percentages of endocardial and pericardial pathological changes are found than at the bedside. The autopsy findings also differ considerably. The reason is probably that various authors evaluate the pathological changes in different ways. There is no doubt that sclerosis develops more easily on a rheumatic basis, and in these situations not the rheumatic but the sclerotic alterations are evaluated. Baggenstoss, Rosenberg and others also emphasized the possibility of rheumatoid cardiac changes [5*a*, *b*].

Vascular system. The vessel alterations may range from the mildest vasculitis—serous inflammation, round cell infiltration, fibrinoid change—to the most serious, necrosing, vessel wall damage. Vasculitis appears as a result of the general reaction of the organism, and according to Kemper et al., and also to others, it is the principal alteration, which is followed secondarily by collagen tissue alteration [47]. According to Epstein and Engleman, however, the vascular alterations commence only during the later stages of rheumatoid arthritis [28]. Paraesthesias presenting during the early stages, and the results of estimations of skin temperature [90], which demonstrated the peripheral skin areas to be colder, reaffirm Kemper's standpoint, while the arteriographic examinations of the peripheries of the lower limbs support Epstein's view. The alteration affects the smallest vessels, i.e. the arterioles and venules. The vasa vasorum and vasa nervorum may also be affected. These alterations may be responsible for the motor and trophic disturbances, and thus for muscle atrophy, and also possibly for bone necrosis.

It has been shown that γ-globulins, probably antibodies, are attached to the endothelium of vessel walls of patients suffering from rheumatoid arthritis. Thus on the appearance of an antigen, an antigen–antibody reaction may occur which is accompanied by inflammatory cell phenomena, and also by a serous inflammation; as a result, disturbance of permeability will occur. Thus the vessel wall damage can truly be regarded as a primary event, leading also to altered permeability of membranes.

Lung and pleura. Since 1947 numerous publications have dealt with this question, and in general five main types are distinguished.

1. Pleuritis with or without effusion
2. Rheumatoid pneumoconiosis (Caplan's syndrome)
3. Non-pneumoconiotic rheumatoid nodules
4. Diffuse interstitial fibrosis and interstitial pneumonia
5. Disease process affecting the intima of small pulmonary arteries and arterioles which leads to pulmonary hypertension.

1. By biopsy performed to confirm the rheumatoid origin of a pleural exudate, nodular changes, partly chronic, non-specific inflammatory processes are found.

The extremely low sugar content of the exudate is regarded as typical, but not of a verifying value. Rheumatoid factor positivity may be misleading, as it is not absolutely typical of rheumatoid arthritis, since latex positivity has been found in other situations as well (e.g. in bacterial pneumonias the incidence is 41 per cent, in cases of carcinoma 20 per cent, in tuberculosis 14 per cent). The presence of rhagocytes may refer to rheumatoid disease. A pseudochylous effusion may also occur in the pleural cavity. In a true chylous effusion, the possible causes are trauma, tumorous compression, internal occlusion, thrombosis of the innominate or subclavian vein, filariasis, while with a pseudochlyous exudate, tuberculosis, syphilis, diabetes must be excluded.

2. In Caplan's syndrome, the development of round shadows in the lungs following the inhalation of dust can be considered along the following immunological lines [79]: proteins are adsorbed onto the surface of the quartz crystals; they undergo structural alterations and act as antigens producing immunological reactions. In experimental silicosis, antibodies against lung tissue can be demonstrated, and both the morphological and clinical pictures correspond to those of immune processes. In the lungs round shadows varying between 0.5–5 cm in diameter are distributed. Cavitation and calcification also occurs. 40 per cent of patients presenting with such lung signs have rheumatoid arthritis. Patients presenting with such lung pathology but without arthritis show a positive Waaler–Rose test in 50 per cent of cases, while patients with the typical lung and joint picture have a 100 per cent positivity rate.

3. Granulomatous lung lesions may also develop without dust exposure, which histologically closely resemble the structure of Meynet nodules. Both types of lung change may precede the development of the joint inflammation.

4. Numerous authors have noted diffuse pulmonary fibrosis and fibrotizing pneumonia associated with rheumatoid arthritis. Histologically two types may be present:

(*a*) cellular thickening of the alveolar wall with expressed tendency to fibrosis;

(*b*) inflammatory exudation, with a proteinous oedema, mononuclear cells in the lumen of the alveoli, and surrounded by a diffuse capillary network.

5. The characterization as a separate type is debatable, as with every rheumatoid alteration there may be an accompanying lesion of vessels of varying degree, from mild vasculitis to necrotizing vessel wall destruction.

Haemopoietic organs. Typical of the blood cell elements are anaemia, normal number of leukocytes, or occasionally a slight leukopenia. The anaemia is normochromic or hypochromic and the serum iron is decreased. It cannot be influenced by oral iron therapy, particularly during the stage when the disease is progressive. According to experience obtained so far, the anaemia cannot be affected during the active inflammatory stages; maybe a role is played in its development by the tropin effect of rheumatoid factor and C reactive protein. This could be one explanation for the poor response to therapeutic measures, since in this stage the erythrocytes progressively disappear from the blood [82].

Kidney. Its involvement is not one of the signs of the early stages. As a complication, glomerulonephritis may also develop. When the joint inflammation has been established for a longer time, and in serious forms, involvement of the kidneys is more frequent. Nephrotic syndrome can occur in the later stages of the process, and finally, as a result of generalized amyloidosis, an amyloid kidney will also develop. (Amongst the causes of death in rheumatoid arthritic patients, besides cardiac insufficiency, amyloidosis holds an important place.)

Spleen and lymph nodes. A small degree of splenic swelling is a frequent symptom in inflammations of joints. The enlargement of the lymph nodes generally presents around the neck and the axillary zones. A leading sign of Still's disease, i.e. juvenile rheumatoid arthritis, is splenic enlargement and lymphadenopathy. Occasionally the disease may start prior to one year of age [45]. The earlier the age of onset, the more likely are sytemic manifestations to occur. The joint disorders, in general, soon lead to serious deformities and subluxations. Several types are classified. Still reported the swelling of lymph nodes and spleen, as being characteristic; it is more correct also to reserve the term Still's disease for this form. Twenty per cent of juvenile cases are not seropositive. Felty's syndrome is adult rheumatoid arthritis with marked splenic enlargement, partly with moderate lymphadenopathy and hepatic swelling. The haematological picture is typified by anaemia and granulocytopenia. These cases are strongly seropositive.

The salivary and lacrimal glands. Alterations of these in association with joint inflammations are seen in Sjögren's syndrome (see Chapter 39). It is in fact rheumatoid arthritis accompanied by keratoconjunctivitis sicca, rhinitis, pharyngitis, laryngitis sicca, xerostomia, and anacidity. The salivary glands are palpably enlarged. In 80 per cent of these cases the sera contain anti-nuclear factor and rheumatoid factor as well as antibody against the duct epithelium of the salivary and lacrimal glands. The LE cell phenomenon may also occur.

Gastrointestinal tract. Hypoacidity or anacidity may point to the involvement.

Eye. Involvement is not frequent, particularly with episcleritis, conjunctivitis and iritis.

Liver. It is not involved in characteristic changes, but in accordance with the inflammatory features, the liver function tests are frequently positive.

AETIOPATHOLOGICAL CONSIDERATIONS

In rheumatoid arthritis, besides rheumatoid factor, LE cells may also be found. Publications up to recent years still included a percentage of 10–20 per cent for the presence of LE factor in the serum of rheumatoid arthritic patients. More recent publications all report smaller percentages: according to Lenoch and Vojtisek only 3.6 per cent in 1,000 rheumatoid arthritic patients [54], to Delbarre et al. [22] only 1 per cent, while Schulhof et al. [74] reported no cases at all of LE cell phenomena when using the *in vivo* LE cell method.

The aetiology of rheumatoid arthritis is not known. It can be regarded today as a disease with a multiple aetiology. We have no such clinical or laboratory data that would prove one definite cause for the disease, therefore, in each instance the stimulating factors related by the patient (effects of cold, trauma, etc.), infection, the constitution, and an inherited tendency should be carefully weighed and the endocrine factors as well as the influence of the nervous system should not be disregarded either.

Data on coccal or viral infection in the precursor period may be frequently found while in other cases an elevation of ASLO titre or antistaphylolysin titre draws attention to it [21*c*, 59*a*, *b*]. Joint inflammations commencing after infection, showing a typical picture of infective arthritis and initially responding to antibiotics, may subsequently develop into typical rheumatoid arthritis.

Besides direct infection, infectious foci may also have some significance. The foci, from the pathological point of view, are secondary tissue alterations, following an initial infection, which show a picture of inflammation and tissue destruction. Their contents may be bacteria or their toxins, viruses and tissue detritus. Their significance, apart from the local reaction, may be found in distant effects. The various concepts of the effects of foci may be summarized as follows:

1. According to the classic Rosenov–Billing concept, bacteria enter the bloodstream from the enclosed focus periodically (bacteriaemia).
2. According to the Slauck-type toxin concept, only the release of toxin is involved.
3. According to the allergic concept, either the bacterial substances or degradation products of the foci act as allergens.
4. The neural concept.

A careful recording of the history is indispensable in the investigation of focal infections: tiredness, insomnia, a rising temperature, palpitations, migrating pain, disturbance of digestion. In such cases a thorough search for infectious foci is necessary since after their removal a remission is more readily available.

Summing up, the inclusion of rheumatoid arthritis in the group of autoimmune diseases is indicated by the presence of autoantibodies. It is assumed that an unknown factor, or factors, initiate the attack on the organism. Following the unknown noxious effects 7S globulins become autoantigenic. As a result, plasma cells commence production of 19S globulin. The 7S and 19S globulin complexes are phagocytosed by the synovial leukocytes, and thus the 'RA cells' or 'rhagocytes' are formed.

We are now faced with the question as to the significance and the role of this phenomenon in the disease process. Phagocytic activity plays a very important role in cellular defence, partly against the cause of the disease, partly in the removal of destroyed cells or their fragments. Substances featuring in inflammation have

TABLE 38-I

Factors influencing the phagocytic activity of leukocytes

Non-specific factors			Specific factors
Promoting phagocytosis	Inhibiting phagocytosis	Tropin-like effect	
1. Histamine 2. Serotonin 3. Leukotaxine 4. Exudin 5. Lymph node permeability factor 6. Hyaluronidase 7. Nucleic acids 8. Bradykinin	1. Leukopenic factor 2. Leukopenin 3. Necrosin	C-reactive protein: (*a*) bacteriotropin (*b*) cytotropin	1. Bacteriotropin 2. LE factor 3. Rheumatoid factor: (*a*) bacteriotropin (*b*) γ-globulin–rheumatoid factor complex (*c*) cytotropin

modifying effects upon the phagocytic activity of white blood cells. Phagocytic phenomena found in chronic polyarthritis are summarized in Table 38-I.

Both groups of factors (i.e. non-specific and specific) affecting phagocytosis may come into consideration. The non-specific factors released due to the unknown noxious stimulus have partly promoting and partly inhibiting effects. CRP, as a non-specific factor, exercises tropin effects. Of the specific factors, besides the bacteriotrophins and LE factor, rheumatoid factor has also shown itself to have tropin effects. It can be established that the presence or absence of the listed specific and non-specific factors determines the intensity of phagocytosis in the synovial fluid.

In essence, however, the phagocytic activity draws attention to the fact that the organism under attack takes great efforts to thwart the assault by the unknown 'noxious' stimuli.

REFERENCES

1. Astorga, G. and Bollet, A. J.: *Arthr. and Rheum.* **8,** 511 (1965).
2. Bach, G. and Schmidt, J.: *Z. Immun.-Forsch.* **144,** 42 (1972).
3. Bach, J.-F., Debrieu, F. and Delbarre, F.: *Presse méd.* **78,** 301 (1970).
4. Bach-Andersen, R. and Elling, P.: *Ann. rheum. Dis.* **31,** 59 (1972).

5*a*. Baggenstoss, A. H. and Rosenberg, F. F.: *Arch. intern. Med.* **67,** 241 (1941).

5*b*. id., *Arch. Path.* **35,** 503 (1943).

6. Bálint, G.: *Rheum. Balneol. Allerg.* (*Budap.*) **8,** 198 (1967).
7. Bencze, Gy.: Lupus Erythematosus (LE) Cell Phenomenon. Thesis. Budapest 1966.
8. Bencze, Gy. and Lakatos, L.: *Ann. rheum. Dis.* **22,** 273 (1963).
9. Bencze, Gy., Lakatos, L. and Forró, L.: *Rheum. Balneol. Allerg.* (*Budap.*) **2,** 28 (1961).
10. Bienenstock, J., Goldstein, G. and Tomasi, Th. B.: *J. Lab. clin. Med.* **73,** 389 (1969).
11. Bloch, K. and Bunim, J. J.: *J. Amer. med. Ass.* **169,** 307 (1959).
12. Blumberg, B. S., Bunim, J. J., Calkins, E., Pirani, C. and Zvaifler, N. J.: *Arthr. and Rheum.* **7,** 93 (1964).
13. Bollet, A. J.: *Postgrad. Med.* **40,** 391 (1966).
14. Bonomo, L., Lospalluto, J. and Ziff, M.: *Arthr. and Rheum.* **6,** 104 (1963).

15*a*. Bozsóky, S.: *Orv. Hetil.* **101,** 1773 (1960).

15*b*. id., *Rheum. Balneol. Allerg.* (*Budap.*) **1,** 129 (1960).

15*c*. id., Serological Diagnosis of Rheumatoid Arthritis. Thesis. Budapest 1962.

15*d*. id., *Orvosképzés* **44,** 49 (1969).

15*e*. id., Rheumatoid Factor—Rheumatoid Arthritis. Thesis. Budapest 1970.

16. Bozsóky, S., Farkas, K., Richter, P., Weisz, M., Bálint, G., Mituszova, M. and Gömör, B.: *Rheum. Balneol. Allerg.* (*Budap.*) **10,** 193 (1969).
17. Bozsóky, S. and Franklin, E. C.: *Arthr. and Rheum.* **9,** 405 (1966).
18. Cammarata, R. J., Rodnan, G. P. and Fennel, R. H.: *J. Amer. med. Ass.* **199,** 455 (1967).
19. Chodirker, W. D. and Tomasi, T. B.: *J. clin. Invest.* **42,** 876 (1963).
20. Christian, C. L.: *J. exp. Med.* **118,** 827 (1963).

21*a*. Cobb, S.: *Arthr. and Rheum.* **8,** 76 (1965).

21*b*. id., *Amer. J. publ. Hlth.* **56,** 1657 (1966).

21*c*. Cole, B. C., Ward, J. R. and Smith, C. B.: *Arthr. and Rheum.* **16,** 191 (1973).

22. Delbarre, F.: *Wien. Z. inn. Med.* **49,** 167 (1968).
23. Dequeker, J., Noyen, R. van and Vandepitte, J.: *Ann. rheum. Dis.* **28,** 431 (1969).
24. Dubois, E. L., Friou, G. J. and Chandor, S.: *J. Amer. med. Ass.* **220,** 515 (1972).
25. Dürrigl, Th. and Zergollern, V.: *Dtsch. med. Wschr.* **97,** 477 (1972).

26. Eberhard, A., Laas, U., Vojtisek, O. and Greiling, H.: *Z. Rheumaforsch.* **31,** 105 (1972).
27. Ennis, R. S., Granda, J. L. and Posner, A. S.: *Arthr. and Rheum.* **11,** 756 (1968).
28. Epstein, W. V. and Engleman, E. P.: *Arthr. and Rheum.* **2,** 250 (1959).
29. Eyquem, A., Guyot-Jeannin, N. and Podliachouk, L.: *Ann. Inst. Pasteur* **96,** 295 (1959).
30*a*. Farkas, K.: *Orv. Hetil.* **100,** 717 (1959).
30*b*. id., *Klinikai pathologia* (*Clinical Pathology*). Medicina, Budapest 1965.
31. Franklin, E. C., Holman, H. R., Müller-Eberhard, H. J. and Kunkel, H. G.: *J. exp. Med.* **105,** 425 (1957).
32. Gáspárdy, G., jr., Weisz, M., Mituszova, M., Bálint, G., Gömör, B. and Bozsóky, S.: *Rheum. Balneol. Allerg.* (*Budap.*) **10,** 1 (1969).
33. Goldfischer, S., Smith, C. and Hamerman, D.: *Arthr. and Rheum.* **10,** 281 (1967).
34. Görgényi, F. and Katona, M.: *Rheum. Balneol. Allerg.* (*Budap.*) **6,** 159 (1965).
35. Harris, J. and Vaughan, J. H.: *Arthr. and Rheum.* **4,** 47 (1961).
36. Heimer, R. and Levin, F. M.: *Immunochemistry* **3,** 1 (1966).
37. Hemmer, P. and Gamp, A.: *Z. Rheumaforsch.* **27,** 261 (1968).
38. Henney, C. S. and Stanworth, D. R.: *Nature* **210,** 1071 (1966).
39. Henney, C. S., Stanworth, D. R. and Gell, P. G. H.: *Nature* **205,** 1079 (1965).
40. Hollander, J. L., Fudenberg, H. H. and Rawson, A. J.: *Arthr. and Rheum.* **9,** 675 (1966).
41. Hollander, J. L., McCarthy, D. J., jr., Astorga, G. and Castro-Murillo, E.: *Ann. intern. Med.* **62,** 271 (1965).
42. Hollander, J. L., McCarty, D. J., jr., Rawson, S. J.: *Bull. rheum. Dis.* **16,** 382 (1965).
43. Kačaki, J. N., Bullock, W. E. and Vaughan, J. H.: *Lancet* **i,** 1289 (1969).
44. Keitel, W.: *Beitr. Rheum.* **12,** 43 (1967).
44*a*. Keith, H. I. and Currey, H. L. F.: *Ann. rheum. Dis.* **32,** 202 (1973).
45. Kellei, V. C.: *Pediat. Clin. N. Amer.* **7,** 435 (1960).
46*a*. Kellgren, J. H.: *Ann. rheum. Dis.* **23,** 109 (1964).
46*b*. id., *Arthr. and Rheum.* **9,** 658 (1966).
47. Kemper, J. W., Baggenstoss, A. H. and Slocum, Ch. H.: *Ann. intern. Med.* **46,** 831 (1957).
48. Kerby, G. P. and Taylor, S. M.: *Arthr. and Rheum.* **10,** 290 (1967).
49. Korossy, S., Csákány, Gy., Bozsóky, S. and Bakos, L.: *Rheum. Balneol. Allerg.* (*Budap.*) **2,** 134 (1961).
50. Lapis, K.: *Orv. Hetil.* **109,** 785 (1968).
51. Lawrence, J. S.: *Arthr. and Rheum.* **6,** 166 (1963).
52. Lawrence, J. S., Behren, T., Bennett, P. H., Bremner, J. M., Burch, T. A., Gofton, J., O'Brien, W. and Robinson, H.: *Ann. rheum. Dis.* **25,** 425 (1966).
53. Legler, F.: *Beitr. Rheum.* **12,** 11 (1967).
54. Lenoch, F. and Vojtisek, O.: *Acta rheum. scand.* **13,** 313 (1967).
55. Malinin, T. J., Pekin, Th. J. and Zvaifler, N. J.: *Amer. J. clin. Path.* **47,** 203 (1967).
56. Masi, A. T.: *Ann. Rev. Med.* **18,** 185 (1967).
57. McCluskey, R. T., Miller, F. and Benacerraf, B.: *J. exp. Med.* **115,** 253 (1962).
58. Messner, R. P., Laxdal, Th., Quie, P. G. and Williams, R. C.: *Ann. intern. Med.* **68,** 746 (1968).
59. Missmahl, H. P. and Rietmüller, G.: *Blut* **15,** 198 (1967).
59*a*. Neumark, T. and Farkas, K.: *Ann. rheum. Dis.* **29,** 653 (1970).
59*b*. Neumark, T., Hollós, I. and Farkas, K.: *Scand. J. Rheumatol.* **2,** 21 (1973).
60. Nordin, B. E. C.: *Lancet* **i,** 1011 (1961).
61. Normansell, D. E.: *Immunochemistry* **8,** 593 (1971).
62. Paltemaa, S.: *Acta rheum. scand.* **14,** 161 (1968).
63*a*. Petrányi, Gy.: Systemic Lupus Erythematosus and the "Rheumatic", "Collagen", "Autoallergic", and "Autoimmune" Diseases. Thesis. Debrecen 1964.
63*b*. id., *Orv. Hetil.* **106,** 1873 (1965).
64. Podliachouk, L., Eyquem, E. and Corvazier, R.: *Ann. Inst. Pasteur* **109,** Suppl. 58 (1965).
65. Rawson, A. J., Abelson, N. M. and Hollander, J. L.: *Ann. intern. Med.* **62,** 281 (1965).

66. Richter, A., Chatel, A. and Mády, Gy.: *Orv. Hetil.* **102,** 208 (1961).
67. Risemberg, A., Gomez, A. and de Rife, U.: *Ann. rheum. Dis.* **28,** 428 (1969).
68. Ropes, M. W., Bennett, G. A., Cobb, J., Jacox, R. and Jessar, R.: *Bull. rheum. Dis.* **9,** 175 (1958).
69. Rottenberger, W. and Thiele, H. G.: *Klin. Wschr.* **48,** 518 (1970).
70. Scheiffarth, F., Warnatz, H. and Essing, H. G.: *Int. Arch. Allergy* **28,** 240 (1965).
71. Schoenfeld, L. S. and Eppstein, W. V.: *Vox Sang.* (*Basel*) **10,** 482 (1965).
72. Schrohenloher, R. E.: *J. clin. Invest.* **45,** 501 (1966).
73*a*. Schulhof, Ö.: *Rheum. Balneol. Allerg.* (*Budap.*) **10,** 209 (1969).
73*b*. id., *X. Congr. Lega Int. Rheum. Roma, 1961.* Vol. I. (*Relationi*). Minerva med., Torino 1961, p. 115.
74. Schulhof, Ö., Vértes, P., Vajda, Gy., Mituszova, L., Weisz, M. and Bakos, L.: *XII. Congr. Rheum. Int. Prague, 1969.* Geigy, Basel 1969. Abstr. No. 344.
75*a*. Singer, J. M. and Plotz, Ch. M.: *Amer. J. Med.* **21,** 888 (1956).
75*b*. id., *Arthr. and Rheum.* **8,** 194 (1965).
76. Smith, C. and Hamerman, D.: *Arthr. and Rheum.* **5,** 411 (1962).
77. Steffen, C., Knapp, W., Thumb, N., Schuster, F., Bösch, J., Brunner, H. and Eibl, M.: *Z. Immun.-Forsch.* **143,** 252 (1972).
78. Steinbrocker, O., Traeger, C. H. and Battermann, R.: *J. Amer. med. Ass.* **150,** 659 (1949).
79. Szinay, Gy.: Data on the Morphology of Collagen Diseases. Thesis. Budapest 1967.
80. Tapanes, F. J., Rawson, A. J. and Hollander, J. L.: *Arthr. and Rheum.* **15,** 153 (1972).
81. Tichy, H., Seidel, K. and Heidelmann, K.: *Lehrbuch der Rheumatologie.* 2nd ed. Volk und Gesundheit, Berlin 1962.
82. Vajda, J. and Bakos, L.: *Rheumaforsch.* **21,** 400 (1962).
83. Vaughan, J. H., Barnett, E. V., Sobel, M. V. and Jacox, R. F.: *Arthr. and Rheum.* **11,** 125 (1968).
84. Vaughan, J. H., Jacox, R. F. and Noel, Ph.: *Arthr. and Rheum.* **11,** 135 (1968).
85. Weiss, L. and Dingle, J. T.: *Ann. rheum. Dis.* **23,** 57 (1964).
86*a*. Weissmann, G.: *Arthr. and Rheum.* **9,** 834 (1966).
86*b*. id., *Ann. Rev. Med.* **18,** 97 (1967).
87. Williams, R. C., jr. and Kunkel, H. G.: *Ann. N. Y. Acad. Sci.* **124,** 860 (1965).
88. Willkens, R. F. and Healey, L. A., jr.: *J. Lab. clin. Med.* **68,** 628 (1966).
88*a*. Wright, D. G. and Malawista, St. E.: *Arthr. and Rheum.* **16,** 749 (1973).
89. Zvaifler, N. J.: *J. exp. Med.* **134,** 276 (1971).
90. Zselyonka, L. and Razgha, A.: *Vascular Function Studies on Rheumatic Subjects.* S. Belák Memorial Issue. Mérnökök Nyomdája, Budapest 1948, p. 98.

CHAPTER 39

SJÖGREN'S SYNDROME

by

GY. LUGOSSY

INTRODUCTION

In 1933 Sjögren [49] described the syndrome which was later named after him. The symptoms originally reported were chronic inflammation of the lacrimal and salivary glands with half to two-thirds of the patients suffering from rheumatoid arthritis or other connective tissue disease. In the so-called sicca syndrome only the first two features are present. Sjögren maintained that the changes of the lacrimal and salivary glands were caused by a chronic inflammation and that the disease was associated with endocrine dysfunction. The possible role of an immunopathological mechanism has lately been suggested [47*b*].

CLINICAL PICTURE

The clinical picture in Sjögren's syndrome is variable.

OCULAR SYMPTOMS

The earliest, and for a long time only symptom is the almost complete failure of lacrimal secretion. As a result, the condition of the cornea called keratoconjunctivitis sicca (KCS) by Duke-Elder develops. The underlying cause is atrophy of the lacrimal glands characterized by a slow onset, chronic course and recurrence. Objective eye symptoms include hyperaemia of the conjunctiva, corneal vascularization, papillary hypertrophy, viscous lacrimal secretion and reduced tear formation.

The usual diagnostic procedures in KCS are Schirmer's test, bengal rose staining and slit-lamp examination.

ORAL SYMPTOMS

Atrophy of the lacrimal glands is followed by a reduction in the secretory activity of other glands of epithelial origin resulting in the dryness of the related mucous membranes. In this way rhinitis, pharyngitis and laryngitis sicca may accompany the involvement of the cornea. The recurrent, gross, relatively rough and painless enlargement of the parotid and submaxillary glands [55] can often be observed simulating Mikulicz's disease [36].

At the early stage of xerostomia the small amount of saliva produced is viscous, yellowish-brown with pH values about 5.3; it contains neither mucin nor ptyalin, nor peroxidase [13]. In fully developed cases there is no salivary secretion, the mouth is dry and a burning sensation is constantly felt. The tongue is red and dry, and is painful on moving and mastication. In addition to xerostomia, other oral symptoms, e.g. hypaesthesia or paraesthesia may also be present [58].

In single cases epistaxis of the ear, nose and throat, nasal septal perforation, sinusitis, serosus otitis media were also reported. The gastrointestinal tract may show symptoms of dysphagia, nasopharyngeal webs and atrophic gastritis.

BONE AND JOINT INVOLVEMENT

These symptoms occurring in the great majority o patients with Sjögren's syndrome include arthralgia, exacerbations suggestive of acute polyarthritis usually with the characteristic signs of rheumatoid arthritis like contractures, limitation of movement and deformities. Calcification of the periosteal tissues especially in the paravertebral regions are common [57]. Excessive fragility of the teeth may be noted.

SYMPTOMS OF THE UROGENITAL TRACT

KCS occurs predominantly in women. It usually develops during or after the menopause. In a relatively large patient material average age was found to be 56.2 years [58]. The ocular and oral symptoms often show a periodicity related to the menstrual cycle with exacerbations occurring before menstruation. Comparing the time of onset of sicca complaints, menopause and polyarthritis, it was found that in the great majority of cases the sicca symptoms were the last to appear and in no case were they the first manifestations [58].

Dryness and atrophy of the vulval and vaginal mucosa may give rise to painful conditions (vulvo-vaginitis sicca atrophicans). Similar manifestations in the urinary tract may be responsible for urethritis and/or cystopyelitis. Renal tubular defects and interstitial nephritis have also been reported. Perianal xerosis is frequent causing pruritus and tenesmus.

SKIN SYMPTOMS

Due to atrophy of the sweat-glands and sebaceous glands, the skin appears dry, thin, seborrhoeic and desquamative; the patient looks older than his age. The nails are brittle. Scleroatrophic areas with telangiectasis and pigment disorders have also been observed. Sclerodermiform appearance of the changes sometimes suggests sclerodermia [27, 28, 29, 44, 48]. Vasomotor disorders, acrocyanosis, Raynaud's phenomena are frequent on the extremities [6, 16]. The hair may become thin, some women patients grow bald.

HAEMATOPOIETIC SYMPTOMS

Purpura (often hyperglobulinaemic) has been observed at different stages of the disease [18, 29, 46]. Pernicious anaemia and other haematological disorders (e. g. thrombocytopenia, leukopenia) associated with the disease are of interest from the aspect of a possible autoallergic pathogenesis. Williamson et al. [63] reported that 77 patients with pernicious anaemia and 20 with idiopathic Addison's disease were screened for keratoconjunctivitis sicca by Schirmer's tear tests, staining of the conjunctiva and cornea by rose bengal dye, and slit-lamp examination. The incidence of keratoconjunctivitis sicca in these patients was not higher than in 72 hospital controls. Sialography was performed on four patients who had xerostomia but no abnormalities were detected.

MISCELLANEOUS SYMPTOMS

Nervous system disorders (e. g. cranial nerve lesions, peripheral neuropathy) and *psychic alterations* have been observed in patients with lymphocytic lymphoepithelial sialadenitis, part of whom suffered from sicca syndrome [23]. Thus nervous disorders may have a pathogenetic role in sialadenopathy, which is present in sicca syndrome and is a major symptom of other diseases of rheumatic origin.

Respiratory system symptoms include tracheitis, bronchitis, pneumonitis, atelectasia, pleural effusions and diffuse interstitial pulmonary fibrosis.

AETIOPATHOGENESIS

Besides genetic factors, the role of various endogenous and exogenous factors has been considered. Lately an immunopathological interpretation of the disease has gained ground.

GENETIC FACTORS

History of patients with Sjögren's syndrome mostly contains references to familiar occurrence of other rheumatic diseases. Disorders of phenylalanine and tryptophan synthesis found in rheumatic subjects is attributed to a hereditary defect of metabolism [39]. Changes in the tryptophan and tyrosine content of the saliva occur as a result [64]. It has been suggested that genetic factors may be responsible for the different immune serological abnormalities observed in the clinical subgroups of Sjögren's syndrome [11].

ENDOCRINE DISORDERS

Sjögren himself called attention to the possible role of disturbances of hormonal regulation because the first symptoms usually corresponded to the start of the menopause. It seems that the hormonal milieu or aging at least contribute to the aetiopathogenesis of Sjögren's syndrome [23, 59].

EXOGENOUS FACTORS

Several investigators [2, 15, 24] attributed a role to vitamin deficiency. The fact that some symptoms of Sjögren's syndrome are similar to those observed in A-avitaminosis would suggest the aetiological role of A-hypovitaminosis. However, serum A-vitamin levels were found to be normal in patients with Sjögren's syndrome.

Based on observations made in experimental immunosialadenitis [20, 33] it has been assumed that tuberculotic infection plays the same role as Freund's adjuvant and promotes the autoimmune process [23].

It is generally accepted that the composition of the commensal oral flora is controlled by complex interactions among the oral microorganisms themselves, the host tissues, and the mechanical washing action and antimicrobial activity of saliva. If one of these factors is greatly altered—for example, the difference in the oral flora of patients with xerostomia (significantly greater numbers of *Candida albicans, Staphylococcus aureus,* and coliform bacilli)—the chronic inflammation of dry mucosa will ensue [33*a*].

A possible virus origin of the disease has also been suggested. Virus-like structures [47*c*] and endoplasmic structures [26*a*] have been found in the endothelial cells, pericytes and lymphocytes of biopsy specimens taken from the parotid gland and kidney.

THE ROLE OF AUTOALLERGY

Changes of the salivary glands and lymphoid tissues are of interest in view of the pathogenetic relation between Still's syndrome, Felty's syndrome and Sjögren's syndrome [17].

Recent clinical, pathological and immunological findings indicate the frequent association of Sjögren's syndrome with other autoimmune disorders, e.g. with systemic lupus erythematosus [4, 7, 8, 22*a*, *b*, 30, 34, 37, etc.], progressive systemic sclerosis [21, 24, 47*a*], polyarteritis nodosa [6, 12, 19, 38, 43], and Hashimoto's thyroiditis [47*b*, 59] (Fig. 39-1).

Organ-specific antibodies (e.g. anti-thyroid globulin, anti-thyroid microsome, anti-mitochondrial, anti-gastric-parietal-cell, anti-salivary-duct-cell antibodies) and non-organ-specific autoantibodies (anti-nuclear factor, antibodies to denatured DNA, precipitating autoantibodies, rheumatoid factor, complement fixing antibodies, LE-cell factor) have been demonstrated in the sera of patients having Sjögren's syndrome [3, 9, 11, 14, 22*b*, 25, 26]. Various pathomorphological and immunological findings are also available which seem to support the autoallergic origin of Sjögren's syndrome.

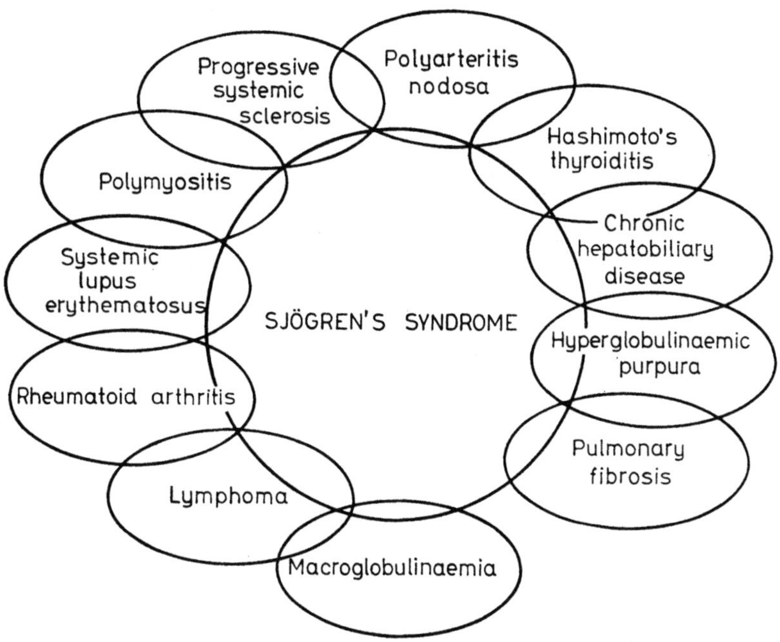

Fig. 39-1. The spectrum of disorders associated with Sjögren's syndrome (Shearn) [47*b*]

PATHOMORPHOLOGY

The relationship between the glandular lesions and rheumatoid arthritis in Sjögren's syndrome remains unclear. Histological examination of the lacrimal glands has shown marked connective tissue proliferation, areas infiltrated by numerous lymphocytes and plasma cells with only isolated residues of tubuli. In the majority of cases lymphocytes dominate in the inflammatory cell population of lymphoepithelial sialadenitis [23]. In KCS the corneal epithelium becomes considerably flattened, the number of cellular layers is decreased, and in several places the superficial layer becomes detached and forms small filaments [32]. Lip biopsies show in labial salivary glands extensive lymphoid cell infiltration [3*a*, 7*a*, 14].

Radnót [41*a*, *b*], Morgan and Castleman [37] and more recently Hollósi [23] investigated the pathomorphological picture of Sjögren's syndrome. Some authors pointed to the primary role of lymphoid tissue inclusions of the salivary glands in the development of lymphoepithelial formations [1, 54]. Changes in the lacrimal glands were found to occur less frequently than in the salivary glands. Alterations in Sjögren's syndrome differed considerably from the lymphoma-like infiltrations. The clinico-pathological resemblance suggested that salivary gland enlargement associated with lymphoepithelial lesion without systemic symptoms was a sub-type of the classical Sjögren's syndrome.

Immunoglobulins, different from the circulating antibodies, have been demonstrated in lymphocytes in the interstitium of the salivary glands using immunofluorescent technique. These globulins differed from the humoral antibodies both in their chemical structure and immunological properties [56]. Under the light microscope the lymphocytes and plasma cells producing these specific globulins did not differ morphologically from the corresponding cells of peripheral lymphatic organs or from those coming from the bone marrow subsequent to an inflammatory reaction.

Focal lymphocytic sialadenitis was observed in patients with rheumatoid arthritis. This lesion has been called 'a miniature Sjögren's syndrome' [60], although some authors could only demonstrate the phenomenon in part of their patients [61].

The syndrome presents a broad spectrum of lymphoproliferation, from benign disease, through non-malignant extraglandular lymphoproliferation ('pseudolymphomas'), to frankly malignant disease, either macroglobulinaemia or lymphomas [14].

Ten per cent of the patients suffering from Sjögren's syndrome were reported to develop in the course of the disease reticulosarcoma or Hodgkin's disease [45, 52]. Benign lymphoepithelial lesion may become transformed into malignant lymphoma [10, 23]. Chronic lymphoid hyperplasia and plasma cell activity of the salivary and lacrimal glands elicit the production of multiple circulating antibodies, excessive proliferation and malignant transformation of lymphoid cells, the formation of certain immunoglobulins or abnormal globulins. The factors responsible for the neoplastic transformation of the hyperactive immunologically competent cells are unknown, the pathogenetic role of X-ray therapy has been postulated [10].

Important observations have been made on the pathomorphology of the nervous symptoms occurring in Sjögren's syndrome. Lymphocytic infiltration could not only be demonstrated in the affected perivascular areas, but also perineurally. This finding can be of great importance from the aspect of the trophic lesions [29] of the skin and accessory organs as well as of the glands situated in the mucous membranes. Neurogenic trophic lesions could also explain the reduced functioning of the endocrine glands [50].

IMMUNOLOGY

Clinicopathological evidence and the association of Sjögren's syndrome with other autoimmune diseases, the pathomorphological changes observed in the lacrimal and salivary glands as well as serological findings directed attention to the immunopathological features of the disease. Studies utilizing biopsy specimens from the lower lips demonstrated the local synthesis of large amounts of IgM and IgG and rheumatoid factor in salivary glandular tissue [3*a*]. Precipitating antibodies against lacrimal and salivary gland extracts [26] and the almost identical histological picture observed in Sjögren's syndrome and Hashimoto's thyroiditis indicated its organ-specific autoallergic nature. Subsequent investigations have, however, revealed that precipitating and complement fixing antibodies in patients with Sjögren's syndrome are, in fact, not organ-specific because they also reacted with e.g. kidney and thyroid extracts [3]. Other authors have found high anti-nuclear antibody and rheumatoid factor positivity in a considerable number of patients [5, 11]. The presence of rheumatoid factor was demonstrated autoradiographically by interaction between anti-IgG–IgG complexes and labelled immunoglobulins [3*a*].

Cells bearing IgG, IgA, IgM and IgD were identified with monospecific fluorescent antisera in Sjögren's syndrome. In five of seven patients the frequency of cells identified with at least two anti-heavy-chain reagents was elevated. The sum of the number of cells binding individual anti-heavy-chain sera was about four times greater than the apparent number of B lymphocytes as identified both with an anti-Fab reagent and by the binding of aggregated γ-globulin. These data indicate that individual B lymphocytes in some patients with Sjögren's syndrome bear multiple classes of heavy chains, an abnormality that has been noted by others in some patients with lymphoma. This association is of interest since there is a spectrum of benign to malignant lymphoproliferation in Sjögren's syndrome [57*a*].

Heaton [22*a*, *b*] demonstrated that rheumatoid factor was positive almost as frequently in Sjögren's syndrome as in rheumatoid arthritis (Table 39-I). This fact supports the view that Sjögren's syndrome is actually a form of rheumatoid arthritis. In Hashimoto's thyroiditis it was only the thyroid autoantibody that occurred in high titres. In both SLE and Sjögren's syndrome positivity to all four autoantibodies was relatively frequent indicating that Sjögren's syndrome was an incipient or mild form of SLE [22*a*].

TABLE 39-I

Per cent frequency of autoantibodies in autoimmune diseases (after Heaton) [22*b*]

	Anti-nuclear factor	Rheumatoid factor	Autoimmune complement fixation test	Thyroid antibody
Hashimoto's thyroiditis	8	2	5	100
Rheumatoid arthritis	14	80	10	11
Systemic lupus erythematosus	98	40	37	25
Sjögren's syndrome	49	82	49	52

In experimental immunosialadenitis elicited in rabbit [8], cat [33] and rat [20] no vascular or neural lesions were observed despite the appearance of immunoglobulins in the glands. Thus, the immunopathological characteristics of experimentally induced immunosialadenitis and human lymphocytic lymphoepithelial sialadenitis were analogous only in some respects.

Immunofluorescent autoantibodies against salivary duct epithelium were demonstrated in 15 per cent of the patients with Sjögren's syndrome without rheumatoid arthritis or other connective tissue diseases; in 65 per cent of the patients with verified Sjögren's syndrome and associated rheumatoid arthritis; in 26 per cent of patients only suffering from rheumatoid arthritis [31]. However, in the latter group of patients the presence of autoantibodies could be related to a presumable KCS due to decreased lacrimal secretion and to symptomatic xerostomia. Thus, autoantibodies against salivary duct epithelium may indicate a subclinical form of Sjögren's disease [31].

In Sjögren's syndrome, the earliest glandular infiltration by lymphoid cells surrounds the salivary ducts, which are also the target of the organ-specific anti-salivary-duct autoantibody found in some patients with this disorder. A sensitizing antigen localized in ductal epithelial cells may elicit both humoral and cell-mediated immune response. In a study using coded specimens from patients with Sjögren's syndrome, sera were tested for anti-salivary-duct autoantibody, and lip biopsies were graded for the degree of lymphoid infiltration and destruction of labial salivary gland. Significantly less cellular infiltration was found in patients who had anti-salivary-duct antibody compared to those who lacked this antibody. In Sjögren's syndrome, the group of anti-salivary-duct negative patients had greater destruction and more severe xerostomia. The possible role of anti-salivary-duct antibody as a blocking antibody is suggested [3*a*, *b*, 14*a*].

As multiple serum antibodies could be demonstrated in both Sjögren's syndrome and SLE, they are both looked upon as rheumatic diseases [53] with an immunological specificity to a number of cell constituents. The main difference between Sjögren's syndrome and SLE lies in the absence of the SLE skin manifestations and the extremely rare occurrence of kidney disease in the former. However, several forms of renal defects occur in patients with sicca complex, as are e.g. hyposthenuria, Fanconi's syndrome and tubular acidosis.

Studies were made to demonstrate precipitating antibodies against six tissue antigens in patients with Sjögren's syndrome. The antigens used were native and heat-denatured DNA, calf thymus nucleoprotein, nuclear extract reacting with the sera of SLE patients, rat liver ribosomes and human spleen cytoplasm extract. Reactivity to heat-denatured DNA was the highest in the group suffering from renal disorder; sera of none of the patients reacted with native DNA and only that of one patient with nucleoprotein.

The serum protein pattern in Sjögren's syndrome has been studied. Benign, idiopathic, rudimentary and malignant parapoteinaemias (with monoclonal immunoglobulin components) have been found mostly with IgM; occasionally there has been Bence–Jones proteinuria [34*a*]. Only very sensitive immunoelectrophoretic methods are able to show up these minor components.

Kryoglobulinaemia and rheumatoid factor are most frequently demonstrable. IgM paraproteins have anti-IgG and/or anti-rheumatoid-factor properties and are demonstrable as kryoglobulin if brought into reaction with IgG. No satisfactory proof has been found to indicate the pathogenic role of different autoantibodies (some of which occur together with paraproteins) in Sjögren's syndrome.

Leukocyte migration inhibition test was positive in 93 per cent of Sjögren-syndrome patients and only in 31 per cent of rheumatoid arthritis [7*a*]. Keratoconjunctivitis sicca was found to occur in 31 per cent of patients with autoimmune hepatitis. Leukocyte migration inhibition positivity occurred in 60 per cent of these. A good correlation was found between the degree of lymphocyte infiltration in the labial salivary gland and the reactivity of parotid extract.

According to Cummings et al. [14] genetic factors leading to an immunological imbalance between cell-mediated and humoral responses to viral antigens might play a role in the pathogenesis.

Whaley et al. [62] studied the immune response in patients having Sjögren's disease. Several patients failed to respond to 2-4, dinitrochlorobenzene sensitization and exhibited poor secondary responses to tetanus toxoid. Mantoux responses, however, were diminished only in patients with the sicca syndrome. Estimation of RNA/DNA ratios of peripheral blood lymphocytes showed increased ratios in groups of patients responding poorly to DNCB and tetanus toxoid. The patients with elevated ratios had an absolute or relative increase in the number of large lymphocytes circulating in the peripheral blood. It is suggested that failure to respond to DNCB may be due to a deficiency of uncommitted small lymphocytes.

PROGNOSIS

The prognosis in Sjögren's syndrome depends, to a large extent, on the nature of associated disorders. According to Shearn [47*b*] it is difficult to make an accurate prediction for the individual patient. In any case, Sjögren's syndrome with or without associated autoimmune disease carries an increased risk of early death, especially from infection, malignant lymphoma, and probably also renal and hepatic failure.

THERAPY

Corresponding to the variability of symptoms, their origin and the immunological manifestations, a variety of therapeutic approaches have been attempted. Nevertheless, the results can hardly be regarded as satisfactory. Chemotherapeutic stimulation of lacrimal and salivary secretion did not prove effective. Prolonged vitamin A therapy, ACTH and cortisone treatment either produced transitory improvement or were ineffective.

Bonnet [10] surveyed the most important current measures applied in the treatment of keratoconjunctivitis sicca. Some of the earlier methods, which have proved their efficacy, are still in use. For a long time, hydroxychloroquine was the only drug applied as general treatment. Good results are expected from immunosuppressive drugs by some authors [14]. Cyclophosphamide has been found to bring about histological improvement and to diminish immunoglobulin synthesis, but the sicca symptoms diminished in half of the cases only [3*a*]. Combined therapy (azathioprin + prednisolone + chloroquine) has lately been suggested [14*a*]. Disappearance of the symptoms shows a reversed order compared with the sequence of their appearance. The benefit derived from the combined therapy has been attributed to the synergistic effect of the individual drugs acting on the various symptoms of the disease which are not uniform either pathogenetically or in their time of appearance. Local symptoms are treated with injections into the lacrimal gland of soluble corticosteroids [10].

Based on experimental results, sex-hormone therapy was attempted. Lacassagne [28] was the first to demonstrate sexual dimorphism in the mouse submaxillary salivary gland. The tubular system in the male was found considerably more developed than in the female. On the effect of castration the tubuli of the male salivary gland became similar to those of the female. Radnót and Németh [42] observed enlargement of the lacrimal glands in response to androgen administration. Histological studies revealed hyperactivity of the parenchyma in the females and the castrated male rabbits. According to Wallner [58], it is not the oestrogen but progesterone that is necessary for the maintenance of the exocrine glandular system. The absence of progesterone production may lead to the development of sicca symptoms; hormonal substitution therapy may bring about improvement. In Wallner's cases the subsidence of the ocular and oral symptoms was accompanied by an improvement in the objective ophthalmological findings, i.e. the values of Schirmer's test, the staining of the cornea with bengal rose and the slit lamp picture. An improvement of xerostomia, the burning of the tongue and of the labial and angular symptoms was also seen. These data indicate that it is not the disease specificity but the organ specificity of the androgen and progesterone preparation that underlies their action.

Messner and Leibowitz [35] reported that keratoconjunctivitis sicca in a patient with advanced rheumatoid arthritis was treated with topical application of 20 per cent acetylcysteine. Previous treatment with various conventional ocular lubricants had been unsuccessful. Acetylcysteine therapy prevented mucus accumulation and resulted in clearing of conjunctival injection, relief of foreign body sensation and blepharospasm, and a marked improvement in visual acuity. A therapeutic trial with a hydrophilic contact lens also produced considerable symptomatic relief. However, this device was not as effective as acetylcysteine administration either in alleviating symptoms or in preventing mucus accumulation.

For evaluating the results of therapy Talal [51, 52] recommended repeated lip biopsies.

REFERENCES

1. Albrecht, H. and Arzt, L.: *Frankf. Z. Path.* **4,** 47 (1940).
2. Allington, H. V.: *Arch. Derm. Syph.* **62,** 829 (1950).
3. Anderson, J. R., Gray, K. G., Beck, J. S. and Kinnear, W. F.: *Lancet* **ii,** 456 (1961).

3*a*. Anderson, L. G., Cummings, N. A., Asofsky, R., Hylton, M. B., Tarpley, T. M., jr., Tomasi, T. B., Wolf, R. O., Schall, G. L. and Talal, N.: *Amer. J. Med.* **53,** 456 (1972).

3*b*. Anderson, L. G., Tarpley, T. M., Talal, N., Cummings, N. A., Wolf, R. O. and Schall, G. L.: *Clin. exp. Immunol.* **13,** 335 (1973).

4. Bain, G. O.: *Canad. med. Ass. J.* **82,** 143 (1960).
5. Beck, J. S., Anderson, J. R., McElhinney, A. J. and Rowell, N. R.: *Lancet* **ii,** 575 (1962).

6. Beiglböck-Hoff: *Dtsch. med. Wschr.* **77,** 1 (1952).
7. Bencze, G.: Systemic Lupus Erythematosus. Dissertation. Szeged 1960.
7*a*. Berry, H., Bacau, P. A. and Davis, J. D.: *Ann. rheum. Dis.* **31,** 298 (1972).
8. Beutner, E. H., Djaninan, A. Y., Geckler, R. C. and Witebsky, E.: *Proc. Soc. exp. Biol. (N. Y.)* **107,** 486 (1961).
9. Bloch, K. J., Wohl, M. J., Ship, II., Oglesby, B. B. and Bunim, J. J.: *Arthr. and Rheum.* **3,** 287 (1960).
10. Bonnet, M.: *Ann. Ocul.* **203,** 775 (1970).
11. Bunim, J. J.: *Ann. rheum. Dis.* **20,** 1 (1961).
12. Cardell, B. S. and Gurling, K. J.: *Path. Bact.* **68,** 137 (1964).
13. Creyx, M. and Levy, J.: *Bull. Soc. méd. Hôp. (Paris)* **64,** 169 (1948).
14. Cummings, N. A., Schall, G. L., Asofsky, R., Anderson, L. G. and Talal, N.: *Ann. intern. Med.* **75,** 937 (1971).
14*a*. Cziráki, L. and Szemere, P.: *Orv. Hetil.* **115,** 796 (1974).
15. Degos, R.: *Bull. Soc. méd. (Paris)* **60,** 25 (1944).
16. Ellman, P. and Weber, F. P.: *Brit. med. J.* **304,** 4598 (1949).
17. Farkas, K.: *Klinikai pathologia (Clinical Pathology).* Medicina, Budapest 1965.
18. Gougerot, H.: *Bull. Soc. franç. Derm. Syph.* **32,** 376 (1925).
19. Haas, E.: *Virchows Arch. path. Anat.* **320,** 264 (1951).
20. Haferkamp, O.: *Virchows Arch. path. Anat.* **335,** 298 (1962).
21. Harrington, A. B. and Dewar, H. A.: *Brit. med. J.* **2,** 1302 (1951).
22*a*. Heaton, J. M.: *Brit. med. J.* **1,** 466 (1959).
22*b*. id., *Proc. roy. Soc. Med.* **55,** 479 (1962).
23. Hollósi, K.: Data on the Pathomorphology and Pathogenesis of Neurovegetative and Rheumatic Sialadenopathies and of Sjögren's Syndrome. Thesis. Budapest 1967.
24. Holm, S.: *Acta ophthal. (Kbh.)* **33,** Suppl. (1949).
25. Hughes, G. R. V. and Whaley, K.: *Brit. med. J.* **4,** 533 (1972).
26. Jones, B. R.: *Lancet* **ii,** 773 (1958).
26*a*. Kerl, H. and Auböck, L.: *Hautarzt* **24,** 95 (1973).
27. Kirkham, T. H.: *Brit. J. Ophthal.* **53,** 131 (1969).
28. Lacassagne, A.: *C. R. Soc. Biol. (Paris)* **133,** 180 (1940).
29. Leriche, R.: *Presse méd.* **55,** 389 (1947).
30. MacLean, A. L.: *Bull. Johns Hopk. Hosp.* **76,** 179 (1945).
31. MacSween, R. N. M., Goudie, R. B., Anderson, J. R., Armstrong, E., Murray, M. A., Mason, D. K., Jasini, M. K., Boyle, J. A., Buchanan, W. W. and Williamson. J.: *Ann. rheum. Dis.* **26,** 402 (1967).
32. Manschot, W. A.: *Trans. ophthal. Soc. U. K.* **80,** 137 (1960).
33. McCabe, B. F.: *Laryngoscope* **71,** 396 (1961).
33*a*. MacFarlane, T. W. and Mason, D. K.: *J. clin. Path.* **27,** 416 (1974).
34. McLenachan, J.: *Trans. ophthal. Soc. U. K.* **76,** 413 (1956).
34*a*. Meiers, H. G., Voigtmann, G., Haensch, R. and Hornstein, O. P.: *Hautarzt* **25,** 118 (1974).
35. Messner, K. and Leibowitz, H. M.: *Arch. Ophthal.* **86,** 357 (1971).
36. Mikulicz, J.: *Beitr. Chir.* (Festschr. für Th. Billroth) 610 (1892).
37. Morgan, W. S. and Castleman, B.: *Amer. J. Path.* **29,** 471 (1953).
38. Mühler, E.: *Münch. med. Wschr.* **103,** 504 (1961).
39. Nishimura, N., Yasui, M., Okamoto, H., Kanazawa, M. and Kotaye, Y.: *Arch. Derm.* **77,** 255 (1958).
40. Offret, G. and Forest, P.: *Bull. Soc. Ophthal. France* **1,** 759 (1950).
41*a*. Radnót, M.: *Klin. Mbl. Augenheilk.* **103,** 120 (1939).
41*b*. id., In *Die pathologische Histologie der Tränendrüse.* Karger, Basel 1939.
42. Radnót, M. and Németh, B.: *Ophthalmologica (Basel)* **129,** 376 (1955).
43. Ramage, J. H. and Kinnear, W. F.: *Brit. J. Ophthal.* **40,** 416 (1956).
44. Richard, A., Cernea, P. and Puig, G.: *Rev. Stomatol.* **49,** 502 (1948).
45. Rothman, S., Bloch, M. and Hauser, F. V.: *Arch. Derm. Syph. (Chic.)* **63,** 642 (1951).
46. Roy, G.: *Presse méd.* **78,** 146 (1948).
47*a*. Shearn, M. A.: *Ann. intern. Med.* **52,** 1352 (1963).
47*b*. id., *Sjögren's Syndrome.* Saunders, Philadelphia 1971.

47*c*. Shearn, M. A., Tu, W. H., Stephens, B. G. and Lee, J. C.: *Lancet* **i,** 568 (1970).
48. Sheldon, J.: *Proc. roy. Soc. Med.* **32,** 255 (1938).
49. Sjögren, H.: *Acta ophthal.* (*Kbh.*) **11,** Suppl. 1 (1933).
50. Szántó, L., Farkas, K. and Gyulai, E.: *Orv. Hetil.* **95,** 413 (1954).
51. Talal, N.: *Ann. intern. Med.* **75,** 946 (1971).
52. Talal, N. and Bunim, J. J.: *Amer. J. Med.* **36,** 529 (1964).
53. Talal, N., Zisman, E. and Schur, P. H.: *Arthr. and Rheum.* **11,** 774 (1968).
54. Thomson, A. S. and Bryant, H. G.: *Amer. J. Path.* **26,** 807 (1950).
55. Tichy, H.: *Lehrbuch der Rheumatologie.* 2nd ed. Volk und Gesundheit, Berlin 1962.
56. Tomasi, Th. B., jr., Tan, E. M., Solomon, A. and Orendergast, R. A.: *J. exp. Med.* **121,** 101 (1965).
57. Touraine, A.: *Presse méd.* **58,** 405 (1950).
57*a*. van Boxel, J. A., Hardin, J. A., Geen, I. and Paul, W. E.: *New Engl. J. Med.* **289,** 823 (1973).
58. Wallner, E.: Clinical and Therapeutical Observations in Sicca Syndrome. Thesis. Budapest 1968.
59. Walser, A., Ivankovic, M. and Bour, M.: *Schweiz. med. Wschr.* **95,** 763 (1965).
60. Waterhouse, J. P. and Doniach, I.: *J. Path. Bact.* **83,** 255 (1962).
61. Whaley, K., Chisholm, D. M. and Downie, W. W.: *Acta rheum. scand.* **14,** 298 (1968).
62. Whaley, K., Glen, A. C. A., MacSween, R. N. M., Deodhar, S., Dick, W. C., Nuki, G., Williamson, J. and Buchanan, W. W.: *Clin. exp. Immunol.* **9,** 721 (1971).
63. Williamson, J., Paterson, R. W. W., McGavin, D. D. M., Greig, W. R. and Whaley, K.: *Brit. J. Ophthal.* **54,** 31 (1970).
64. Zipkin, I.: cited by 22.

CHAPTER 40

AUTOIMMUNE DISEASES OF THE SKIN AND SKIN DISORDERS WITH DIVERSE IMMUNO-PATHOLOGICAL ABNORMALITIES

by

S. KOROSSY

INTRODUCTION

Skin autoimmune state means specific humoral (autoantibody-mediated) or cell-mediated sensitization to constituents (autoantigens) of the skin. Autoantibody–autoantigen reactions causing tissue damage (cytotoxic effect) may be regarded as hypersensitivity reactions. Such damages of the skin, if leading to any clinical manifestation, are called skin autoimmune diseases [263]. In clinical practice this term is used in a wider sense including diseases associated with the presence of autoantibodies which probably play a role in the pathogenesis of the actual illness which, however, has not so far been proved.

Whitefield [614*a*, *b*, *c*] was the first, in the early nineteen-twenties, to suggest the autoallergic origin of some skin diseases. He started from three observations. (*i*) Trauma or intensive local treatment in eczematous areas is often followed by the spread of the eczema to the entire body. (*ii*) Serous discharge from eczematous foci may induce, after a short incubation period, eczema in intact skin areas. (*iii*) Haematoma in the skin may be followed by papulous and urticarial eruption. He postulated a 'hypersensitivity to self components' in such cases.

In non-organ-specific autoimmune diseases (e.g. SLE), it may happen that autoantigens from organs localize in the skin and react immunologically to cause dermatitis. In the first part of this chapter the autoimmune reactions are dealt with in which the humoral or cell-mediated autoimmunity is obviously organ- or tissue-specific for the skin.

Although there are in the skin a number of potential organ-specific autoantigens, difficulties in their extraction have hindered their investigation [122]. Keratin in the form of keratene or metakeratin is able to induce species- and substance-specific antibodies in rabbit [468]. Investigating the water-soluble antigens of normal human skin, up to 10–12 antigens were found possessing electrophoretic motility from albumin to γ-globulin [602*a*]. There were found 4–5 organ-specific skin antigens which in the immunoelectrophoretic analysis were localized in the zones of α-, β- and γ-globulins. Other authors [18] found three precipitating antigens, believed to be epidermal skin-specific in skin homogenates. The sera applied in these investigations had been repeatedly absorbed with other tissues. In similar tests with extracts of callus and psoriatic scales, four antigens were found, three of which were also demonstrable in the normal stratum corneum [445*b*].

Recent studies with the immune adherence test performed with sections of human skin and unabsorbed or absorbed human serum have indicated that two water-phase antigens are present in the normal stratum corneum [387]. Normal stratum corneum and callus may differ serologically. Indirect haemolysis tests with pepsin-digested immunoglobulins showed binding by their Fab portion, indicating an antigen–antibody reaction. However, the antigenic stimulus that had induced these antibodies in healthy subjects has remained unknown. Humoral antibodies to antigens that are present in the cytoplasm of normal adult epidermal cells were found in 17 per cent of normal persons, 21 per cent of patients with various dermatoses, 32 per cent of those with malignancies and 27 per cent of patients with malignant melanoma [84]. Human dandruff contains a water-soluble substance, antigen dandruff, which precipitates with some, but not all, human sera [538]; it has not been found to occur in other body tissues and is not related to the Australia antigen.

Cross-reactions were found between human epidermal and house-dust antigens [19]. In atopic individuals, cutaneous tests with these two antigens showed a correlation, and a cross-absorption between them was apparent, but there are discrepancies as regards the molecular weights of the peak activities. Electrophoretically, the protein fraction of the epidermal antigen having a mol. wt. of 19,000 showed three sharp bands.

Some of the tissue-specific antigens appear to be both tissue- and species-specific, whereas others may also be present in heterologous stratified epithelial or smooth-muscle cells.

Collagen has proved antigenic [498] and basement membrane (BM), reticulin, elastin, melanin and subcellular components as yet undefined must also be considered potential antigens [621]. Hyaluronic acid has been reported to be non-antigenic [480].

Of the above-mentioned antigens keratin is the only organ-specific antigen of the skin. Since it is poorly soluble in physiological solutions and is mainly confined to degenerated cells and dead squamae, the antibodies to keratin are probably harmless [445*a*]. The interepithelial cell substance is epithelial tissue-specific, but not organ- or species-specific [445*a*].

Immediate hypersensitivity to sweat and hair extracts has been described [39]. Elevated anti-sweat precipitins (IgG) were demonstrated in many skin disorders (erythema multiforme, atopic dermatitis, nummular eczema) [455*b*].

Epidermal constituents are prevented from becoming autoantigens by several physiological mechanisms: (*i*) The basal cells eventually leave the organism as squamae, consequently, the proteins of the epidermis cannot play a role in self recognition. (*ii*) In the epidermis there are neither lymphatics nor blood vessels and the BM may prevent epidermal antigens from reacting with immunocytes. However, the demonstration of serum proteins in the epidermis has shown that the BM must be permeable for some proteins. On the other hand, haptens (mostly chemicals) causing exogenous eczema after having coupled with protein, cross the skin and do react with immunologically component cells. It seems that it is not an anatomical segregation but immunological tolerance due to self recognition which has to be broken through.

The nature of the epidermal autoantigen is still unknown. Immunofluorescence studies have shown that the majority of humoral antibodies taken up by the epidermis are localized on the epidermal cell surface, on the desmosomes, in the intercellular cement substance, in the BM and in the cytoplasm of skin adnex cells. Thus, the antigens are to be sought there.

The skin autoantibody and autoantigen may possess special organ-, tissue-, species- and even individual specificity [106*b*] as demonstrable by serum absorption tests [448]. It was supposed that the skin autoantigen might be an altered form or precursor of keratin, a structural protein known to be synthesized locally. This is supported by the fact that foetal skin, which is not keratinized, does not react with the cytotoxic antibody [447]. It is not clear whether the degree of degradation by which keratin becomes antigenic in lower animals does in fact occur in the human organism spontaneously and whether the cytotoxic antibodies occurring in the serum of patients with disseminated eczema is specific for keratin [448].

One should reckon with a number of non-organ-specific skin antigens [445*a*], e.g. intracellular nuclear and cytoplasmic antigens exposed in damaged cells, interepithelial substance, non-cellular antigens formed by changes in plasma components (aggregation or degradation of γ-globulin forming determinants reacting with rheumatoid factors, anti-nuclear antibodies anti-masked determinants), etc.

Recently it has been postulated [14] that T lymphocytes play a key role in preventing autoimmunity, and that diseases associated with a depression of cell-mediated immunity may lead to an autoimmune process. There are circumstances in which the physiological barrier protecting non-tolerated tissues is injured by a primarily non-immunological event, e. g. traumatic tissue damage, infection, drugs, resulting in a progressively destructive process, e. g. in the eye, in the testis and in the central nervous system. Possibly self identity can be lost when tolerated tissue is damaged by virus, mycoplasma, bacterium, chemicals, enzyme or autologous serum factor at sites of chronic inflammation; as a result, the epidermal structure may be destroyed and degraded, or denatured proteins and polysaccharides of new antigenic properties may arise [573, 621]. If the organism fails to eliminate the damage of malfunctioning cells, the originally normal constituents will be recognized by the immunologically competent system as foreign; the resulting humoral antibody or primed lymphocyte will react with cell debris, bound or denatured globulin and may even cross-react with molecularly similar unchanged tissue substances, thus aggravating and prolonging the tissue damage. It is also possible that 'masked antigens', occult proteins (e.g. protein–carbohydrate conjugates) become accessible or are released.

It has been suggested that the antigenic properties of the skin may be age dependent. In guinea pigs of different age groups a common antigenic component has been demonstrated with passive cutaneous anaphylaxis test [180] besides a number of age dependent antigens. In old animals skin antigens seem to decrease in number. Since T cell functions often decline in old age, relaxation of T cell control may be a factor in the appearance of autoantibodies in ageing individuals [13]. The same subject may develop sensitivity to two or three organs on the basis of a shared antigen possibly deriving from common embryonic origin of the tissues [621]. For instance, immunoelectrophoresis of rabbit anti-dog-lens antibody revealed an antigen common to the crystalline lens and the skin; this finding explains the association of juvenile cataract with atopic dermatitis [216]. In volumes 7 and 8 of the present work the reader can find numerous examples suggesting that tolerance to self antigens can be broken by immunizing the individual with a foreign antigen which has determinants in common with the 'self' antigen [309] and thus one should reckon with cross-reactivity based on foreign antigens sharing antigenic determinants with tissue antigens.

Overlap of antigenicity between, e.g. a bacterium and tissue cell may result in autosensitization [445*a*]. The cell-wall antigen of type 17 group-A Streptococcus is, e. g. related to heart and kidney tissue antigens. The lipopolysaccharides of *E. coli* 014 cross-react with human colon [391*a*]. As to the role of viruses there are many peculiar problems [167*a*]. Enveloped virions (e.g. herpes virus and myxovirus virions) incorporate host antigens, and thus the membranes of infected cells acquire virus-specific antigens [13, 234*b*]. Hence, host and viral antigens occur in the same functional unit so that helper effects may permit immune responses to self-constituents. On the other hand, some RNA viruses, especially oncornaviruses, are capable of suppressing the host's immunoreactivity.

Furthermore, one should reckon with the breakdown of immunological tolerance due to hapten-tissue combination; simple chemicals (drugs or metabolites) bound as haptens to skin-identifying protein carrier molecules may induce antibodies reacting not only with the hapten-host protein conjugate but also with the carrier molecule itself [13, 114, 142*a*,*b*, 513].

Since conditions allowing antibody formation through helper effects occur frequently, T cell control may also operate [13]. In such cases contact dermatitis may be, to some extent, an autoimmune disease [621].

Some skin diseases may be associated with an abnormal thymus function and/or lymphoreticular tumours (e.g. lymphosarcoma, leukaemia, benign lymph node hyperplasia). These may lead to antibody formation and/or a mutation or disinhibition of a cell population. Such association of diseases may also be due to medical interventions, such as immunosuppressive therapy. It has been proposed [408] that lymphoma may represent an unrestricted and uncontrolled proliferation of cells belonging to the immune system. Therefore, an emergence of 'forbidden' clones producing autoantibodies is not unexpected. Alternatively, such clones might emerge as a result of spontaneous mutation. The forbidden clones are as a rule eliminated by the homeostatic mechanism, whose failure may allow the clones to survive. The depression of cell-mediated immunity in Hodgkin's disease is well known, and a co-existence of e.g. pemphigus and Hodgkin's disease has been observed [548].

Human thymic and peripheral lymphocytes are able to react as antigen binding lymphocytes with autoantigens [166*c*]. Such lymphocytes, presumably B cells, are increased in number in patients with autoimmune disease. Self-tolerance is due to the control by continually present antigen-reactive lymphocytes, whereas autoimmune disease represents an escape from this control. It is reasonable to put the question [166*c*] how to explain that normal newborns and adults with peripheral autoantibodies may remain symptomless, though, their immunologically competent cells must have been exposed to these antibodies. The formation of autoantibodies requires co-operation of T and B lymphocytes; when these antigens circulate in a low concentration T lymphocytes do not react with them even if sensitized B lymphocytes are present in the usual number [166*c*]. Evidence has accumulated that these are able to produce antibody against the antigen in question. Some peripheral lymphocytes from normal persons are able to bind autoantigen. These were identified as B lymphocytes with immunoglobulin on their membranes. The number of such cells was found increased in autoimmune disease. In formation of antibodies against autoantigen, T cells which do not react with the antigen may have a helper effect.

The histopathological lesions and clinical manifestations in animals with organ-specific cellular hypersensitivity and associated experimental autoimmune disease resemble in many respect the human autoimmune conditions. In spite of this, the involved pathomechanisms may be different. This becomes evident, among others, from the fact that experimentally induced organ-specific cellular hypersensitivity is generally not associated with demonstrable autoimmune tissue damage, unless Freund's adjuvant is used. Thus, although organ-specific, cellular hypersensitivity has been found to be a probable causative factor behind tissue damage and clinical symptoms in animal experiments, it has as yet been difficult to substantiate a pathogenetic analogy to autoimmune disorders in man [36].

Animal model experiments with homologous or autologous cutaneous extracts incorporated in complete Freund's adjuvant [602, 618] have not readily confirmed the role of autoimmunity in the pathogenesis of dermatitis. The injected material is eventually surrounded by macrophages, lymphoid and plasma cells. Autosensitization may result because the activated lymphoid cells at the site do not pass through the thymus and thereby escape destruction and inhibition [445*a*]. They survive and thus produce antibody or specifically activated lymphocytes. The situation may be complicated by the presence of bacterial antigens [448]. Animals immunized with sterile foetal skin developed neither dermal nor delayed hypersensitivity [605]. The most suggestive evidence for the experimental production of an immunologically induced generalized dermatitis in which cutaneous antigens participate is in the graft-versus-host reaction [554]. However, the skin inflammation in this situation almost certainly involves transplantation antigens present in other organs as well. It is therefore unlikely that transplantation immunity would play any role in human dermatitis [448]. The concept that autoimmunity to skin could result in rejection of autografts is of interest. Such a possibility arises, e.g. in chronic ulcerations of legs resistant to grafting, the colon ulcerations associated with certain systemic diseases, and pyoderma gangraenosum. An appropriate fractionation of the crude tissues now in use and repeated testing of positive sera in standardized tests are expected to tell which tissue fraction may be involved as antigen in a given disease state [621].

One shuld reckon with the existence of an underlying defect, a so-called autoimmune diathesis. This defect indicates a potential disease which may be brought about by various trigger factors. A possible association with any HL-A specificity of diseases of supposed autoimmune character has been investigated by the microdroplet lymphocyte cytotoxicity test. A susceptibility gene linked to an HL-A antigen has been supposed for numerous diseases. Associations have recently been found for HL-A antigens in pemphigus vulgaris (HL-A10, W-5, W-15) and dermatitis herpetiformis (HL-A1, HL-A8). Two possible mechanisms of association might be assumed [335*b*]: (*i*) a close linkage between a gene governing the immunological responsiveness to disease and HL-A gene, or (*ii*) cross-reaction between the HL-A antigen and the aetiological agent (streptococci or viral envelope antigen). Among environmental factors, attention has been called to infectious agents, such as mycoplasmas, viruses, bacteria, UV radiation, drugs, etc. The high incidence of autoantibody-like factors in such diseases might be considered side-effects of genetically determined tissue damages [445*b*].

In the pathogenesis of autoimmune diseases two factors play a major part, viz. an organ-specific antigen and the characteristic structure and function of the organ, including the ultrastructure and the dynamic functions of the vascular bed. The transportation of various substances through the endothelium and BM is different in various organs.

The normal skin does not synthesize immunoglobulins, whereas damaged skin may produce any of IgG, IgA, IgM and IgE, even in a pattern different from that characteristic of the mucosa adjacent to the skin [350]. Immunoglobulins are produced by plasma cells and lymphocytes, but not by other types of cells. Immunoglobulin-positive cells have been found by fluorescence microscopy (epi-illumination, blue-narrow excitation light) in skin lesions of patients with bullous pemphigoid, dermatitis herpetiformis, mycosis fungoides, atopic dermatitis and lichen planus, but not in the normal skin [350]. The affected skin showed mainly IgG-positive cells, whereas in normal mucous membranes, except for the oral mucosa, IgA-positive cells predominated [350]. The immunoglobulin-positive cells were morphologically plasma cells or lymphocytes; they occurred scattered in the dermis of the skin and in the lamina propria of mucous membranes. The results were supported by tissue culture experiments.

In the course of autoimmune diseases various humoral organ-, epithelial-, tissue- and non-tissue-specific antibodies are produced which react with cellular elements of human tissues, or with subcellular components. Some of these are organ-specific. The latter may, e.g. be indirectly cytotoxic by forming complexes with the exposed antigens that may result in Arthus-type or cell-mediated reactions and thus perpetuate and exacerbate an existing inflammation [445*a*]. IgG was detected in intercellular spaces of the horny layer of the normal skin, too [435], but the reaction was less intense there than in the diseased skin. In contrast, IgM and IgA could not be detected in the normal skin.

The antibodies to keratin present in the IgG and IgM fractions of many human sera, though activate C, seem to be non-cytotoxic (see p. 108). Neither rheumatoid factor nor anti-nuclear antibody produces disease when transferred to healthy recipients. Presumably the natural skin antibodies to stratum corneum antigens are hetero- or autoantibodies without any damaging effect [3*b*, 342]. A comparative *in vitro* study of anti-rat-skin and anti-rat-lymphocyte donkey sera showed that both sera exerted similar cytotoxic effects upon rat lymphocytes [118]. The anti-skin sera differed from the anti-lymphocyte sera in that they did not suppress blast transformation induced by PHA, concanavalin A or lipopolysaccharide.

As to the role of C in the pathogenesis of autoimmune diseases the reader is referred to Chapter 15 of Vol. 1 and to the respective chapters dealing with the individual diseases. It seems justified to mention that various C components are synthesized by macrophages, and, probably, by other cells [350]. The concomitant occurrence of C fragments in or around skin lesions indicates that C is occasionally activated in or on these tissue constituents. Whether this is the cause or the result of skin lesions remains unanswered. The concomitant occurrence of immunoglobulins and C may indicate that the former have played a role in the activation process. Other pathways are also possible, e.g. C may be activated by enzymes in autoimmune disease. The biologically active C fragments or components may explain the accumulation of granulocytes.

It is important to distinguish between cause and effect. The antibodies either in the role of autoantibodies or as non-antigen induced aggregates are primarily involved in the pathogenesis of autoimmune diseases, but possibly, as a part of a secondary immunological mechanism, they may be directed against antigenic debris of degenerated tissue constituents (scavenger role).

The presence of humoral antibodies or even fixation of autoantibodies alone have failed to provoke any pathological reaction *in vivo* [445*b*], for (*i*) these antibodies if transferred from patients to normal subjects cause no disease; (*ii*) cannot be demonstrated in every patient and occur in some normal individuals; (*iii*) the antibody titre is independent of the duration and severity of the illness; (*iv*) most of these antibodies are not organ-specific and may be found in several diseases without affecting the organ. It is not clear whether these autoantibodies must be considered a normal immunological consequence of the death of cells or of a damage of cells with a clearing function [339].

Alternatively, a major proportion of the cutaneous damage might be attributed to cell-mediated immunity. An influx of small round cells, presumably specifically sensitized lymphocytes, is considered an evidence for an immune response [621]. Plasma cells and histiocytes in the infiltrate represent a further evidence for the primarily immediate-type inflammatory response [621]. Lymphocyte infiltration is a prominent feature of acute and chronic eczematous dermatitis, just as it is of chronic thyroiditis and certain other human diseases in which autoimmunity is thought to play a prominent role. The possible role of cell-mediated immunity in infantile eczema has been considered [248]; it was demonstrated that peripheral blood lymphocytes from patients with this condition undergo transformation in response to a cutaneous antigen extract. The cytotoxicity mediated by specifically sensitized lymphocytes is a more intricate problem [445*b*]. The damage may be demonstrable by the release of radioactive insotopes icorporated in the target cell membrane. Discrepancies may result from variations in the ratio of specifically sensitized lymphocytes to target cells and in the time interval between the sensitization of the donor animal and the harvest of the lymphocytes. However, the possible role in the mitogenic response of bacterial antigens in skin has not been excluded. Studies on the toxic effect of native autologous human sera on epidermal cells in tissue culture [16] have proved that such effects show close correlation with increasing age and the extent of the skin disease and may be due to an antibody-like substance. Cells from human epidermis showed some capacity for stimulating blood lymphocytes of other donors [536]. This stimulation was weaker than observed with PHA or staphylococcal filtrate or the stimulation obtained with equal numbers of X-ray irradiated lymphoid cell line cells. Epithelial cells are effective targets for murine lymphocyte stimulation *in vitro* [215]. The magnitude of the response to incompatible epithelial cells was equal to or slightly greater than that following incubation with lymphoid cells. Lymph node lymphocytes appear slightly more reactive to epithelial cells than comparable preparation of spleen cells. This model was used to show whether differentiation of skin antigens which are not expressed on lymphoid cells can provoke an *in vitro* allograft reaction. Lymphocytes *in vitro* can acquire the capacity to react with cultivated normal syngeneic fibroblasts [256*b*].

Several authors [391*a*] have dealt with the pathogenetic role of humoral or cell-mediated antibodies. Steffen [555] has differentiated between (*i*) obviously, (*ii*) probably and (*iii*) possibly autoimmune diseases. The following criteria have been proposed which, however, are too strict for clinical use [621]: (*i*) demonstration of antibodies active at body temperature, or delayed-type hypersensitivity; (*ii*) the antigen(s) responsible for the immunological response should be identified and be capable of inducing antibodies and/or delayed-type hypersensitivity in experimental animals; (*iii*) proper stimulation of experimental animals with the antigens should lead to an illness comparable with the disease under study; (*iv*) the disease thus produced in animals should be passive transferable with serum or cells. It will be shown below that clinicians have to make use of indirect evidence, rather than such criteria [621]. For practical purposes it is important to exclude every possible antigen before accepting the autoallergic nature of a disease.

Of the skin diseases dealt with in the first part of this chapter, it is the pemphigus group which most closely approximates the above criteria. Nevertheless, it has not been proved yet that an autoimmune reaction is the direct cause of these diseases. In the second part of the chapter diseases of unknown aetiology are discussed in which, at least at some stages of the disease, an autoimmune character is demonstrable and occasionally contributes to the diagnosis. However, the circumstances which lead to the production of autoantibodies is still unknown.

There are a growing number of diseases in which humoral antibodies to different organ extracts or to more specific components of normal tissues, such as DNA or nucleohistone, have been demonstrated. These diseases may involve almost every organ [621], but the reports are, in general, too isolated to be entirely conclusive. First of all the natural conditions for an organism to develop antibodies to its own tissues should be reconsidered in the sense of the current immunological theory [621].

In the third part of this chapter, skin diseases and systemic diseases affecting the skin are dealt with in the course of which immunopathological abnormalities can be demonstrated at a variable frequency; in respect of these diseases the role of autoimmunity has not been proved, but it seems to be worth while to call attention to their immunological aspects, as this may help in the clarification of their pathogenesis.

The drug therapy of autoimmune and immunopathological diseases will be outlined in connection with the respective diseases. As an introduction, some general measures of care, prevention and rehabilitation are only discussed.

The care of autoimmune patients should be the task of special outpatient departments, where specialists, consultants and an immunological laboratory are available. The period of hospitalization can be shortened in this way [567]. Severe relapses and iatrogenic complications can be prevented by such a systematic follow-up, though prevention is almost impossible unless the aetiology of individual cases is clarified [461].

Rehabilitation of such patients is invariably influenced by their actual status. Patients with fever and pain are not able to work regardless of their occupation. On the other hand, patients with an increased erythrocyte sedimentation rate, dysproteinaemia, mild albuminuria, pain without any objective background or a slight, constant abnormality in the ECG should be encouraged to go back to work, if their job does not require hard physical exertion [461]. Patients with chronic or progressive disease should be adviced to change occupation for lighter work as early as possible [461]. Each case should be treated individually and for this purpose it is advisable to discuss the case with the doctor the patient regularly sees (GP) and/or factory medical consultant. Estimation of the working capacity should be based on the patient's actual status especially on the functional status of the organs affected [461]. Symptoms may be eased by an adequate therapy in spite of existing mild functional defects. To avoid the consequences of organ atrophy, substitution therapy is necessary in cases of torpid course. Functional loading of the involved organs is undesirable.

SKIN DISEASES MOST PROBABLY AUTOIMMUNE IN NATURE

BULLOUS SKIN DISEASES

The pemphigus group

Pemphigus vulgaris (PV). Cutaneous bullae are mostly small and flaccid on skin having a normal appearance (Fig. 40-1). The bulla breaks easily, leaving a denuded area surrounded by a peripheral collar of detached epidermis. The denuded areas, often covered by haemorrhagic crusts, usually show little tendency to healing. The healed bullae leave no scar, but temporary hyperpigmentation is often present. The appearance and the fate of the mucosal lesions (Fig. 40-2) are similar to those of cutaneous lesions. The earliest phenomenon in PV consists of intercellular oedema followed by disappearance of the intercellular bridges in the lower epidermis. The resulting loss of coherence between the epidermal cells (acantholysis) leads to the formation of clefts and then of bullae in a predominantly suprabasal location (Fig. 40-3*a*, *b*). The basal cells remain attached to the dermis like a 'row of tombstone'. The bullae contain acantholytic epidermal cells. At the floor of the bullae, irregular upward growth of papillae, lined by a single layer of epidermal cells, so-called villi, are to be seen. The dermis shows a mild or moderately severe inflammatory infiltrate with fairly numerous eosinophils. The acantholytic cells, also called Tzanck cells, show characteristic changes in shape (Fig. 40-4). The changes are usually considered degenerative in nature, but according to recent investigations the nucleus of the Tzanck cells is rich in DNA and their cytoplasm is rich in glycogen, suggesting that they might be young undifferentiated elements with active protein synthesis [472]. Acantholytic cells occur not only in PV, but also in other vesiculobullous or pustular dermatoses. On the other hand, in older or treated lesions of PV acantholytic lesions may be absent. Immunohistochemical examinations may be helpful in the differential diagnosis between PV, herpes zoster and herpes simplex, as well as aphthosis. In PV the nucleus of the acantholytic cell does not show fluorescence and the fluorescence of the cell membrane predominates [201*b*]. An important role of lysosomes in the pathogenesis has been established [7]. Electron micrographs [316] show oedema in the cell periphery and widening of the intercellular space, furthermore, a significant increase in the activity of hydrolytic lysosomal enzymes in basal and prickle cells; these dissolve the intercellular substance and destroy the desmosomes. In areas where the desmosomes had disappeared, tonofilaments stretching towards the contact areas of the cells may be seen [592]. Owing to the disappearance of desmosomes, tonofilaments take a circumnuclear position [65*a*, *b*]. More frequently [592] desmosomes are present without attached tonofilaments, giving an impression that the initial changes occur in the tonofibrils, which detach from the desmosomes and arrange themselves

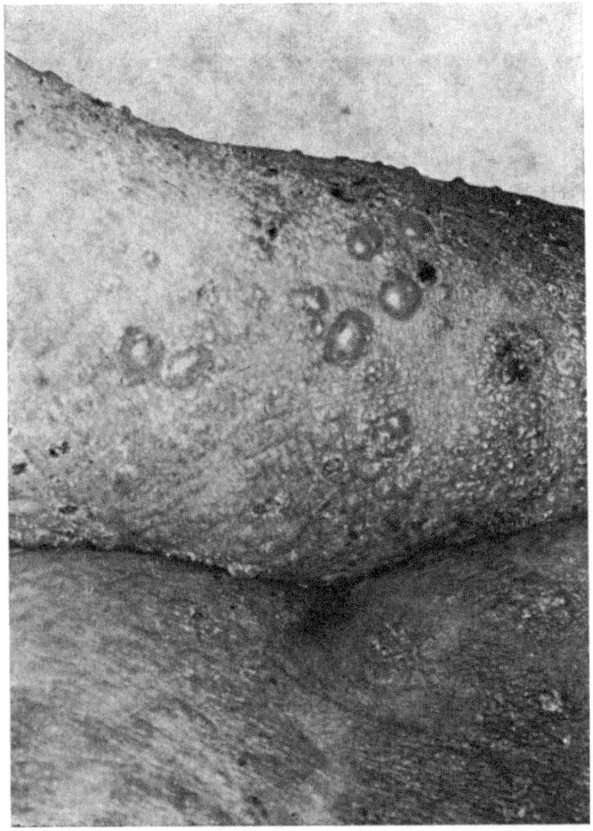

Fig. 40-1. Pemphigus vulgaris. Pinhead- to pea-sized vesicles with serous content on the arm. Note the reaction-free basis. (Courtesy of Professor N. Simon, Department of Dermatology, Szeged University Medical School)

around the nucleus, and that the disappearance of desmosomes is a secondary phenomenon [617]. There is no doubt [316] that the rarefaction of the desmosomes is accompanied by changes in the tonofilaments. In most severe cases the destruction of bundles of collagen and elastic fibres were observed in the papillary layer [7, 316]. It is believed [316] that acantholysis results from an alteration in the cementing intercellular substance. Others have suggested that the intercellular cohesion is governed by the intercellular substance rather than by the desmosomes, for (*i*) the intercellular cohesion is lost and the acantholysis is initiated by an absorption of the intercellular cement substance when the desmosomes are still intact [252]; and (*ii*) treatment of the epidermis with cantharidin, which disrupts desmosomes and tonofilaments is not accompanied by loss of intercellular cohesion (electron-microscopic study) [627].

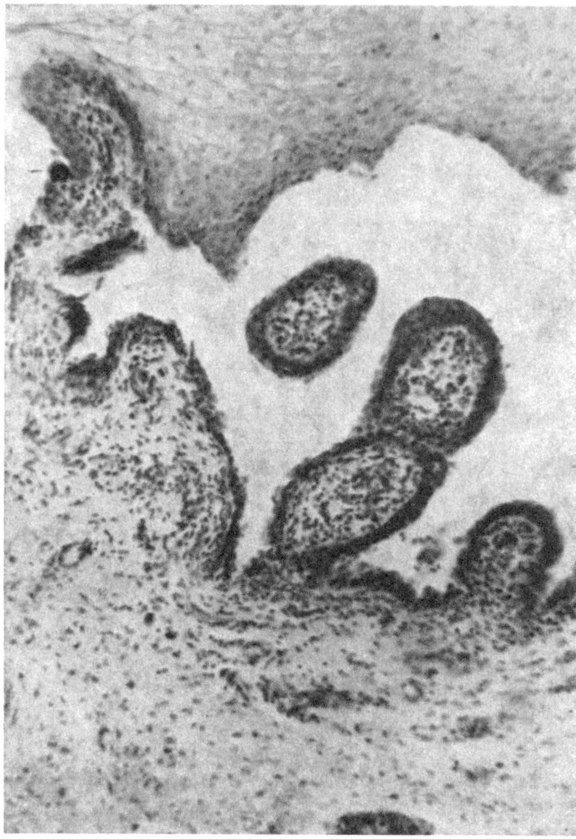

Fig. 40-2. Pemphigus vulgaris. Intraepidermal vesicle on the oral mucous membrane. The connective tissue forming the basis and the connective tissue papillae protruding into the vesicle are bordered by a row of epithelial cells. ×40 (Courtesy of Professor N. Simon, Szeged)

In the active phase of PV, the patients' serum contains 'anti-epithelial', 'anti-epidermal-cell-surface', and 'anti-intercellular-substance' antibodies [2*a*, 17, 31*a*, 40, 41, 78, 81, 155, 201*a*, 288, 303, 305, 318, 507, 563, 581) demonstrable by the indirect immunofluorescence technique. Owing to the fragility of the wall of the bullae, the demonstration of antibodies in its content is rarely successful [31*b*, 108*a*]. Slight or medium amounts of autoantibodies are present in healthy areas of the patient's skin as well [46]. Anti-intercellular-substance antibodies may appear in the serum even in cases when only the oesophageal mucous membrane is affected [483]. Immunoelectrophoretically, the contents of the bullae show a pathological band between the α_2 and γ bands [304].

The serum antibody level as determined by the indirect technique usually runs parallel with the severity and extent of the clinical phenomena [43, 47,

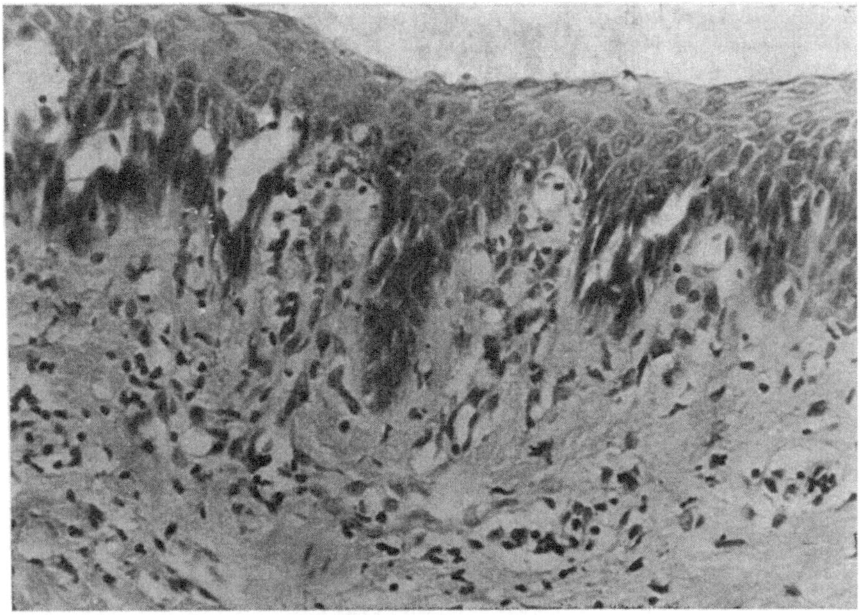

Fig. 40-3*a*. Pemphigus vulgaris. Suprabasal cleft formation in the initial stage. ×20 (Courtesy of Professor L. Szodoray, Department of Dermatology, Debrecen University Medical School)

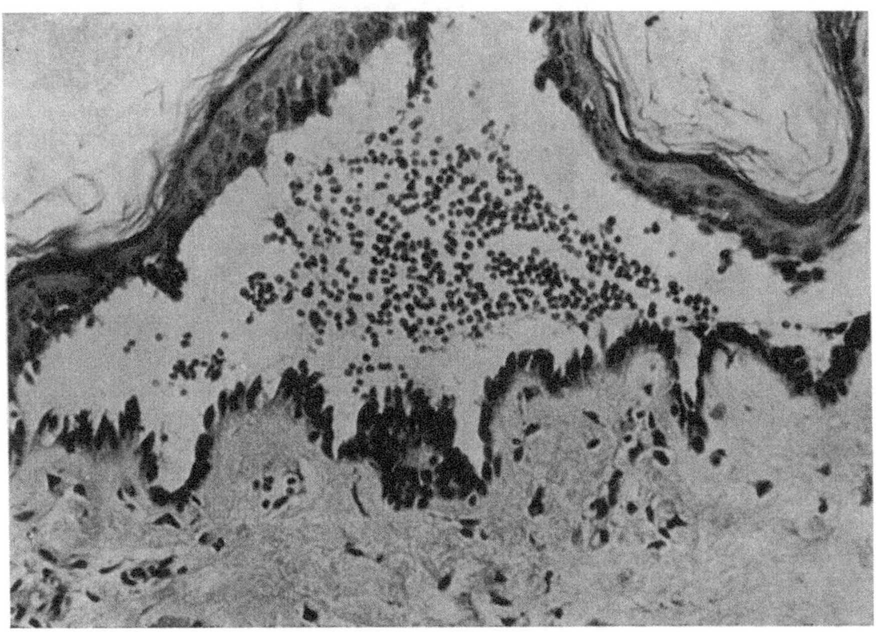

Fig. 40-3*b*. Pemphigus vulgaris. The basal cells on the basis of the vesicle are detached. The basal cells are fixed only to the corium. ×20 (Courtesy of Professor L. Szodoray, Debrecen)

312, 369, 373]; it is high in the eruptive stage, low in the quiescent stage and zero in the long-lasting clinical remission stage. The dynamics of the titre may be of prognostic value [106b, 312]; its increase indicates a potential aggravation whereas its decrease, a remission. Remission with constant titre suggests that the therapy has been insufficient. Antibody titration may be helpful in the determination of the maintenance dose of the drug. During corticosteroid therapy, the titre declines parallel with the total Ig [312]. The serum may be negative for pemphigus antibody during a fresh relapse of PV, whereas taken from the same patient several days later may be strongly positive. In the 'negative fresh relapse' sera antigen–antibody complexes and pemphigus antigen alone can be

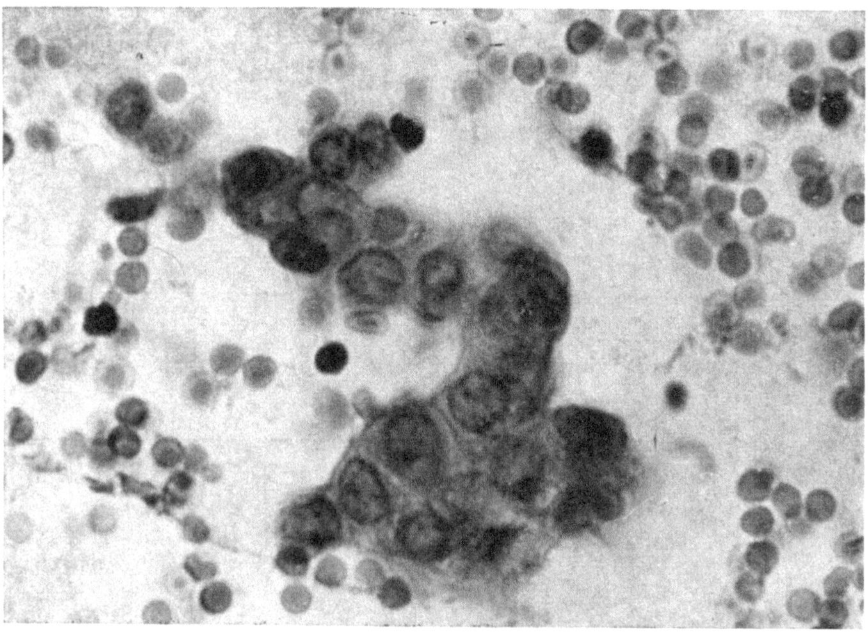

Fig. 40-4. Pemphigus vulgaris. A group of epithelial cells showing ballooning degeneration of variable degree. ×240 (Courtesy of Professor L. Szodoray, Debrecen)

demonstrated by various immunological methods [48]. The correlation between the antibody titre obtained by the indirect immunofluorescence test and the clinical activity has been confirmed by using the passive cutaneous anaphylaxis test carried out with an extract of normal human epidermis as the source of antigen [450].

Ultrastructural examination with ferritin-conjugated anti-human IgG [606], and, recently, combined electron-microscopic and immunocytochemical investigations with peroxidase enzyme-labelled anti-human γ-globulin antibody [199, 303, 626] suggest that the antibodies are deposited in, and confined to, the intercellular spaces of the epidermis, further, that the antibody binds to the surface of the epidermal cells. This is well visible also, when a fresh lesion (Fig. 40-5) or isolated cells that have undergone acantholysis are examined. In direct immunofluorescent studies of bullae and Tzanck smears individual acantholytic cells [144, 201*b*, 472] coated with the typical apple-green, green-white fluorescence have been observed. Some binding occurs not only on the cell membrane, but also around desmosomes [606]. A patient with a malignant lymphoid neoplasm developed PV; the tumour homogenate obtained from the inguinal lymph nodes contained high-titre pemphigus antibodies to stratified squamous epithelium and the tumour tissue produced excessive IgG-type antibodies [505]. It was

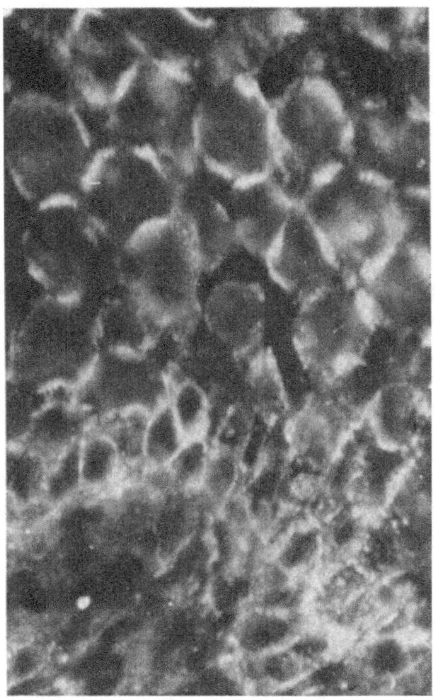

Fig. 40-5. Pemphigus vulgaris. Immunofluorescent technique. Fine granular fluorescence at the intercellular space. Anti-human IgG/FTC. Leitz Ortholux. × 1,000

concluded that the localization of the antibody is disease-specific and the intercellular cement substance must be the primary factor in the development of the lesion. To examine whether pemphigus antibody might be a component of bound immunoglobulins, acantholytic cells from Tzanck smears of PV, stained with FITC-labelled anti-human IgG, were used. Brilliant immunofluorescence was obtained. Incubation of Tzanck smears with citrate buffer of pH 3.0, which dissociates antigen–antibody complexes, markedly reduced the immunofluorescence [432*a*]. The significance of the demonstration of antibodies to epithelium should be emphasized. The fact that, according to comparative mmunofluorescence tests, there are individual differences in the quality of the antibodies is not inconsistent with the disease-specificity of the autoantibody [109].

The diagnostic significance of the demonstration of anti-intercellular-substance antibodies by indirect immunofluorescence is unquestionable if a standardized quantitative technique is used and the result is repeatedly positive [43, 106*b*]. This is true even for histologically atypical cases as well as for cases of mini pemphigus and intraepidermal non-acantholytic pemphigus with spongiosis [580*a*]. The test is negative in a wide variety of other vesiculobullous diseases [43, 108*b*, 289*b*, 303, 581] including childhood pemphigus, benign mucosal pemphigoid, the classical dermatitis herpetiformis of Duhring–Brocq, erythema multiforme bullosum, muco-synechial dermatitis atrophicans of Lortat–Jacob, Hailey–Hailey's disease, transient acantholytic dermatosis of Grover, impetigo herpetiformis, herpes gestationis, Sneddon–Wilkinson's disease, and porphyria bullosa. However, serum samples from patients burned on 20–80 per cent of their body surface and of those with extensive toxic necrolysis may transiently contain anti-intercellular-substance antibodies [1*a*, *b*, 579*c*], thus simulating the usual finding in PV [43]. In cases with Lyell syndrome, mild thermic burning, toxicoderma bullosum arsenicale, myasthenia gravis, squamous cell carcinoma as well as in patients under ALS therapy, low titre intercellular fluorescence may occasionally be demonstrated [1*b*, 303, 579*c*, 580*b*]. Similar pemphigus-like anti-epithelial antibodies have been detected in the serum of patients with benign (hypertrophic) and malignant (carcinomatous) diseases of the prostate by indirect immunofluorescence [1*c*]. Occasionally anti-epithelial antibodies have been described in connection with drug sensitivities (e. g. to the sulphomethoxy-pyridazine preparation Kynex) [43], in patients with morbilliform or maculo-papular eruptions caused by penicillins (especially ampicillin) [183, 184], in a *Trichophyton rubrum* infection [458] and in true PV induced by D-penicillin-amine therapy [265]. It is supposed that in such cases (*i*) the patient is prone to produce autoantibodies [106*b*]; (*ii*) denatured epidermal proteins are rendered more antigenic by coupling with drugs [183]; or (*iii*) the drug reactions induce an abortive form of PV [183].

Direct immunofluorescence test should be performed in strongly suspect cases if the indirect test is negative [81]. A positive result with acantholytic cells is of practical value, for an early recognition of pemphigus oris improves the chances of a successful therapy [201*b*]. In the very rare false negative results obtained with standardized method a special species-, organ- or individual specificity of the antibody may play a role; for instance it may react exclusively with a monkey mucous membrane substance or only with a mucous membrane antigen or with the own epidermis of the patient [106*b*]. If *in vivo* bound immuno-globulins have been demonstrated [590] in both epidermal intercellular spaces and dermoepidermal BM, the direct immunofluorescence test should be supple-mented with an indirect test. In such cases the patient's serum will react with the intercellular spaces, but not with the BM.

The pemphigus autoantibody is — in contrast with the epithelium of ileum, kidney and liver — also skin-(epithelium) specific, i.e. tissue-specific [234*b*, 445*a*]. Slight non-disease-specific fluorescence [47] may appear in cells of the skin adnexae (hair follicles, sebaceous glands, excretory ducts of sweat glands, galactophorous ducts), at the boundary of the cytoplasm, on some cytoplasmic constituents forming a perinuclear ring or even on the cytoplasmic membrane of prostatic secretory epithelial cells [1*c*]. Intercellular deposits have been demonstrated in apparently uninvolved skin of patients with PV, but here the staining reaction is weaker than that observed at or near the bullae. Supposedly, threshold amounts are necessary to induce pathological changes [40].

The autoantibody is not species-specific. Skin and Malpighi-type mucosa layers from man or some mammals may be used as substrate. However, there are differences in sensitivity between the substrates. Pemphigus antibodies show less affinity to the human skin [44, 127] than to the oesophageal mucosa of the rabbit. This is seemingly inconsistent with the pathogenetic role of pemphigus antibodies in the development of bullae.

Pemphigus antibodies are considered to be of the IgG type [305, 312, 626] because in two-thirds of the cases the antibody appears in the top and middle fractions of the ultracentrifuged serum, and also because antibody binding to epithelial cell can be shown in cultures if erythrocytes specifically suitable for the detection of IgG are used. Fibroblastic cell cultures, at the same time, yield negative results. Pemphigus-antibody-positive sera from patients with PV are pathogenic if administered intramucosally into the lip of monkeys. The IgG fraction of sera induces typical lesions, but the lesions differ (non-typical after 22 h) from those elicited by whole serum when studied with the immunofluorescent technique [208]. Since the antibodies bound in the course of the direct immunofluorescence test stain with anti-human IgG, this test is used, and considered conclusive, in the routine diagnosis. In addition to the IgG antibody, IgM-type pemphigus antibodies are present in about half of PV patients [301*a*, 312]. As regards IgG subclasses, stepwise elution form DEAE cellulose columns combined with immunofluorescent staining with monospecific antisera to subclasses have shown [516*b*] that pemphigus antibodies are composed of several subclasses; they were consistently found in three of four DEAE fractions.

To explain the discrepancies between the findings of different authors, numerous factors that may influence the demonstration of the antibodies have been considered [2*c*, 15, 129, 305, 312, 616]. Three types of undesirable or irrelevant fluorescence have been distinguished, viz. (*i*) autofluorescence of tissue; (*ii*) non-specific staining due to the fluorochrome effects of conjugates, a non-immunological adsorption of labelled protein and/or fluorescein to tissue; (*iii*) undesired specific staining, an immunological reaction of unwanted antibodies in the conjugate and/or test sera which react with tissue antigens.

First of all, the blood group substances [15] and the interactions by anti-B and anti-A isohaemagglutinins [234*a*] and the adherence of erythrocytes to stratum corneum [343*a*] should be eliminated by serum absorption, for an interference between auto- and isoantibodies seems to be possible, especially in the case of identical blood group [580*a*]. Blood group antigens are present as surface components in many epithelial and vascular endothelial cells. Sera tested by indirect IF for antibodies reacting with epithelial substance gave positive reaction in 7.4 per cent before, and only in 0.8 per cent after absorption with A and B erythrocytes [438]. The blood group antibodies demonstrated by indirect immunofluorescence were of the IgG class, sometimes of the IgA class, whereas haemagglutinating anti-A and anti-B antibodies belong to the IgM class; this explains the lack of correlation between indirect immunofluorescence and haemagglutinin titres against blood group substances [438]. In order to obtain a correct diagnosis of PV by the indirect immunofluorescence technique, all sera reacting with the epithelial intercellular substance should be re-examined after absorption with A and B erythrocytes. It should be noted that 39 per cent of sera with elevated (1:800–1:1600) antistreptolysin O titres showed a biological false positive indirect immunofluorescence reaction to PV [438].

To eliminate the disturbing non-specific fluorescence in the indirect immunofluorescence test, horizontal sections of the human epidermis are used as substrate [312]. It has been observed occasionally that the antibody was not detectable unless the anti-nuclear factor, the rheumatoid factor and the glomerular BM antibodies, factors which may interfere, had been absorbed [1*c*, 43, 81, 127]. In suspect cases the direct immunofluorescence has been recommended, since *in vivo* the anti-human IgG binds to the intercellular space in contrast to the haemagglutinins of IgM nature. From mixed agglutination the antibody produced against the epithelial cell culture can be separated with absorption from the anti-intercellular-substance antibody [305]. To localize the antigen-bound antibody and the antigen–antibody complexes, investigations have been made with anti-human γ-globulin.

Besides immunoglobulin C or the C factors C1q, C3a and C4, α_2D may bind in different amounts to the same intercellular substance areas of the skin or mucosa [125, 596*a*, *b*]. This can be demonstrated by the direct C staining method suggesting that antibody mediated C deposition and/or the alternate pathway activation may play a role in the underlying mechanism in PV [369]. However, some results speak against the pathogenetic role of C [301*b*]; for example, C staining is not demonstrable *in vitro*, suggesting that pemphigus antibodies are not capable of binding C [302]; furthermore, when the IgG subclass of pemphigus antibodies was investigated by stepwise elution from DEAE cellulose columns and immunofluorescent staining with monospecific antisera, the pemphigus antisera did not fix C even though the antibody activity was composed of all four IgG sublasses [516*b*]. It has been supposed that (*i*) the amounts of the C fixed by pemphigus antibodies are too small to be detected by the *in vitro* test; (*ii*) the anti-intercellular-substance antibodies make only a minute portion of the total pemphigus antibodies observed [302]; (*iii*) there might be more than one subclass of each of IgGl and IgG3; one that fixes C and another that does not; (*iv*) the amounts of the IgG1 and IgG3 antibodies might be too little to fix C, the bulk of the antibodies being IgG4 and IgG2 [516*b*].

Little is known of the nature of the autoantigen characteristic of PV. Its mobility in the ultracentrifuge in serum corresponded to that of serum albumin and was accompanied by IgG [48]. According to Inderbitzin and Katz [288], the epithelial antigen in PV might be a 'hidden' antigen similar to the antigens in the lens tissue, the retina and the testicles, to which no immunological tolerance is developed. It has been supposed that it is a protein or a lipoprotein complex [110]. Being present in the Malpighi layer of every mammalian species [234*c*], it is considered a panantigen. At least three kinds of antigens or antigen determinants may be located on the surface of the epidermal cell; (*i*) pemphigus-specific extract antigen [2*d*, 234*a*], (*ii*) A or B blood group antigen [15, 234*c*,

580*b*], and (*iii*) the common tissue antigen of epidermal cells and T lymphocytes [234*e*, 580*b*].

It seems unlikely that the pemphigus antigen is an HL-A antigen. The HL-A13 alloantigen was found more frequently in patients with PV (28 per cent) than in the control population (4 per cent). However, anti-HL-A sera did not react with the pemphigus intercellular antigen in an indirect immunofluorescence test [311]. Of patients typed for HL-A antigens by the microdroplet lymphocyte cytotoxicity test [337], HL-A10 was present in 61 per cent of unrelated Jewish patients as compared to the 20 per cent of Jewish control patients. In non-Jewish white patients the frequency of HL-A10 was also elevated, but the difference was not significant. A pemphigus susceptibility gene linked to HL-A has been postulated.

Extracts of bovine oesophagus separated by immunofluorescent absorption test contained not only insoluble, but also soluble pemphigus antigens [2*a*]. A saline extract of human epidermis and sera from PV patients gave positive PCA [450]. The variations in solubility of pemphigus antigens suggest that pemphigus antibodies react with an inhomogeneous group of antigens of similar intercellular distribution. According to literary data, the insoluble pemphigus antigens from rabbit oesophagus are polypeptides with some traces of lipid and a mol. wt. of 12,000 [3]. As regards the thermostability of the pemphigus antigens, equivocal data have been published; they have been found stable [1*b*] as well as labile [3, 234*a*]. Antigens reactive with pemphigus antibodies isolated from rabbit oesophagus are soluble in 70 per cent ethanol, but insoluble in water [482]. In contrast, the reactive antigens in the human oesophageal mucosa are saline-extractable and not precipitable by distilled water. Pemphigus antigens in the human oesophagus extract are proteins with an estimated mol. wt. of 68,000; they are readily inactivated in 30 min at 56 °C. Electrophoretically, the antigens migrated in the γ region [562]. These findings suggest the heterogeneity and protein nature of the pemphigus antigens of different sources.

It has been postulated [626] that the intercellular substance (intercellular cement or glycocalyces) acts as a carrier for, or contains, the antigen. From the observations that pemphigus antibodies are of low reactivity with the intercellular substance of the normal human epidermis it may be concluded that alterations of antigenic determinants present in the intercellular spaces of the epidermis of patients with PV occur prior to the antibody fixation [596*b*].

The development of pemphigus antigens in human foetuses aged 9–40 weeks was examined by immunofluorescence [420]. Pemphigus antigen was weakly demonstrable in the epidermal intercellular area at 9 weeks of age and strongly from the 12th weeks on, i.e. before the development of a mature keratinizing epidermis. The early appearance of the pemphigus antigen may reflect its functional importance in intercellular cohesion. It has been suggested that an extracellular carbohydrate coat or glycocalyx, present on the surface of many types of cells, may be responsible for the cell-to-cell cohesion and may play an immunological role. In PV, possibly a change in surface polysaccharide composition results in a reduced adhesiveness of epidermal cells, and simultaneously presents an antigenic stimulus. Using fluorescein-conjugated PHA, Concanavalin A and PHA-P (proteins that bind to saccharides) an intercellular staining pattern apparently identical with that found in various forms of pemphigus was observed

[432*a*, *b*]. The intercellular staining can be inhibited or abolished by certain simple sugars. A similar pattern of staining was produced *in vivo* in mouse and guinea pig skin by intradermal injection of fluorescein-conjugated Concanavalin A [251*a*]. Since Concanavalin A is known to bind carbohydrate group(s) containing α-glycosidic linkages, the reciprocal blocking experiments strongly suggest that pemphigus antibody is directed against a specific moiety (moieties) in the glycocalyx of the human epidermis. The question arises whether sugar residues are abnormal in glycocalyx and thereby elicit autoantibody production.

It has been shown in animal experiments that the antigen is demonstrable in the aqueous and ethanolic extract of the oesophageal mucosa of man, rhesus monkey and cattle. This is suggestive of tissue specificity [1*a*, *b*, 4]. In rabbits hetero-immunized with an ethanol extract of bovine oesophageal mucosa and complete Freund's adjuvant [2*a*, *b*, *c*, *d*, 369] or injected with homologous tissues [234*b*, 287*a*, *b*], production of pemphigus-like autoantibodies was demonstrable. In indirect immunofluorescence tests, the effects of these autoantibodies could not be distinguished from those of the human pemphigus autoantibody. In Ouchterlony's immunodiffusion test they showed common specificities. The tissue- and species-specificity of the autoantibody has also been examined in animal experiments [1*a*, 4, 312]. Positive results were obtained with other tissues (e.g. tongue) which contained a stratum squamosum, but not with kidney, liver and spleen tissue [2*d*]. Heterologous lymph node serum reacted in the immunofluorescent test with the epithelial antigen, but did not react with pemphigus antigen or A or B blood group substances. The experimental pemphigus-like antigens proved not to be species-specific [287*b*].

Little is known of the aetiology of the pemphigus group. Indirect data [319*a*] (virus neutralizing and C-fixing antibodies in the serum) appear to be suggestive of the causative role of viruses (adeno- or papovaviruses), particularly in the Brazilian pemphigus foliaceus [289*a*]. Sera from patients with PV were examined for paramyxovirus antibodies. The frequency of antibodies to SV5 and DU virus as tested by indirect immunofluorescence and virus neutralization was not higher than in various control groups [138*a*]. This, however, does not exclude that (*i*) pemphigus might be caused by some virus other than SV5 or DU; (*ii*) only part of the cases is caused by these viruses; (*iii*) pemphigus antigen might be a virus antigen incorporated in the membrane of cells surviving myxovirus infection. Direct experiments [319*b*] have been less suggestive.

The experiments aimed at the demonstration of the pathogenetic role of pemphigus antibodies have been complicated and have led to inconsistent results. The effect of pemphigus sera on normal human skin as examined in organ cultures [406*a*] was intercellular oedema at 12 h, suprabasilar or diffuse acantholysis between 24 and 72 h and extensive acantholysis at 120 h (H-E stain). Direct immunofluorescence studies showed questionable or weak intercellular staining between 6 and 24 h. When experimentally produced antibody was injected into strongly immunized rabbits intradermally, some authors [287*b*] observed formation of intraepidermal clefts. Others [234*d*] failed to confirm the *in vivo* binding of autoantibodies in the rabbit skin. When serum obtained from patients with PV was injected into monkey skin, the serum was bound intercellularly, but did not cause acantholysis [46, 105, 234*e*], except when high-titre Brazilian pemphigus sera were used in the form of multiple (two or three) intradermal injections [42*b*]. According to more recent investigations [272], repeated intramucosal injections of monkey lip with patient's sera or their IgG fractions was followed by development of intraepithelial lesions. Immunofluorescent–studies have confirmed the binding to the intercellular region of the epithelium. Suprabasal clefts and the disruption of epithelial coherence were considered nonspecific or artefacts. It has been attempted to explain the need for repeated injections by supposing that some time–quantity threshold of antibody binding may be necessary. In man, intradermal injection of pemphigus autoantibodies were followed by some transient abnormalities reminding of experimental pemphigus [4].

It has been supposed that, in the rabbit, migration of the autoantibody from the serum into the epidermis is hindered by a dermal-epidermal barrier [234*b*]. To eliminate this, the skin surface was pretreated with dry ice and by rubbing in of sodium lauryl sulphonate. Some authors succeeded in inducing intraepidermal cleft formation, acantholysis and acantholytic cells swimming free in the lumen using high-titre serum in immunized animals [287*a*, 288, 369]. Others [234*b*] failed to reproduce these results completely. It seems likely [105] that acantholysis needs, in addition to the permeability-increasing factor, enhancing factor(s) present in pathological sera (e.g. of patients with pneumonia or tuberculosis) to develop. (Sera with high-titre pemphigus antibodies mixed with sera of patients suffering from acute bacterial infection were injected into rabbits: intercellular acantholytic lesions developed.) Passive induction of intraepidermal clefts in rabbits by transfer of sera from patients suffering from Brazilian pemphigus foliaceus was also successful [42*a*] if the transfer was immediately followed by treatment with 1 per cent or 2 per cent solution of 2,4-dinitrochlorobenzene. The epidermal changes including microbullae were characteristic of those seen in human PV both in the IF pattern and the histopathological picture, except that typical acantholytic cells did not appear. Human PV plasma transfusion caused neither disease nor lesions demonstrable with immunofluorescence in four rhesus monkeys, in spite of strong binding of antibodies to the epidermal intercellular space [515]. These experiments cast doubt on the direct role of pemphigus antibodies in the pathogenesis of PV. The antibodies of the serum, being possibly related to different antigenic determinants, are inhomogeneous in their biological properties. It may be that the species of antibody that causes the disease is already bound to the intercellular space and humoral antibodies are not responsible for production of lesions.

As triggering mechanism a virus infection [289*b*] may be considered that may start the process in immunologically predisposed subjects. It is remarkable that UV light applied to the normal appearing skin of patients with PV induces immunochemical changes leading to a progressive increase in the *in vivo* binding of IgG and C in the irradiated areas [131].

The role of cell-mediated immunity in the pathogenesis of the PV bullae has also been investigated [405*a*, *b*]. The investigations started from the observation that lymphocytes and lymphoblasts were found in Tzanck smears prepared from mucosal or skin lesions. It should be noted that the Tzanck cells show positive direct immunofluorescence [144], especially membrane fluorescence [201*b*]. The appearance of lymphocytes and lymphoblasts in the tissue cultures might be explainable by assuming that the anti-intercellular-substance antibodies can transform the epithelial cells into Tzanck cells and the epithelial and intercellular substances represent an antigenic stimulus for the lymphocytes. Electron-microscopic study of eosinophil leukocytes in tissues and blister fluid have shown that the matrix of the blister eosinophils may have a granular or microvesicular structure ('matrix transformation') or a change leading to disappearance of the granules ('matrix lysis') [629].

Inderbitzin and Katz [288] suggest that the basic defect in PV is a breakdown of a 'plasma-epidermis barrier'. In their opinion the autoimmune mechanism is based on an antigen–antibody reaction capable of producing an alteration or derangement of cellular metabolism, perhaps a change in the surface polysaccharide composition [432] that could result in a decreased cellular adhesiveness; thus acantholysis would be based on a cytotoxic effect. It should be noted that immune complex formation has not been proved by immunochemical methods in PV. Further evidence against the presence of immune complexes has been derived from the finding that the serum C3 level was found significantly elevated in 40 per cent of the PV cases and in 57 per cent of the pemphigus foliaceus cases [1*c*]. The hypothesis of Inderbitzin and Katz has been supported [40, 172, 289*b*, 626] by the following: the anti-intercellular-substance antibodies behave like autoantibodies; the localization of the antibody reaction corresponds to the primary PV lesion; occasionally, the antibodies have been demonstrated to bind C; the reaction is negative in other diseases; the serum titre is directly related to the severity of the clinical disease; the reappearance of the antibodies in serum may precede that of the histochemical lesion; in rabbits, the epithelial substance may induce the production of antibodies by which acantholysis-like lesions can be elicited; immunosuppressive therapy has been successful. In some cases, association with some other antibody, e. g. anti-nuclear factor, anti-thyroglobulin, anti-thyroid-microsomes, anti-gastric-parietal-cell and anti-muscle antibodies, has been demonstrated [41]. PV has also been diagnosed in certain patients suffering from thymoma [557, 600]. Fifty-nine case reports were collected in which association of pemphigus with thymoma or malignancy was described [335]; in 54 per cent of the malignancies the lymphoid system or the RES was involved. If in the course of postnatal thymic disease, thymitis or thymoma, the thymic milieu has so changed that autoantigens being present in the thymus (in cell nuclei, myoid cells and squamous epithelium: Hassal's corpuscles) exert an immunological rather than tolerogenic effect, autoantibodies may be formed to those constituents. This might explain the association between thymic disease, particularly thymoma, and autoimmune disease [557, 600, 615].

It is to some extent contradictory that, e. g. the pemphigus antibody does not bind C [301*b*]; the so-called autoantibodies cause a direct pathogenic effect in PV by dissolving desmosomal bridges, thereby forming blisters. However, this opinion has not been supported by the latest animal experiments of Grob [234*a*, *b*]. According to Sams and Schur [516*b*], two characteristics of the humoral antibody are difficult to reconcile, viz. (*i*) its failure to confer disease after passive transfer of monkeys [515] and (*ii*) a positive correlation of antibody titre with disease activity. Thus, it is to some degree uncertain [1*b*] that the humoral pemphigus autoantibody is the basic cause of blister formation or must necessarily be pathogenic [339] or that acantholysis is a simple autoimmune sign.

It is possible that the autoantibody is not the cause, but a consequence of the disease, in other words a phenomenon substantiating the immunological events.

Little is known of the autoallergic origin of the other diseases within the pemphigus group. In *pemphigus vegetans* (in Lever's opinion the PV of subjects highly resistant to the disease), and in *familial benign pemphigus* or *Hailey–Hailey's disease* (Fig. 40-6*a*, *b*], which is according to Lever a genodermatosis not belonging to the pemphigus group, the demonstration of autoantibodies

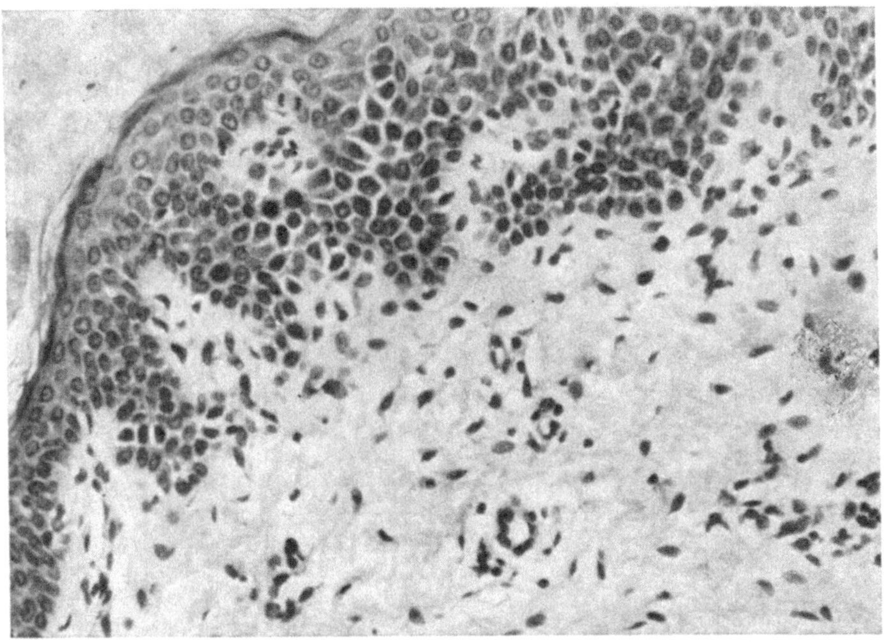

Fig. 40-60. Hailey–Hailey's disease. Extensive acantholysis at the initial stage, the connection between epithelial cells has ceased in a large area. ×60 (Courtesy of Professor L. Szodoray, Debrecen)

to either the intercellular substance or the BM has failed [43, 246, 581]. It has been emphasized that part of the pemphigus vegetans diagnoses are incorrect [106*b*]. In an active clinical case of pemphigus vegetans pronounced changes in the tonofilament-desmosome complexes and migration of eosinophils from dermis to epidermis were observed [238]. Observations with the acridine-orange UV fluorescence and the direct immunofluorescent techniques have shown that the Hailey–Hailey's disease is a distinct disease entity: neither '*cerne de deuil*' in the isolated cells nor fluorescent cell margins are to be seen [571], both being present in PV.

In *pemphigus foliaceus* some authors did [40, 234*b*, 289*b*, 524], others [507] did not succeed in demonstrating anti-epithelial autoantibody. An occasional high titre could be explained with the generalized character of the cutaneous lesions. Subcorneal anti-intercellular-substance antibodies were found in 4 out

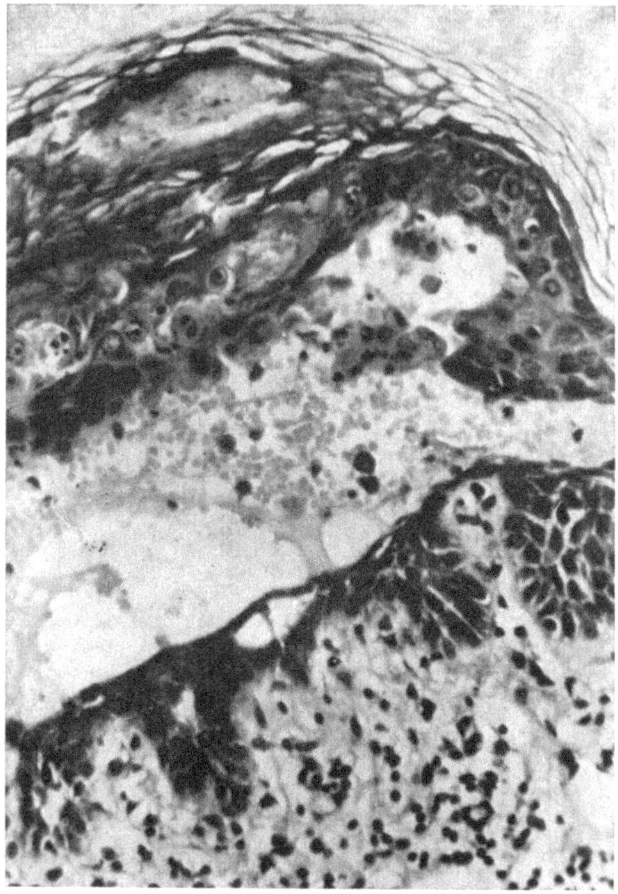

Fig. 40-6*b*. Hailey–Hailey's disease. Numerous dyskeratotic cells (*corps ronds* grains) on the top of the vesicle. ×60 (Courtesy of Professor L. Szodoray, Debrecen)

of 10 patients with definite or suspected pemphigus foliaceus and suggest that this form of pemphigus may be associated with distinctive antibodies [83*b*, *c*]. Direct immunofluorescent studies showed faint linear immunoglobulin deposits at the dermal-epidermal junction. Indirect immunofluorescence tests of sera showed intercellular antibodies reacting solely with antigens in the intercellular substance of the uppermost layers of squamous cells just below the stratum corneum. Familial occurrence has been described [601].

The *Brazilian pemphigus foliaceus (fogo selvagem)* is endemic in certain parts of Brazil. In patients the autoantibody has also been demonstrated [289*b*, 364]. The anatomical site of the lesion (intraepithelial cleavage) and the pathological features (acantholysis) are approximately the same as in PV, but the disease seems to have a different aetiology. Epidemiological observations are suggestive of an infectious (viral) agent.

Pemphigus seborrhoicus sive erythematosus sive Senear–Usher's syndrome. The immunological relationships of this disease are still unclear [552]. Autoantibodies to the intercellular substance occur frequently [436], and those to the BM have also been described [581]; even coexistence has been demonstrated [34, 107*b*, 506], both IgG and C factors (C3, C4) have been found diffusely bound to fibres not only in the intercellular space, but also at the dermoepidermal junction [596*a*, *b*]. Other investigators [213] succeeded in demonstrating linear BM IgG deposits only in the most severely affected area. In this disease the immunosuppressive therapy is more successful than in other diseases of the pemphigus group. The disease may be associated with myasthenia gravis [290, 436], bronchial carcinoma [506] and thymoma [43]. Based on immunofluorescent studies, it was suggested that pemphigus seborrhoicus represents a simultaneous occurrence of PV and SLE [34, 107*b*]. However, most of the authors [213] have failed to detect anti-nuclear antibody in the serum. Based on the electron-microscopic finding that the degree of disappearance of the desmosomes in the blister resembles that seen in early blisters in PV, pemphigus erythematosus was considered a PV which has not developed beyond an initial phase, or an abortive form, or, according to Lever, an early phase of pemphigus foliaceus. The degree of the disappearance of desmosomes in pemphigus erythematosus appears to be less pronounced than in pemphigus foliaceus [592]. Furthermore, it has been supposed [213] that the IgG deposition is not specific, but C and fibrinogen leave blood vessels and accumulate in the epidermal junction as a result of severe alteration (inflammatory infiltration almost exclusively consisting of polymorphs) and the consequent increase of vascular permeability. At present it seems impossible to determine the pathogenesis of the disease.

The various members of the pemphigus group may develop into one another [368*a*]: PV into pemphigus erythematosus, pemphigus erythematosus into pemphigus foliaceus or pemphigus vegetans into PV.

Therapeutic possibilities in the pemphigus group. The prognosis of PV was very grave before the corticosteroid era; nearly all patients died. The earlier the corticosteroid therapy is started the more rapid remission can be expected. Prednisone is the corticosteroid of choice. Its introduction into the therapy has reduced the mortality rate from 90 per cent to 34–44 per cent [495]; mortality as low as 5 per cent has been reported [459] for patients treated with high doses. The initial dose should be high (30–105 mg or even higher, up to 360 mg per day). Then the dose may be reduced in a logarithmic fashion, parallel with the clinical remission [368*a*, 449].

For cytostatic drugs contraindication of, damage by, and/or resistance to, corticosteroids is an absolute indication. The drug of choice is methotrexate (weekly dose, 12.5–25–45 mg, intramuscularly); this drug is dermotropic therefore it can be given as a weekly injection without difficulty [368*c*]. One should reckon with damages including hepatotoxicity, bacterial infection, reactivation of tuberculosis, cerebral thrombosis, erosions of the oral mucosa, etc.; in such cases leucovorin calcium, an antidote of methotrexate, should be given. Azathioprine alone (50 to 250 mg per day) usually gives good results, both clinically and immunologically (decrease in the indirect immunofluorescence titres) [495], but occasionally complications (transient leukopenia, fatigue, etc.) have been observed. In early PV azathioprine alone may control the disease [595]. Administration of cyclophosphamide (100 to 150 mg per day) appears to be particularly favourable [336] when the high maintenance dose of corticosteroid must be reduced. As side-effects reversible alopecia and leukopenia have been reported. 6-mercaptopurine and mechlorethamine are administered less commonly. Their combination with corticosteroids (synergistic effect) enables a reduction of the daily dose of prednisone or a stabilization of the maintenance dose, and increases clinical efficiency. Clinical remission needs at least 3–4 weeks. The result is the best in pemphigus erythematosus. In PV, the cutaneous lesions heal much more readily than the mucous membrane symptoms [368*c*]. It seems to be the most promising if the level of the circulating antibody tends downwards, but inconsistent results have also been reported. Methotrexate alone is usually insufficient to reach bulla stop. In general, long-term therapy is necessary (morbostatic effect), but little is known of the success of such therapies. Relapses should be treated similarly. They can be predicted when the antibody level is rising. As an alternate therapy, parenterally administered gold sodium thiomalate may be considered, though, undesirable side-effects may occur [460]. The corticosteroid-sparing effect of β-adrenergic blocking agents has also been investigated in PV [543]. Propranolol acts on the vasodilator fibres and thus stops the extravasation of plasma into the bullae.

ALS destroys, especially the sensitized, immunoactive lymphocytes, but its side-effects counteract its wide clinical use.

Therapy may be supplemented with anabolic hormones for restoration of the pathologically altered protein metabolism [314].

Bullous pemphigoid of Lever (BP)

A number of synonyms are in current use: benign pemphigus, parapemphigus, old man's pemphigus and dermatitis herpetiformis varians bullosa. The disease occurs predominantly in the old age [104, 289*c*, 301*a*, 368*a*, 581]. Numerous large, initially tense bullae are present, in most cases on erythematous areas, mainly on the groins, on the inner aspects of the thighs and flexor surfaces of the forearms (Fig. 40-7). The oral mucosa is involved in about one-third of cases and lesions in the small-intestinal mucosa are more frequent than believed previously. The blisters break less easily than in PV as the cells of epidermis do not show acantholytic degeneration. The denuded areas of once broken bullae do not tend to extend; they show a good tendency to heal. The degree of itching is variable. The mucosal lesions [394] small in size and few in number are mainly intact blisters. In the course of generalized BP, exacerbations and remissions alternate. Fatal cases are extremely rare. Death usually results from general debility of old patients or from complications, e. g. bronchopneumonia. Histologically [489], the first lesions usually consist of the formation of numerous microvacuoles (Fig. 40-8). Through the coalescence of these, larger vacuoles of subepidermal location (Fig. 40-9), and subsequently subepidermal bullae arise. Early bullae are found fully in subepidermal location [368*b*], but after two days peripheral regeneration of the epidermis begins. In older bullae the

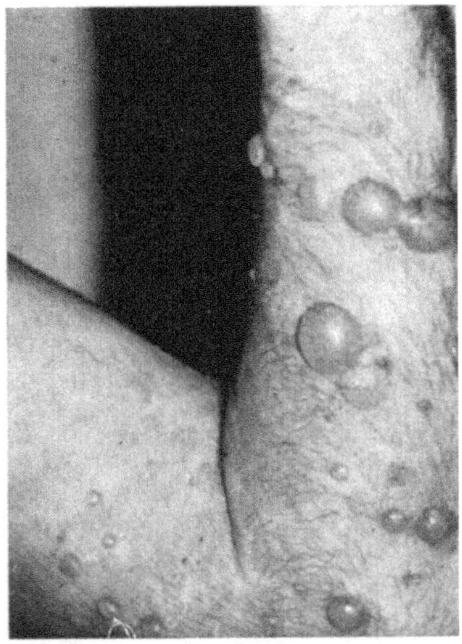

Fig. 40-7. Bullous pemphigoid. Numerous large tense bullae on the upper extremity. (Courtesy of Professor N. Simon, Szeged)

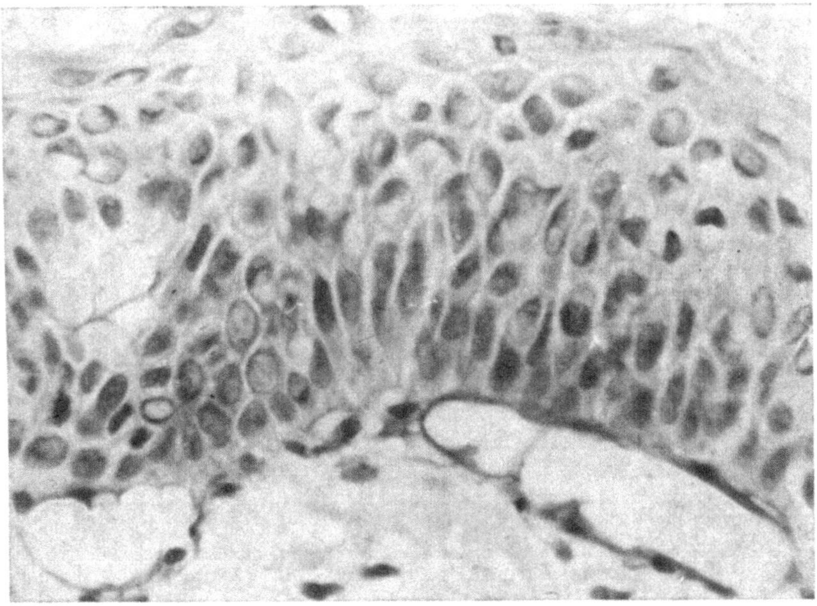

Fig. 40-8. Bullous pemphigoid. Subepidermal vesicle, initial stage. ×160 (Courtesy of Professor N. Simon, Szeged)

epidermal cells may undergo necrosis and then disintegrate; in this way the bulla may eventually become subcorneal in location. The dermis contains only a mild perivascular infiltrate consisting of lymphocytes and eosinophils. In the latter case, the epidermis may show evidence of vasculitis. The primary electron-microscopic changes occur in the dermis [98, 103].

In general, three stages of blister formation can be distinguished [521]. The first stage is characterized by a marked oedema in the dermis and epidermis and rather pronounced cellular infiltrate in the dermis; projections of basal cells are in contact with infiltrate cells. (Amorphous or fibrillar protein precipitates occur not only in BP, but also in dermatitis herpetiformis, in suction blisters

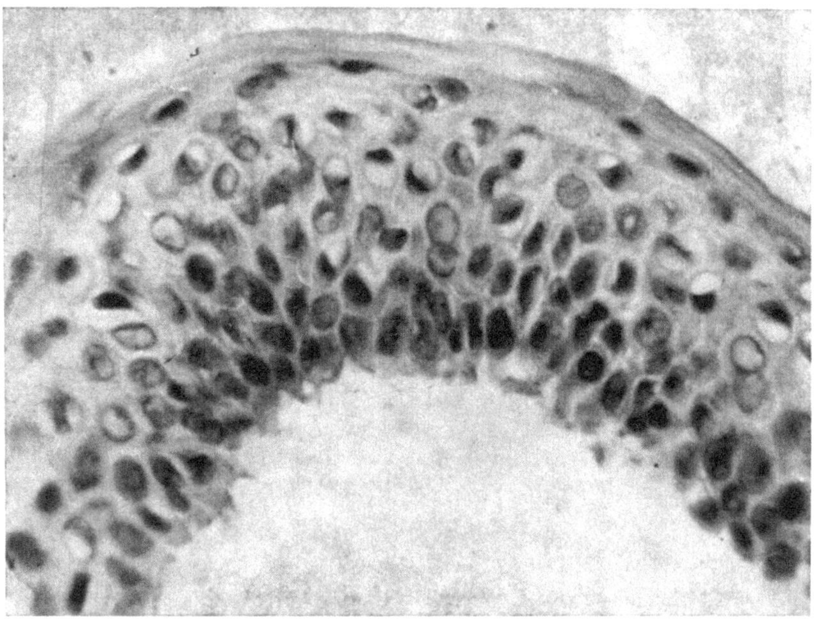

Fig. 40-9. Bullous pemphigoid. A developed subepidermal vesicle. All layers of the epidermis are to be found on the top. ×400 (Courtesy of Professor N. Simon, Szeged)

and in allergic vasculitis.) In the second stage the changes in the BM consist of either thickening or smudging with or without interruptions in continuity. The basal lamina shows discontinuities. Some of the basal cells develop degenerative cytoplasmic changes. Eosinophils migrate into the epidermis and degranulate. In mature blisters of the third stage the basal lamina is usually lacking. Electron-microscopically, BP seems to be indistinguishable from dermatitis herpetiformis [521]. Nevertheless, BP can be considered a disease entity.

In about three-quarters of the cases a linear homogeneous band of anti-BM-zone autoantibodies is demonstrable in acute-phase serum samples by the indirect immunofluorescent technique [17, 47, 108*a*, 126, 155, 267, 276, 289*c*, 300, 355*a*, 369, 421, 485, 507, 563, 579*d*, 606]. Sometimes autoantibodies can be demonstrated in blister punctates, too [106*b*, 301*c*, 608]. The antibody titres of serum and blister punctate are different in most cases [608]. Binding of autoantibodies in the BM zone has been shown by an immunohistochemical technique (peroxidase-labelled antibody method) as well [199]. BP is the only disease with subepidermal bullae in which autoantibodies have been found in the serum, a fact that may be very helpful in differentiating BP from erythema multiforme and dermatitis herpetiformis [368*b*]. The autoantibody is organ-specific, not species-specific [312, 421]. Antibody may be fixed *in vivo* to the BM zone of several organs of epithelial origin (skin, oesophagus and vagina) [355*a*]. Simian oral or oesophageal mucosa appears to be the substrate of choice for routine tests for these antibodies. Demonstration of an interdependence between antibody titre and clinical picture has usually failed [507]; such a correlation may exist in untreated cases. The duration of the disease and extension of the lesion should also be considered in this respect. Thus, patients with extensive lesions of more than one-month duration usually have high titres, in contrast to those with fairly extensive eruption but of less than one-month duration [368*b*]. Treatment with high doses of corticosteroids or with methotrexate, as a rule, reduces the titre [368*b*, 608]. As a result of low-dosage corticosteroid therapy, the clinical picture may improve without a considerable change in the antibody titre [608]. Occasionally autoantibody may remain demonstrable after the skin phenomena have disappeared, especially if the patient's own epidermis is used as antigen [289*c*]. Negative results may be explainable by differences in species, organ and individual specificities [289*c*]. Biological false positive reactions can be excluded by applying an adequate immunofluorescent technique (with special regard to the conjugate) [289*c*].

Immunoelectrophoresis may show a slightly raised IgA level and a low IgM level; the C level is usually below the normal [608]. The autoantibody is of the IgG class [312]. In the direct immunofluorescence test, IgG gives a selective homogeneous band in the BM zone [104, 267, 507, 579*d*, 606] (Fig. 40-10). Thus, BP is characterized by the presence of both circulating and tissue-fixed BM-zone antibodies [355*a*]. In the surrounding area and in the uninvolved skin, only a fraction of the IgG antibody reacts with the fixed BM antigen [58]; the direct immunofluorescence test, e.g. with tracheal substrate, may even be negative [442]. In the case of a lower titre the bond is narrow and a fine IgG deposit is detected in the junctional zone [128]. Furthermore, IgG bound *in vivo* [46, 108*a*, 300] and C, more precisely C3a and C4 [126, 267, 276, 301*c*, 302] were found in the BM zone, along the border line of skin papillae but seldom in the roof of the bullae consisting of the lower strata of the epidermis. The specificity of the reaction has been checked by a blocking test. However, the immunoglobulin and C fixation in the BM zone is not disease-specific, for it may be present in lesions of chronic discoid lupus erythematosus as well as in the clinically intact skin of patients suffering from SLE [289*c*]. In such cases the clinical picture and the indirect IF method may be useful in the differential diagnosis. IgD deposits in blood vessel walls of the affected skin and their surroundings was demonstrable by immunofluorescence studies in one-third of the cases [126], but the presence of IgD appears not to be characteristic.

The role of C has recently been examined in detail [355*a*]. It was found that C was consumed within the blister cavity, perhaps by activation of the alternate pathway. The eluted IgG antibody did not fix C *in vitro*, but C3 was fixed to the BM zone *in vivo*. Presumably, this was accomplished via the alternate pathway, since C3PA was also demonstrated. Total C, C3PA and individual C components were depressed in the blister fluid, suggesting local activation of the C cascade. At sites of the BM zone staining with fluorescein-conjugated anti-β1C/β1A after addition of human C with *in vivo* bound Ig was demonstrable, but it was not demonstrable with *in vivo* fixed C [267]. This might indicate that either antigen–antibody complexes are unsaturated *in vivo* or the fixed C disappears. These results suggest that BP serum contains autoantibodies with non-C-fixing and C-fixing activity. BM antibodies were fractionated by ion-exchange chromatography and the individual fractions were examined with fluorescing

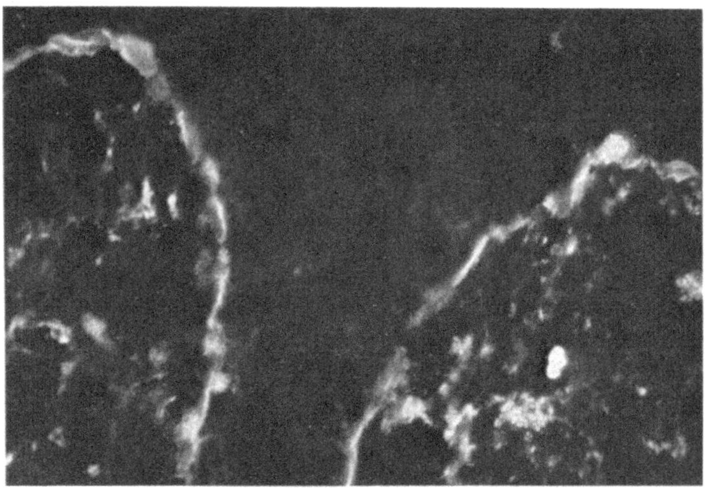

Fig. 40-10. Bullous pemphigoid. Discontinual linear fluorescence in the basement membrane zone. Elastic autofluorescence in the corium. Leukocytes and mainly perivascular immunoglobulin complex deposits. Anti-human IgG/FTC. Leitz Ortholux. ×500 (Courtesy of Professor N. Simon, Szeged)

conjugates of antihuman IgG and β1C/β1A [516*a*]. The IgG subclasses of BP antibodies have been investigated using stepwise elution from DEAE cellulose columns and immunofluorescent staining with monospecific antisera [516*b*]. The antibody activity in non-C-fixing BP sera was confined to the third and fourth peaks and was exclusively IgG4. On the other hand, antibody activity in C-fixing BP sera was found in all four peaks, except C-fixation to the first peak, which contained IgG3.

Apparently Fe^{2+} ions are necessary for the reaction between anti-BM antibodies and the antigens on the BM [57] as proved by the following experiment. When treated with EDTA, the IF staining on the BM with a BP serum disappeared. This effect was reversed by adding Fe^{2+}. A series of other cations proved to be ineffective.

Antibodies to thyroid gland, cytoplasm and gastric parietal cell antigen may occasionally occur in BP sera [421]. The antibodies of certain patients do react with their own skin *in vitro*, but do not *in vivo* [267, 300]. This might be due to the poor sensitivity of the applied method or to the possible existence of a barrier inhibiting the antigen–antibody reaction *in vivo*.

It is still questionable whether the BP antibody is directly responsible for the lesions. Transferred antibody was found to bind to the BM in the monkey skin, but produced no lesions there. This might be explained by the antibody being unable in itself to cause lesions, or by its not being identical with the antibody bound to the skin and thus causing tissue damage. The conjugate BP serum had not been blocked by the treatment with eluates [355*b*]. Direct immunofluorescent testing of several organs revealed anti-BM-zone antibody only in the skin, in the oesophagus and in the vagina [355*b*], but anti-BM-zone antibody was also eluted from the trachea with citric-acid-buffer of pH 2.2 and the thus eluted antibody was similar to the fixed BP antibody in terms of IgG subclass, tubular pattern and inability to fix C. However, the two antibodies did not share equal affinity for the antigenic suite. C studies revealed activation of both the classic and alternate pathways within the tissue and a reduction of all C components in the blister fluid [355*b*].

The nature of the antigen(s) is unknown. The development of BP antigens in human foetuses aged 9–40 weeks has been examined by immunofluorescence [420]. The fluorescence corresponding to BP antigens was weak and patchy at 12 weeks and bright linear fluorescence of the BM zone appeared consistently only from the 23rd week on. The lack of correlation between classical BM and BP antigenicity indicates some degree of independence between these structures [420]. In preliminary studies [421] a protein moiety appeared to be an integral component of the antigen. BP is sometimes associated with internal tumours, less frequently with lymphoreticular proliferation [106*a*, 107*a*], whence a causal relationship between these conditions has been considered [170, 557]. These observations point to the possiblity of two distinct groups of autoantigens or of two different mechanisms of inducing the formation of autoantibodies in these diseases.

More recently [561] isolation of the active antigen of the human cutaneous BM, strictly speaking, a molecular component that manifests immunochemical activity and thus may represent the natural or self antigen, has been reported.

Numerous authors [108*b*, 369, 514, 616] have spoken for the autoimmune pathogenesis of BP, supported by the following observations: (*i*) patients possess a serum IgG antibody to their own skin BM; (*ii*) this IgG3 subclass antibody is capable of binding C *in vivo*; (*iii*) both the antibody and C (C3, C4 fragments) have been found at the exact sites of BP lesions; (*iv*) in the inflammatory infiltrate polymorphonuclear leukocytes predominate; (*v*) BP has a chronic clinical course. Additional evidence for an immunological pathogenesis has also been called up: (*i*) clinical improvement may occur in response to corticosteroid and/or methotrexate therapy [421]; (*ii*) blood eosinophilia and infiltration of the bullae and BM zones by eosinophils suggest the presence of immune complexes [378]; (*iii*) the disease may associate with other autoimmune diseases; (*iv*) autoantibodies to other organs also occur.

Some authors [129, 368*b*, 579*c*] are more cautious as regards the causative role of autoantibodies demonstrable in the serum because (*i*) the passive transfer of the disease with anti-BM-zone antibodies has failed; (*ii*) the correlation between the disease activity and antibody titre is questionable; (*iii*) the binding of both Ig and factors C3a and C4 to the BM zone may be an *in situ* immune reaction, but alternatively it may result from a secondary local accumulation of the transudate; (*iv*) even the C-fixing activity within the tissue may be non-specific as in the case of heat-aggregated γ-globulin; (*v*) the fact that immunoglobulin binds to the BM zone in both the affected and unaffected skin indicates that the binding of the antibody in itself is not sufficient to cause visible lesions in the skin [267]; (*vi*) discrepancies have been observed between the results of the *in vitro* and *in vivo* C-fixations as well as between the anti-BM-zone antibody level and the IgG level [301*a*].

The elective fixation of the antibodies at the precise site of bullous detachment has nevertheless remained an important argument suggesting that the auto-antibodies represent at least one of the pathogenic factors.

The mode and the cause of the production of autoantibodies are still unknown. There are two main hypotheses.

1. The production may be the result of an autoimmunity arising as a result of disfunctioning of the immune regulation system; this would be in accordance with the simultaneous appearance of other antibodies. Early during the attack the IgM level is rising, which is followed by a rise in the IgG parallel with an increase in the BP antibody level [608]. An objection to this hypothesis is that (*i*) in the serum the changes of IgG concentration of the dynamics of the antibody titre are poorly reflected; (*ii*) it is difficult to demonstrate that the autoantibodies actually cause lesions. Also, the hypothesis does not define the mechanism that leads to the disfunctioning of immune regulation.

2. The second hypothesis, which leaves the initial aggression to be elucidated, postulates that the production is secondary, an epiphenomenon following the release of autoantigens from the destroyed BM. The anti-BM-zone antibody is produced partly in the middle part of the dermis due to stimulation of immunologically competent cells inside the round-cell-infiltrated lesions [608]. Part of these antibodies are bound in the area of the lesion and in its immediate vicinity, the rest migrate into the vesicle and the serum [608]. It should be noted that the anti-BM-zone antibody titre begins to rise during, not prior to, the attack. This suggests that the antibody production is stimulated by the skin phenomena themselves; subsequently, in turn, the specific antibody in the serum determines the activity and the dynamics of the disease. The second hypothesis is more consistent with the clinical and biological facts.

For practical purposes it is of importance that the anti-BM-zone antibodies are considered specific for BP, therefore, their demonstration by positive immunofluorescence using anti-IgG and anti-C3 antisera is a great diagnostic aid, especially in cases without demonstrable circulating antibody [81].

The observation that polymorphonuclear leukocytes are present in the lesions and C is not fixed by the eluated IgG antibodies *in vitro* suggests several possibilities [516*b*]: (*i*) the inflammatory lesions of BP may be the results of different mechanisms including mechanisms activated by different immunoglobulin classes; (*ii*) immunoglobulins could activate a non-C-fixing system or (*iii*) the immunoglobulins bound to BP skin are secondary to damage to the BM zone and are not pathogenic. Which of these possibilities is the correct one, is still unknown. It is also unclear why there is no clinical difference between cases with C-fixing and those with non-C-fixing antibodies. All these antibodies may simply be secondary to primary damage caused by another mechanism as evidenced by the observation of transient pemphigus antibodies following thermal burns [579*c*].

Therapy is essentially similar to the therapy in the pemphigus group. Without corticosteroid therapy up to 50 per cent of the patients, mainly in the elderly age groups, may die. Spontaneous remission may occur, but this is, as a rule, followed by relapse. If the eruption is severe, the therapy is started with large daily doses of prednisone; Lever [368*b*] recommends 180 mg per day. The daily dose can be reduced as soon as the lesions have shown the expected healing. Since in old subjects corticosteroids are apt to cause serious side-effects, the combination of prednisone with cytostatics (Lever prefers methotrexate) [368*b*] may be necessary. Separation of the epidermis from the dermis to produce blisters by means of suction is a quantitative method for studying epidermo-dermal adherence *in vivo*, a monitor of the effect of treatment [120].

Benign mucous membrane pemphigoid (BMMP). (Synonyms: cicatricial pemphigoid, ocular pemphigus, pemphigus conjunctivae, essential shrinking of the conjunctiva, muco-synechial dermatitis atrophicans, etc.) Electron-microscopically the basal lamina appears to be discontinuous in the dermoepidermal junction; severe oedema in the adjacent dermis and lesions of the connective tissue fibres are characteristic of the disease [91]. In contrast to BP, circulating anti-BM-zone antibodies could not be demonstrated by indirect immunofluorescence in the serum in the majority of cases [35, 45, 191, 233, 289*c*, 327]. Direct immunofluorescent staining revealed the presence of tissue-fixed linear homogeneous BM-zone IgG deposits in fresh skin and mucous membrane lesions, with staining characteristics similar to the deposits in BP [35, 138, 191, 233, 267, 274, 327]. Occasionally the deposits contained also IgM, IgA or C3. In addition, deposition of IgG was demonstrated [140] at the dermo-epidermal junction, along the BM zone surrounding hair bulb and on the BM zone of apocrine glands. Benign non-acantholytic pemphigus of the buccal mucosa may be accompanied by the appearance of serum antibodies to components of the BM zone. These antibodies are absent in the muco-synechial dermatitis atrophicans of Lortat-Jacob (pemphigus of the eyes) [484]. The classification of BMMP into the BP group is inconsistent with the lack of demonstrable humoral antibodies to the BM zone in the majority of the cases. It is, however, possible that antibody is present, but not demonstrable by immunofluorescence (improper antigen, interference or prozone phenomenon, improper technique). It might be another explanation that in an early phase of the disease the bulk of the humoral antibody identical with that being fixed to the BM-zone antigen is undetectable in the circulating blood. As a third possibility, it has been suggested that only a small amount of antibody is produced and is therefore unable to enter the circulation. It has been emphasized that the situation may be analogous to that in discoid lupus erythematosus, in which tissue-fixed anti-nuclear antibody is demonstrable consistently, whereas humoral antibody only rarely [35]. Atrophy and scarring are usual in both diseases. It is of interest in this respect that two cases were described in which mucosal ulcerations and conjunctival lesions resulted in scarring, and serum antibodies to the intercellular area of the epithelium were demonstrable; in the same cases immunofluorescence studies revealed bound IgG at the BM zone of the involved ocular and oral tissues [132]. It is difficult to explain why this disease differs from BP in its sites of predilection, chronicity and sequelae. Some authors believe this to be a *form fruste* of BP or the benign end of a spectrum with predilection for mucous membrane and a tendency to scarring. The similar binding sites and the different clinical course seem to be suggestive of an IgG distinct from those supposed to have a pathological role in BP. The reaction of IgG with apocrine and hair-follicle BM may represent a less specific but more affinitive antibody as compared to that found in BP. It should be clarified whether there is any correlation between the humoral antibody titre and the activity of the disease. It is also to be cleared up whether BMMP is a clinically unique pathological entity separate from BP.

Corticosteroids are of poor efficiency, while methotrexate therapy has shown partial success. Azathioprine might be more beneficial [140].

Dermatosis bullosa chronica benigna juvenilis [299]. (Synonyms: chronic non-hereditary blistering disease in children, *Duhringsche Krankheit bei Kindern*, benign chronic bullous dermatosis of the childhood.) Its main characteristics are large tensile blisters on intact or erythematous skin on the lower half of the trunk, on the median surface of the thighs and on the lumbar region; mucous membranes are not involved [33]. Histological examination shows subepidermal blister without microabscesses [289*c*]. Electron-microscopically it is characterized by destruction of the BM and its substitution with a fibrillar substance [66*a*]. The disease resists sulphapyridine therapy but responds to sulphone. The immunofluorescence pattern is usually different from those of both BP and dermatitis herpetiformis papulovesiculosa [33, 66*a*, 289*c*, 299]. Occasionally the findings resemble those obtained in BP of adults [32], i.e. IgG and C may be found in the junctional zone and in the upper layers of the dermis, with [32, 185] or without [174] antibodies against the BM zone. In other cases the clinical, histological and immunopathological picture may imitate dermatitis herpetiformis and respond well to sulphapyridine [289*c*]. Depending on the different observations, this condition has been regarded as a childhood BP [314*a*], or a bullous childhood variety of dermatitis herpetiformis [66*a*]. It is questionable whether the disease is a nosological entity [33] or whether it should be considered a syndrome of mixed aetiology [289*c*].

PV and BP may occur concurrently. The use of immunofluorescent studies is promising as to the detection, analysis and classification of atypical cases of bullous diseases [624*a*]. Occasionally the same patient had two different types of blisters, some resembling those of PV, presenting as flaccid bullae on seemingly unchanged skin, others were tense and partially haemorrhagic, reminding of BP. The histological findings in subepidermal bullae in some lesions and suprabasal blisters in others confirmed the clinical and immunological duality. In a case [109*a*] the early clinical, histological and immunological findings showed typical PV, but later the patient developed additional features of frank BP associated with circulating antibodies to both the intercellular and BM zone and IgG deposits demonstrable by direct immunofluorescence. It seems therefore possible that patients may suffer from an underlying immunological disturbance that can give rise to one, two or even more types of autoimmune response or autoimmune disease [109*a*].

It may occur at almost any age, most frequently in adult males; it is characterized by bilateral symmetry of lesions, itching and burning, chronicity, recurrence, and a polymorphism (Fig. 40-11) owing to continual appearance of fresh and disappearance of old lesions. Acute erythematous and urticarial lesions develop from groupings of papules and minute, clear, relatively tense vesicles. There may be developing postinflammatory pigmentations [104, 276, 368*a*,

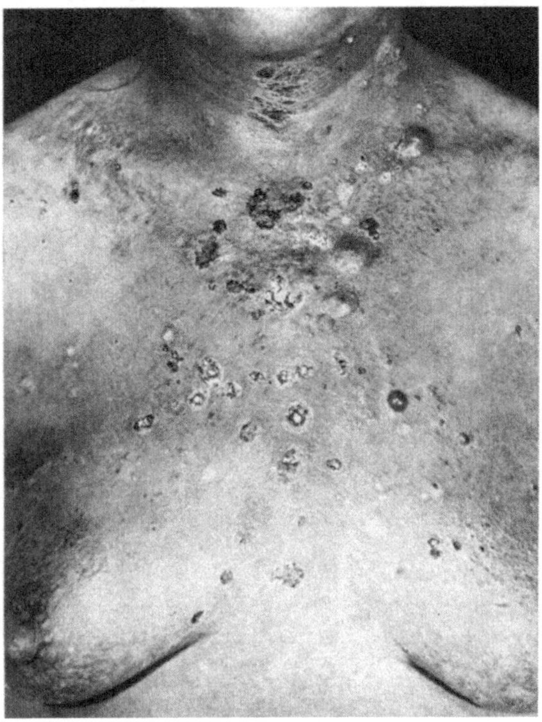

Fig. 40-11. Dermatitis herpetiformis. Polymorphous skin lesions on the chest (Courtesy of Professor L. Szodoray, Debrecen)

581]. In typical cases, the oral mucous membranes are not or very rarely involved [196]. The early histological picture [112, 388, 466, 486] is characterized (Fig. 40-12*a*, *b*) by a small amount of nuclear debris just below the BM and cuffing with lymphocytes and histiocytes of the underlying venular bed. Subsequently, dermal papillary microabscesses (Piérard) composed of neutrophils become progressively prominent and confluent, eventually resulting in dermoepidermal separation (Fig. 40-13). The presence of polymorphonuclear leukocytes is considered an important differential diagnostical sign [594*b*]. The resultant fully developed subepidermal vesicles may show, at times, a small intact papillary microabscess at their margins. Numerous eosinophils appear by the fifth day.

Electron-microscopic studies [202, 237, 486] revealed, perhaps due to immunoglobulin deposition at this level, the presence of glycogen and lipid particles in the basal cells at the dermoepidermal junctional zone, rarefaction of half desmosomes, which might be the cause of supralaminar disjunction and alterations in the basal lamina including its discontinuity and thickening. Epidermal cellular changes, consisting of a reduction in the epidermal pegs and a decrease in organelles, were confined to the basal regions of the basal cellular layer. In the erythematous skin, epithelial basal cells and the basal lamina appeared separated

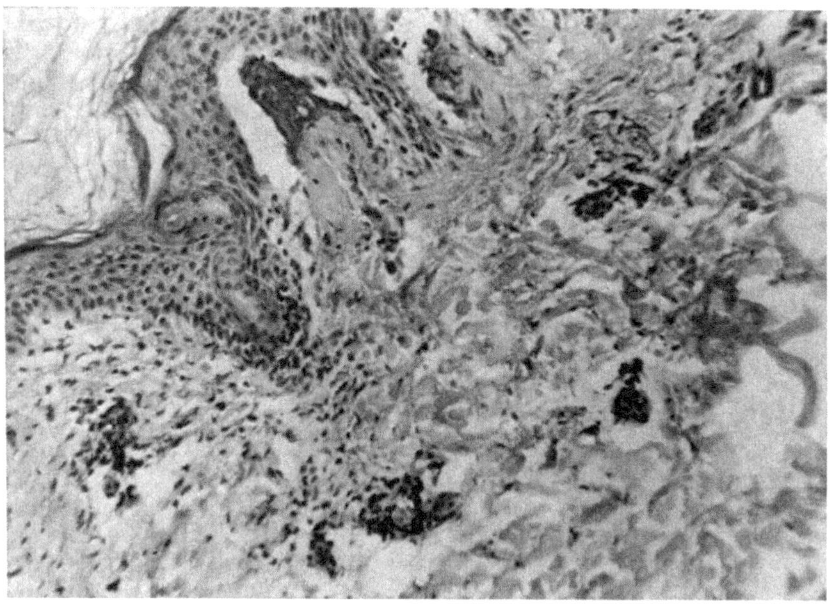

Fig. 40-12*a*. Dermatitis herpetiformis. Subepidermal vesicle developing multilocularly. ×40 (Courtesy of Professor N. Simon, Szeged)

from each other. In the vesicles, fibrin with its typical cross-binding pattern was seen. Paper electrophoresis showed an extremely low protein concentration and a significantly reduced albumin content [169].

In 70–95 per cent of the cases, the process in the skin may be associated with pathological changes of the mucous membrane of the small intestine: a patchy enteropathy mainly in the proximal parts [203, 227, 381, 395, 593]. Clinical signs of malabsorption are usually absent or very mild. Histologically [227, 550*b*, 593] and electron-microscopically [550*b*], the picture of the lesions of the mucous membrane is indistinguishable from that found in coeliac disease of adults or in idiopathic steatorrhoea. Small-intestinal abnormalities may vary from mild to severe. Mitochondrial changes and partial vacuolation of the endoplasmic reticulum, even the disappearance of microvilli have also been reported.

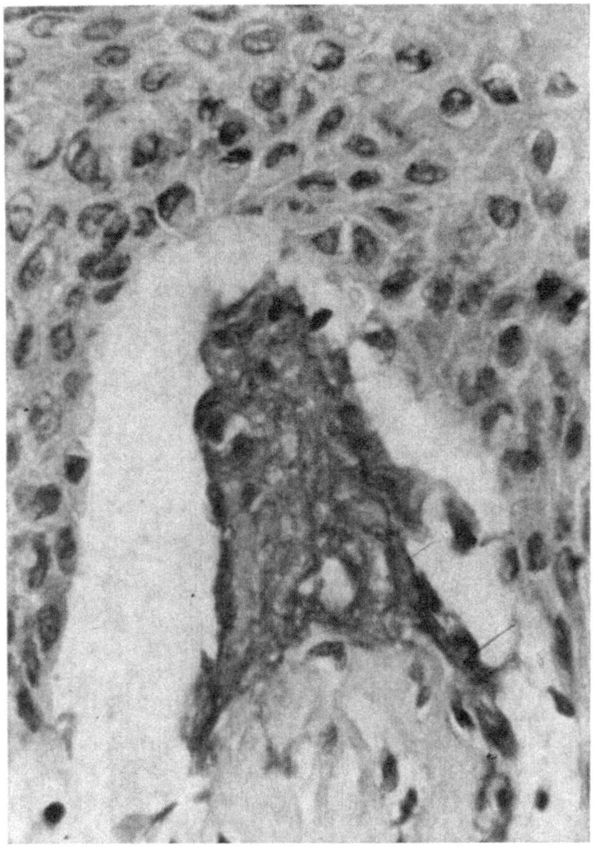

Fig. 40-12*b*. Dermatitis herpetiformis. Papillary fibrin deposition at the initial phase of vesicle formation. Enlarged from Fig. 40-12*a*. ×160

The aetiology of DH has not yet been cleared up. Formerly it was thought to be a bacterial or parasitic disease. HL-A typing showed that 89 per cent of the patients were HL-A8 positive [395*a*].

Its pathogenesis also awaits clarification in view of the many conflicting data. Simultaneous endogenous infective focal events occur frequently, drug allergy less frequently [368*a*]. Exacerbation of the disease has been reported due to halogen drugs [276] and, also, as a paraneoplastic syndrome. Seventy-two cases associated with malignancies have been reported [393]. Treatment of pulmonal epithelioma often caused regression of the symptoms. The role of humoral factors has also been considered [485]. However, the attention is now being focussed on the immunological aspects. Immunoelectrophoretically, reduction of the IgM and C levels, and rarely a raised IgA level have been found [608].

The early studies using the indirect immunofluorescent test yielded contradictory results. Some authors [78, 154, 579*b*] succeeded in demonstrating anti-

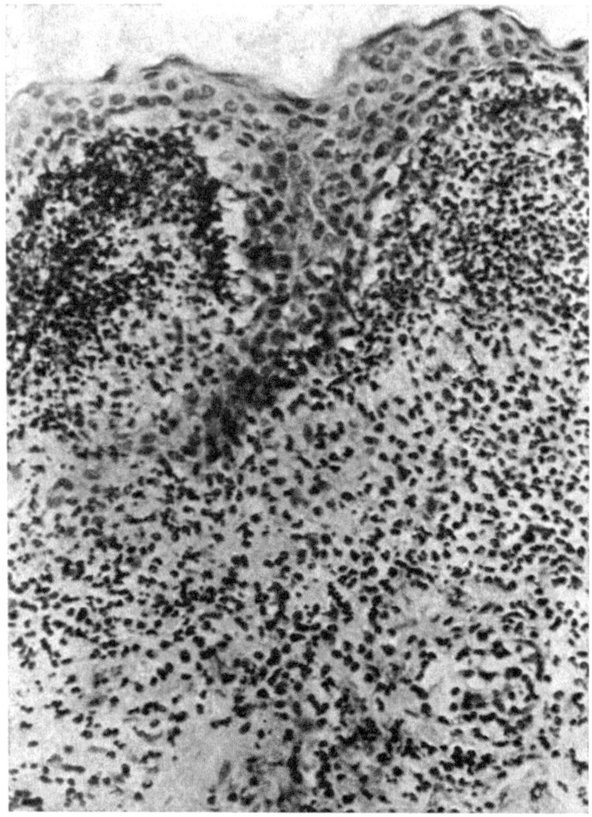

Fig. 40-13. Dermatitis herpetiformis. Owing to the microabscesses filling up the papillae, the epidermis has separated from the corium. ×60 (Courtesy of Professor L. Szodoray, Debrecen)

BM-zone antibodies with all of their characteristics (organ specificity, but no species specificity, etc.), while others [104, 108*b*, 276, 552] observed no immunofluorescence in the vesicular lesions. In positive cases, the character of the immunofluorescence remained unchanged during remission and relapse [104]. The contradiction may originate in the fact that many authors do not accept Lever's dualistic conception [368*a*] based on immunological criteria, suggesting that the designations, 'bullous pemphigoid of Lever', 'dermatitis herpetiformis bullosa', 'pemphigoid' and '*syndrome de pemphigoide bulleuse de Brocq–Lever*' refer to the same disease entity, whereas 'dermatitis herpetiformis', 'dermatitis polymorpha' and '*syndrome de dermatite herpétiforme de Duhring*' are names of another entity. Accepting this conception, both the negative and the positive results can be explained, for DH is characterized by the absence of humoral anti-BM-zone antibodies [79, 580*c*, 581]. However, the opponents of the conception

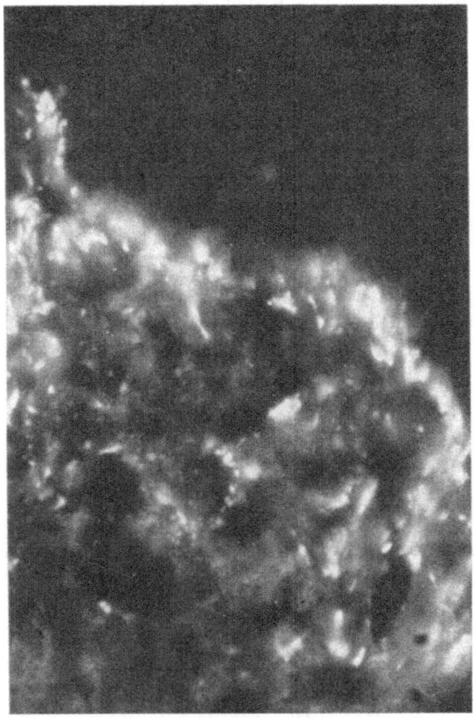

Fig. 40-14. Dermatitis herpetiformis. Coarse granular fluorescence of mainly IgA nature localized to thenei ghbourhood of the dermo-epidermal junction. Perivascular precipitate in the connective tissue. Anti-human IgA/FTC. Leitz Ortholux. ×1,000 (Courtesy of Professor N. Simon, Szeged)

point to the absence of anti-BM-zone antibodies in about a quarter of typical BP cases as well.

On a clinical basis, several authors distinguish, in addition to the 'pemphigoid' and 'herpetiform' forms, a third one, called *'une variété intermédiaire'* [60*a*] or 'mixed bullous disease' [26*a*], for some patients develop in consecutive attacks, sometimes simultaneously, both pemphigoid blisters and erythematovesiculous herpetiform plaques. The indeterminate or hybrid nature of these cases is supported by the histological picture and their response to therapy [26*a*].

Direct IF test has shown, in the majority of the cases (83 per cent), granular and diffuse deposits of IgA in the circumvesicular area, and papillary or continuous deposits in the dermal papillae of apparently normal skin (Fig. 40-14) and/or in the blood vessels of the dermis [104, 129, 155, 203, 276, 530, 594*a*, 608]. IgA deposits are rarely demonstrable in elastic fibres [608]. IgG is less frequently deposited [154, 276, 608] at the sites of predilection. Fibrin [424], fibrinogen [608], in more than 50 per cent of the cases C3, less frequently C1q are present in the involved skin [273, 528, 531, 594*a*, 608]; these usually correspond in location to the IgA deposits [528]. C is activated in the involved and uninvolved skin irrespective of therapy [531]. The IgA, probably in an aggregated form, activates C via the alternate pathway [528]. Where C1q was detected, the presence of IgA was associated with that of IgG and IgM, both of which activate C in the 'classical' pathway [528]. More recent immunofluorescent studies [530] confirmed by immunoelectron microscopy have shown that IgA deposits occur only in a fibrillar or microgranular pattern, always along the subepidermal fibres of the connective tissue in the dermal papillae. IgA deposits in continuous line and IgG deposits below the BM are rare findings [528]. IgM deposits in the dermal papillae occur more frequently [528]. The presence of IgD in affected skin appears not to be typical of DH [126]. DH seems to be characterized by concomitant occurrence of IgA and fibrinogen deposits in papillary microabscesses, in the absence of anti-BM-zone antibodies [126]. A negative indirect immunofluorescence associated with positive direct immunofluorescence in a form of granular immune complex deposits in the endothelium of the upper dermal capillary [608] may speak against the assumption that the deposited IgG would be directed against some dermal tissue structure. As to the pathogenesis of the mucous membrane lesions of the small intestine and their relationship with the dermal process, no conclusions can yet be drawn from the growing number of data.

The autoantibody reactivity to the gastric mucosa of patients suffering from DH is different from that of patients with atrophic gastritis or SLE [563]. In DH, the titre is usually lower, and binding takes place on every epithelial cell of the gastric mucosa, whereas in atrophic gastritis and SLE the titre is higher and binding takes place mainly on the cytoplasm of parietal cells. It has been evidenced by numerous observations that the orally ingested heterogeneous antigen may raise the IgA level, first of all in the gastric juice and also in the peripheral blood [591]. Since polymerized IgA has a mucous membrane protecting effect [29], detailed investigations in this field would be of high importance.

Elevated IgA and IgM levels were found in the jejunal juice in DH [403]; this is suggestive of a disturbance of the gastrointestinal secretory immunoglobulin system. The levels tend to be higher in achlorhydric patients. The higher serum IgA and reduced IgM levels showed no correlation with the small intestinal immunoglobulin concentrations. Furthermore, no correlation was demonstrable between the histological picture on the one hand, and Ig levels and bacterial colonization of the small intestine on the other. Comparative studies [352] have shown a marked increase in IgM-containing cells without any correlation with the IgM content of jejunal juice in DH and adult coeliac disease, distributed throughout the lamina propria, with the highest density at the bases of the villi. There was no correlation between plasma cell abnormalities and either jejunal morphology or treatment with gluten-free diet. The intraepithelial lymphocyte count was significantly raised in gluten-sensitive enteropathy [204] of patients with DH, and the infiltration lessened after three years of gluten-free diet. Normal looking mucosa with raised intraepithelial lymphocyte counts was often associated with low folate levels in serum. In one-third of the cases examined by splenic scan, a definite splenic atrophy was found, but this showed no relationship with any other parameter (biopsy, folate, status, reticulin antibody, treatment) [462]. Recent studies [203] have shown low erythrocyte folate levels in 26 per cent of patients with DH; the positive cases had IgA deposits in uninvolved skin, and enteropathy. Low serum folate levels were found in 81 per cent; of these patients 74 per cent had IgA deposits in uninvolved skin and enteropathy, and proved to be Dapsone (diaminodiphenylsulphone-N-acetate) responsive.

Biochemically [551], the disaccharidase activity in the homogenized biopsy material of the small intestine, an inconsistent finding [550*b*], might point to intracellular metabolic disorders.

Anti-jejunal-mucosa organ-specific antibodies could be demonstrated, but no anti-jejunal-epithelium-cytoplasm antibodies, characteristic of steatorrhoea [154].

Circulating immune complexes of 8–10 S and C-fixation supposedly containing IgG were detected by an anticomplementary method in sera from 80 per cent of patients on a diet containing gluten and in only 36 per cent of those on gluten-free diet [419]. By the C1q subcomponent method immune complexes were detected in 12 per cent of DH patients and in one-third of patients with either Crohn's disease, coeliac disease or ulcerative colitis. Supposedly, the immune complexes are formed in the intestines in response to gluten and are transferred to the skin, where they may cause damage [419]. Their presence in the skin lesions might be compatible with the presence of C [273, 594*a*] and fibrin [424]. It has been supposed that the complexes include a part of the gluten molecule. It was also assumed that gluten would play a central role in the pathogenesis of DH [419], but the precise mechanism by which the small intestine is damaged by gluten remained unknown. Although gluten could damage the small intestine by direct contact, damaging to the skin needs a toxic factor having entered the blood stream [419].

The so-called unitary concept [205] is based on several observations. (*i*) A strict long-term (5 months or more) gluten-free diet benefits the skin lesions in almost every case and has enabled reducing or even stopping Dapsone therapy. (*ii*) Electron-microscopic investigation shows subepidermal membrane-bound vacuoles in normal skin of patients whose eruption has been treated with Dapsone, but similar vacuoles were not present in patients on gluten-free diet, suggesting that the skin lesions and the gut lesions are gluten dependent and that both lesions are part of the same disease process. Association of DH, steatorrhoea and malignancy has been described in two cases [218]. (*iii*) HL-A8 phenotype was found in 58–84 per cent of DH patients with associated villous atrophy [211, 311*a*, 613]. In gluten-sensitive enteropathy and adult coeliac disease HL-A8 had been found with similar frequency. In contrast, only 33 per cent of the patients without gastrointestinal disease and 17–33 per cent of the control normal population carried the same phenotype. It has been suggested that the immunological phenomena reported in DH with associated villous atrophy could be under the control of an 'immune response' (IR) gene.

According to others, the skin and gut lesions of DH patients seem to be pathogenetically distinct and that the skin lesions are unrelated to gluten sensitivity. This concept is based on the following observations: (*i*) no precipitating gluten-antibodies were found in the sera of patients [227]; (*ii*) histological changes in the skin of DH patients are different from intestinal changes in gluten-sensitive enteropathy; (*iii*) Dapsone controls the skin disease, but has no effect on the gastrointestinal disease; (*iv*) the gut defects respond to gluten withdrawal, whereas in respect to the response of the skin condition there are inconsistent views [218, 227, 605].

Alternatively, the complexes might be related to part of the reticulin molecule. Circulating anti-reticulin antibody occurs in DH and coeliac disease [527, 529]. When IgA was present in the uninvolved skin, anti-reticulin was demonstrable in 19 per cent [203]. The anti-reticulin antibody titre falls slowly in patients on gluten-free diet, parallel with the clinical healing. Furthermore, cross-reaction has been demonstrated between fraction III of gluten and reticulin [530]. This cross-reaction helps to explain the localization of the skin lesions deep in the basal lamina, which is rich in reticular fibrils [281]. It is, therefore, possible that the connective tissue is damaged by gluten primarily and complexes may be formed from the damaged connective tissue secondarily if healing takes a long time [419].

On the basis of the staining patterns, anatomical distribution and species specificity, five types of anti-reticulin antibodies can be distinguished; these react with distinct antigens of intra- and extracellular mesenchymal components [491]. Antibodies to all these antigens have been found in DH (47 per cent) and coeliac disease (44 per cent), and less frequently (17 per cent) in Sjögren's syndrome. The antibodies appear to be stimulated by bacterial or nutritional antigens and are likely to represent anamnestic responses [491].

In spite of all these, it is not clear whether immune complexes exert a direct pathogenic effect or are secondary to the disease process. IgA and C3 have been found in the small intestine of patients with intestinal lesions [535]. It has yet to be explained why IgA binds to the reticulin of dermal papillae in DH but not in coeliac disease. The associated immunological anomalies are variable. There is no significant increase in anti-nuclear antibodies [527], but anti-thyroid antibodies are encountered at an abnormally high frequency [563, 579*c*]. Antibodies of anti-vascular specificity have also been detected [527].

The differential diagnosis of DH is made difficult by the occurrence of intermediary, transitional or mixed cases, most frequently in children with variable clinical and histological pictures. There may be large bullae or a vesiculo-papular eruption with or without microabscesses; the response to sulphapyridine or sulphones may be as dramatic as in typical DH, whereas the immunological features may be of the BP-type (linear IgG and IgA deposits) [79, 128, 276, 289*d*]. In such cases the vesicles should be examined immediately after their appearance and repeatedly thereafter. The blister of BP is unilocular spreading by cleavage between the BM and the plasmic membrane. The blister characteristic of DH arises in the papillar dermis and attacks the BM later [79]. Although in the vast majority of BP and DH cases there are differentiating features, an overlap of the clinical and immunological findings may occur [289*d*]. Repeated prospective clinical and laboratory studies over long periods of time with use of standardized criteria may be decisive in such cases [276]. A case designated 'acantholytic herpetiform dermatitis' [152] was described. In this case the clinical features resembled DH and the disease was responsive to Dapsone. Repeated biopsies showed a mixture of features suggestive of both DH and PV. Electron-microscopic studies suggested PV. The patient's serum showed the serological signs of PV (intercellular IgG was demonstrated by direct immunofluorescence).

In classical DH the disruption of the basal lamina and the blister formation may be secondary, due to local mechanical disruption [486], or a papillar depolymerization of hyaluronic acid may be the initial lesion [424]. The first step may be formation of a fibrin thrombus in the venous apices of the capillaries of the stratum papillare. Accumulation of eosinophils and polymorphs in microabscesses may be due to the chemotactic properties of the C locally activated by immune complexes. Whether reticulin is abnormal in these conditons or is an 'innocent bystander' of antibodies has remained uncertain. The fluorescent globular deposits, even though stained specifically, might be simply extravascular deposits, playing no pathological role, and perhaps represent a physiological process of immunoglobulin transudation in the skin. For this reason the results of the direct immunofluorescent test can only be interpreted in combination with a clear-cut clinical context. Furthermore, it has been shown recently that the postulated difference between BP and DH, namely linear in contrast to granular IgA deposits, is in fact not a clear-cut difference [579*c*]. The participation of immune complexes and of the C system in DH is regarded by several authors [594*b*] as merely a working-hypothesis.

The immunological origin of DH might be supported [166*b*] by (*i*) the occurrence of circulating anti-nuclear factors, and thyroid microsomal and gastric parietal antibodies; (*ii*) quantitative changes in the serum immunoglobulin levels; (*iii*) IgA deposits in the skin; (*iv*) the typical histological appearance of the skin lesions with eosinophils, abundant polymorphs and 'polymorph dust' resembling the changes seen in leukoclastic angiitis, on the one hand, and the Arthus phenomenon on the other; (*v*) humoral antibodies to the BM of the normal jejunum and fixed antibodies in the same region. It is possible that the renal lesion (glomerulitis) [145] develops on the basis of immune complex formation, but it is not clear whether immune complexes play an essential role in the disease. Thus, both the aetiology and the pathogenesis of DH need further systematic research.

Sulphapyridine, sulphones (diaminodiphenylsulphone, e.g. Dapsone) and sulphoxone (e.g. Diasone) have proved to be effective in relieving the symptoms and suppressing the eruption [587]. The dosage required for suppression is variable and should be individualized; if necessary, the dose may be increased to the tolerable maximum. On improvement, it should be reduced to the optimum maintenance dose. The possible side-effects of the drugs require close surveillance. Sulphapyridine therapy may be accompanied by anorexia with nausea and vomiting, headache, fever, leukopenia, haemolytic anaemia, agranulocytosis, hepatitis and renal damage [380]. The main side-effects of sulphones are haemolysis, methaemoglobinaemia, Heinz body formation and the sulphone syndrome characterized by fever, exfoliative dermatitis, liver necrosis with icterus, and lymphadenitis [148]. Some patients do not tolerate either sulphapyridine or sulphones, and for them systemic corticosteroids may be the only treatment. The enteropathic conditions may respond to a gluten-free diet, but the cutaneous eruptions must be treated with sulphones or sulphapyridine.

BCG immunotherapy has opened a new way in the therapy of vesicular diseases. The idea was based on the high frequency (93 per cent) of negative tuberculin tests in the 'pemphigoid', 'herpetiform' and 'intermediary' forms of vesicular diseases, and that the positive tuberculin reaction often reproduced clinical features of these diseases [60*a*]. On intracutaneous BCG vaccination 11 out of the 15 vaccinees became symptomless [60*b*].

SKIN DISEASES HAVING AUTOIMMUNE FEATURES

IMMUNOLOGICAL CONSIDERATIONS IN THERMAL INJURY

An extensive deep burn presents an ideal situation for bacterial invasion and, at the same time, alters normal immunological processes. The stress of a major traumatic episode, the systemic action of bacterial toxins absorbed through the burn wound, and the presence of necrotic tissue on the wound surface may lead to immunological defects, the immunological responsiveness may be affected and, mainly in the development of the paracombustional syndrome, autoimmune abnormalities can be expected.

Humoral antibody response. In severely burned patients, the serum protein abnormalities are the most pronounced on the 2nd or 3rd day following combustion [325*b*]. Serum protein electrophoresis showed prolonged hypalbuminaemia, hyper-α_2-globulinaemia and hypo-γ-globulinaemia [490]. There is a pronounced decrease in total serum protein, serum albumin and serum immunoglobulin levels, depending upon the extent and degree of the tissue damage and on individual factors [20, 361]. In a case the IgG, IgA, IgM, IgD and IgE levels fell to 30, 44, 39, 35 and 22 per cent of the average normal value, respectively. The fall of the immunoglobulin levels, due to the increased permeability of the microvasculature, lasts 3–10 days. It cannot be compensated even with large doses of γ-globulin or plasma infusion [325*b*]. In some cases cleft IgG molecules have been demonstrated. Both IgG and IgM are lost in the burn wound, reaching their lowest levels in the serum on the first few days; both return to normal levels during the second week and usually remain elevated thereafter [361]. The IgA level may rise, in small children less intensively than in adults, sometimes reaching 200–300 per cent of the normal value. IgD shows great individual variation. The IgE level rises after a short decline [325*b*]. IgG and C-fixing peripheral or membranal anti-nuclear autoantibodies masquerading as intercellular antibodies have been observed by indirect immunofluorescence in autologous skin specimens of two patients after thermal injury [3*a*].

The ability of synthesizing specific antibody to a given antigenic stimulus has been examined both in burned patients and experimental animals. The degree of antibody response depends upon many factors including the time interval between thermal injury and administration of the antigen, size of the burn, dose and character of the antigen and route of administration. Some authors obtained no evidence of impairment of the humoral immune response following thermal trauma [361]; according to others, the primary and/or secondary immune response to heterologous erythrocytes was absent or markedly reduced in severely burned patients [11]. The secondary response to tetanus toxoid was, however, accelerated and accentuated [11, 361]. The responses to somatic bacterial antigens were approximately normal. Good clinical results have been achieved by active (re-)immunization with vaccines containing a variety of microorganisms, first of all Pseudomonas species [9, 182, 297, 504]. As the interval between burn injury and the first injection of vaccine was increased, a progressive decrease in responsiveness was observed. There was no rise in the titres of naturally occurring antibodies, viz., isoagglutinins [361].

Serum complement levels have been found markedly diminished in both humans [188] and experimental animals [10, 293]. Parallel with other serum proteins, the lowest values are reached on the second or third day and the normal value is restored during the second week [8]. The same is characteristic of the C1 and C2 components [325*b*]. C3 and C4 remain at low levels until complete recovery. These observations are consistent with the presence of immune complexes, but do not exclude an autoimmune process. Furthermore the presence of C-fixing antibodies and the *in vivo* binding of C following thermal injury may offer some explanation to the increased susceptibility to infection and general depression of host defense mechanisms observed in burn patients [3*a*].

Abnormalities of cell-mediated immunity. Patients who have sustained a burn of more than 20 per cent of their body surface showed a depression of cell-mediated immunity, persisting for at least three weeks after the injury [94]. A significant lymphopenia and depletion of small lymphocytes deriving from secondary lymphoid tissues and the thymus are usual concomitant phenomena. Rebound hyperplasia of the thymus may be observed during recovery several months after the injury. Increased levels of circulating adrenocortical steroids, lymphopenia and markedly reduced delayed-type skin reactions are characteristic of the period of stress [10]. Allogeneic skin grafts applied to non-burned areas immediately, or to burned areas several weeks after injury, show prolonged survival [10, 28, 101]. The length of graft take depends upon both the degree of histocompatibility difference and the extent of the burn [101]. Further phenomena having been reported are disfunction or depletion of T cells, decreased delayed-type skin reaction [482], depression of the ability of spleen cells to induce graft-versus-host reaction [423], altered PHA response of lymphocytes [390] and a decreased ability of lymphocytes to stimulate or respond in mixed cultures [508]. As regards the reactivity of the lymphocytes *in vitro* after skin burns, an increased PHA reactivity of burned rat lymphocytes has been observed following less severe burns, the effect reaching its maximum 4 days after the injury [171*a*]. After 20 per cent third-degree skin burn rabbit spleen and peripheral blood lymphocytes demonstrate significantly depressed reactivity *in vitro* to PHA, in correlation with the lower blood plasma IgG level [431*a*]. The burned and normal skin saline-extracted protein antigens do not stimulate lymphoblast transformation *in vitro*. In burn patients shortly after the thermal trauma a temporary increase in PHA responsiveness has been observed but, at the same time, the response to antigens and allogeneic lymphocytes was diminished [360*a*]. Unilateral mixed lymphocyte culture tests revealed a decrease in both the responding and the stimulating capacity of lymphocytes of burn patients. The observed alterations in lymphocyte reactivity were somewhat more pronounced and lasted longer in the severely injured patients. All parameters resumed normal values after 4–6 weeks. This altered responsiveness might be based on a shift of lymphocyte subpopulations in the circulating pool in favour of the B cells [360*a*]. A factor was demonstrated in the serum of acute burn patients, which was *in vitro* cytotoxic to rabbit cardiac fibroblasts and inhibited the migration of human lymphocytes [244*a*]. The acute burn serum inhibitor can be isolated from the affected skin; according to adsorption tests it is bound to lymphocytes and may be regarded as a glycoproteid having toxic effect. The *in vitro* rosette inhibition test is not suitable for a direct measure of the immunosuppression of lymphocytes in burned patients [102].

Autoimmune phenomena. Since thermal injury denatures proteins, it is not surprising that in burned patients antibodies are present which react with altered skin components [66, 397]. Such antibodies which may cross-react with the original native structure [360] have been found from the 12th to the 30th day in the serum of burned patients and experimental animals [580*c*]. Humoral autoantibodies directed against a variety of antigens, including those in skin [40, 481, 579*b,c*, 580*b*], collagen [66], erythrocytes [21, 162, 307, 401, 402], leukocytes [283, 476], nuclei [283, 481, 579*c*], immunoglobulins [97, 283, 481] and BM of the skin [579*c*] have been observed after thermal injury. In the serum of burned guinea pigs, heterophilic antibodies were found. Macromolecular protein fractions, with a relatively high content of specific antigenic components (determined by the double immunodiffusion test) were isolated from the burned skin of Wistar rats by gel filtration and ion exchange chromatography [418*b*]. It has been supposed that fibrinogen might be the antigen component of the burned skin [306*b*]. Immunization against the blood-group antigens A and B may also occur [287*a*, 579*c*]. Anti-nuclear factor was found in 31–35 per cent; rheumatoid factor was detected with the sheep cell agglutination test in 32 per cent and with the latex fixation test in 67 per cent [283, 481]. In immunoelectrophoresis only anti-IgG produced a new arc; the corresponding antigenic component seems to be comparable with an enzymatically produced $F(ab')_2$ fragment [223]. In addition to dysproteinaemia, paraproteinaemia (cryoglobulinaemia, amyloidosis) may occur [455]. The cryoglobulinaemia is secondary, its level fluctuates and seems to be dependent on the degree and extent of the burn as well as on the disturbances of protein metabolism. With cryoglobulinaemic sera cryophagocytosis can be induced [455]. The staining patterns of direct immunofluorescence are weakly positive for several weeks. According to Beutner [40], IgG does not bind to the intercellular substance *in vivo*. The antibody does not fix C *in vitro* [481]. It has been shown recently that binding of the human antiglobulin to the dermoepidermal structure shows three different patterns [306*a*]: (*i*) as a network to the intercellular space of the stratum spinosum or to the two or three cell layers covering the BM; (*ii*) to the BM; or (*iii*) to the vessel walls in the stratum papillare.

Indirect immunofluorescence showed pemphigus-like antibodies in 52 per cent and basement-layer-staining antibodies in 22 per cent [481], the former being different from true pemphigus antibodies in their failure to bind *in vivo* [271]. Of the sera from thermally injured patients tested with indirect immunofluorescence on guinea pig epithelium, 35 per cent showed humoral pemphigus-like antibodies of different immunoglobulin classes [360]; 4 per cent of the same sera contained an antibody directed against epithelial cytoplasm. Biopsies of normal skin revealed the presence of IgA localized in an intercellular substance in 50 per cent of the cases; 35 per cent revealed IgG antibodies directed against some substances lying between the parenchymal cells of the adrenal gland.

In 13 per cent, antiglobulin was demonstrated and in 9 per cent of these cases the antiglobulins appeared to be so-called anti-antibodies. No correlation could be found between the antibodies detected and the extent of the burned area or other clinical parameters. In view of the known existence of common antigens on the BM of different tissues, the renal disfunction in burned patients [89, 328] may be explained on the basis of cross-reacting antibodies. The absence of the titre rise of some naturally occurring antibodies favours the idea that the rise in immunoglobulin levels is due to a specific reaction of the humoral immune system and not to a non-specifically increased synthesis of immunoglobulins in general [361]. Presumably the lymphocytes are stimulated by the tissue degradation, or the adjuvant effect leads to the stimulation of pre-existent forbidden clones and thus to the appearance of auto-antibodies [481], a third possible explanation, the tissue destruction itself may be supposed to raise the titres of natural anti-tissue antibodies.

The recent widespread use of porcine and canine xenografts to replace human allografts has made reasonable to study the immune response to these antigens. After repeated applications of xenografts, patients produce antibodies specific for the foreign skin and its blood constituents.

The clinical significance of these antibodies in producing autoimmune disease in the burned patient is uncertain. Anyhow, antibodies against denatured collagen might contribute to some components of the paracombustional syndrome, e. g. the hypertrophic scar, blister formation on autografts, and pruritus.

Although prolonged graft survival can be expected in case of compatible or identical major histocompatibility antigens [101], even the histocompatible grafts are eventually rejected, and there remains the necessity to treat the recipient with immunosuppressive drugs to achieve permanent coverage.

In burned animals, graft survival was significantly prolonged by immunosuppression [334], which, however, markedly increases the risk and severity of bacterial and fungal infections. Gram-negative bacteria and *Candida albicans* are the most dangerous microbes in this respect. Among the immunosuppressants, ALS is used most widely. Pretreatment of the recipient with donor antigens to induce tolerance and thus prolong graft survival is a procedure still at an experimental stage.

AUTOALLERGIC ECZEMA, AUTOSENSITIVE DERMATITIS

The main antigenic factor inducing autosensitization (autoeczematization) of skin should always be sought in the altered skin. Crural eczema, passive oedema, varicosity, post-thrombotic condition, etc. may stimulate tissue changes resulting in antigens which are then recognized by the organism as foreign. The antigens originating from interactions between skin proteins and microorganisms are dealt with in the appropriate chapter of this book (Chapter 70, Vol. 7). Autoantigens have been sought in heterogenized epidermis, especially cutis protein in absorbed tissue decomposition products in devitalized skin as well as in epidermal cells floating in inflammatory exudate. Autoantigen production may be induced by factors loosening the skin, the use of water-impermeable ointments, occupational microtraumas and occasionally, intensive scratching or irradiation.

Epidermis-specific haemagglutinating and *in vitro* cytotoxic antibodies have been a rare finding in generalized eczema and exfoliative dermatitis [447], especially in the period of dissemination.

According to Parish [445*b*] the characteristics of the autoantibodies to skin are as follows: (*i*) rare incidence (demonstrable in 4.9 per cent of patients with acute generalized dermatitis following or during periods of exacerbation of a chronic localized eczema or varicose ulcer); (*ii*) species specificity (man); (*iii*) organ specificity (skin); (*iv*) antigen site (subcorneal); (*v*) it is demonstrable in the IgG fraction; (*vi*) it fixes C *in vivo*; and (*vii*) is cytotoxic *in vitro*. If injected into the skin, it causes a weal and flare reaction, occasionally followed by a small indurated lesion. The antibody in the presence of C caused vacuolation and death of epidermal cells in explants of skin and organ cultures. An autoantibody was detected with Boyden's passive haemagglutination test, using an antigen–antibody complex in serum samples of patients suffering from eczema [308]. In some patients with acute widespread dermatitis, C-fixing antibodies to skin have been encountered but rarely [621]. The possible significance of circulating antibodies is still unclear [446]. Their formation may be a harmless consequence of the inflammatory process. Epicutaneous application of eczematous focal debris appears to be a more reliable test [501]. The so-called 'homo-epidermis extract' may contain an active principle of the skin and thus may give positive results in the majority of the cases [445*b*]. There have been few reports on *in vitro* detectable delayed-type autosensitization to skin. It was claimed [247, 248] that extracts of skin induce mitosis in cultures of leukocytes from patients with infantile eczema, but this has never been confirmed. The examination of the real antigen is hindered by a number of factors; for instance, IgG and IgM autoantibodies to the intercellular substance of the stratum corneum are demonstrable in the serum of healthy adults. These antibodies are, at least partly, diaplacentar [341*a*, *b*, *c*]. Immunization of experimental animals with heterologous, and sometimes homologous, skin extracts or skin homogenates was followed by the appearance of humoral antibodies [503*a*], occasionally accompanied by a dermatotoxic effect [502, 503*b*], but skin-specific sensitization inducible by intra- or even epicutaneous test was observed very rarely [326]. Sensitization by pretreatment of the skin surface with freezing and thawing has also been reported [431]. All these results are more or less objectionable. In spite of this, it cannot be excluded that autoantibody production may be stimulated by heterologous, or altered homologous, human skin tissue. It may be noted that precipitating, passive cutaneous anaphylactic and fluorescent antibodies were demonstrated in 38, 62 and 56 per cent, respectively, of patients with dermatitis dysseborrhoica; as antigen autologous seborrhoeic scale was used [249].

AUTOIMMUNE PROGESTERONE URTICARIA AND DERMATITIS

Progesterone is derived largely from the corpus luteum but is also an important intermediate in adrenal steroidogenesis. Autoimmune progesterone urticaria and dermatitis is a hormone dependent mechanism due to cell-mediated immunity against endogenous progesterone. It is distinguishable from the exogenous sensitization induced by progesterone therapy and from the dermodromes of pregnancy including impetigo herpetiformis, herpes gestationis and papular dermatitis of pregnancy [50]. The means by which endogenous progesterone becomes antigenic is unknown. It is possibly related to the production of some altered form of the hormone in these individuals. The fact that relapses occur in the premenstruum and the disease subsides during menstruation suggests that it is related to hormonal events [159*c*]. Since at the same time the body temperature rises, herpes simplex flare-up should be excluded. Serial herpes simplex antibody titrations and testings with exogenous progesterone should be done. The clinical symptoms are rather variable. Grouped vesiculo-bullous dermatitis has often been observed [269, 298, 534], less frequently pruritus and/or maculopapular eruption [579*a*] and urticaria [176, 210, 243, 418, 588, 630], exceptionally ulcerative stomatitis [38], and acneiform eruption with an eosinophilic infiltration in every layer of the skin [50] occur. The symptoms may appear recurrently in the premenstruum [210, 269, 298, 588], less frequently during pregnancy [50], post partum or after spontaneous abortion. After the skin phenomena have disappeared, the process can be reproduced by an intramuscular injection of progesterone [176, 534, 588] or a contraceptive mixture [50]. Intracutaneous skin testing with aqueous progesterone produces a delayed-type hypersensitivity reaction [50, 298, 630] with histopathological features apparently identical with those present in the naturally occurring disease [50]. Immediate-type skin reaction has only been observed very rarely [176]. Positive immunofluorescence in luteinizing cells of the corpus luteum has been reported [176]. In some cases an increased plasma oestradiol, a reduced progesterone level, an accelerated ^{47}Ca turnover and/or raised serum IgG and IgM levels were demonstrated [50]. Attempts to detect anti-progesterone serum antibodies have failed [50], but successful passive transfer of skin sensitivity has been described [176]. The indirect basophil degranulation test has been found either positive [298] or negative [534]. The lymphocyte transformation test was consistently negative [109]. For therapy 40 U cortropin and 100 mg minocycline daily is usually given [159*c*].

SECONDARY ERYTHRODERMAS

Severe cases of chronic eczematous dermatitis or psoriasis may rapidly turn into a secondary exfoliative erythroderma, without any change in management or other precipitating factor. Continuous exoserosis and desquamation involving the whole body surface lead to a severe protein and iron loss, hypoproteinaemia, dyssiderosis, hypalbuminaemia, hyperglobulinaemia and a parallel liver damage. Such an erythroderma is hardly distinguishable from those often associated to lymphoma, microbial, or drug-allergic events or erythrodermas of unknown origin. The lack of identification with the original disease and the extremely chronic (self-perpetuating) course suggest that secondary erythrodermas might represent a true organ-specific hypersensitivity [357, 455, 542, 621]. The clinical picture is characterized by a universal erythema with desquamation, excoriations and crustations secondary to scratching as well as alopecia and onychodystrophy owing to an involvement of hair and nail matrices [621]. The metabolism of the skin is tremendous. It has been postulated that eosinophilia in secondary erythroderma might be an indicator of the acute destructive phase of inflammation and lymphocytosis a sign of proliferative process indicating the adequate immunologic responses of the patients [493*c*]. In the infiltrate of the skin (Fig. 40-15) lymphocytes and plasma cells predominate and the increasing number of plasma cells correlates with chronicity [621]. In the serum and in lymph node extracts the γ-globulin level is raised (37 per cent and 64 per cent, respectively), presumably due to an enhanced activity of the large pyroninophilic cells. It might be supposed [493*b*] that the excess globulin contains auto-antibodies to denaturation products of the connective tissue of the skin. Homologous and heterologous DNA as well as antigens from the normal skin and from the patient's own affected skin were used as antigens in Boyden's test, in immunodiffusion tests and in the 'friable bodies' test [493*b*]. Titres of sera from patients with secondary erythrodermas as measured with own affected skin as antigen were found to be significantly higher than those obtained with antigens from other sources. It may be supposed that humoral antibodies are formed as a response to the allergic inflammation of the skin and to products of pathological protein metabolism. The phenomenon of macrophage aggregation activity in sera of patients with exfoliative erythroderma may result from overproduction of mediators of cell-mediated immunity [344*a*]. Macrophage aggregation factor is spontaneously released by lymphocytes obtained from patients. Detection of this factor may contribute to an understanding of the pathogenesis.

Saline extracts of scales from patients with erythrodermia psoriatica contained IgG, IgM, IgA and C [344*b*]. The extracts agglutinated rabbit erythrocytes to higher titres than those obtained from patients with other forms of psoriasis. In addition, the extracts obtained from erythrodermia psoriatica scales contained antibodies to stratum corneum, and anti-human IgG. In saline extracts of thoroughly washed tissues antibodies could not be demonstrated. However, eluates prepared from the tissue sediments at 56 °C contained anti-IgG antibodies to stratum corneum and C3. Apparently, there is a passive transepidermal diffusion of serum protein into psoriatic lesions, and specific antibodies are bound in the parakeratotic stratum corneum. According to a hypothesis of Krogh and Tonder [344*b*], anti-IgG factors and C are fixed by immune complexes, and these immunological phenomena may be involved in the pathogenesis of erythrodermia.

LYMPHOCYTIC INFILTRATION OF THE SKIN (JESSNER–KANOFF)

(Synonyms: lymphocytic lupus erythematosus, non-scarring type of cutaneous lupus erythematosus, non-atrophic cutaneous lupus erythematosus.) This clinical picture is similar to chronic discoid lupus erythematosus in the following: clinical resemblance, tendency to anti-nuclear antibody response, relatively high frequency of the occurrence of the anti-nuclear factor, similarity of the nuclear immunofluorescent pattern (homogeneous and/or thready) [82*a*]; photosensitivity often occurs. Occasionally a γ-globulin band has been demonstrated at the dermo-epidermal junction [82*b*, 340], but this could not be confirmed [572, 583]. Other characteristics of the disease are suggestive of an autonomy [583]: hyper-

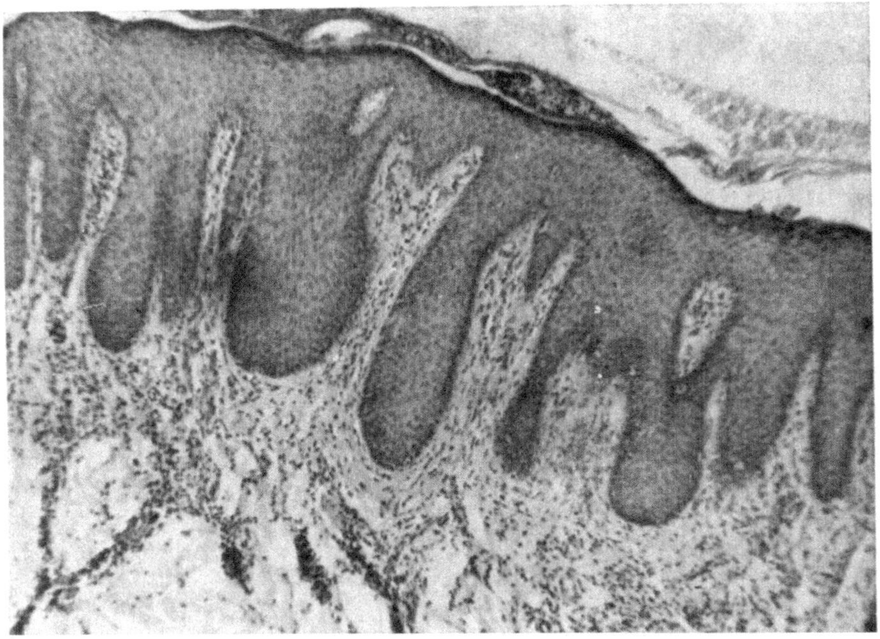

Fig. 40-15. Secondary erythrodermia. Little cellular exudate in the parakeratotic stratum corneum. Irregular acanthosis in the epidermis. Note the oedematously rarified upper part of the corium and the inflammatory infiltration at the same place. ×20 (Courtesy of Professor L. Szodoray, Debrecen)

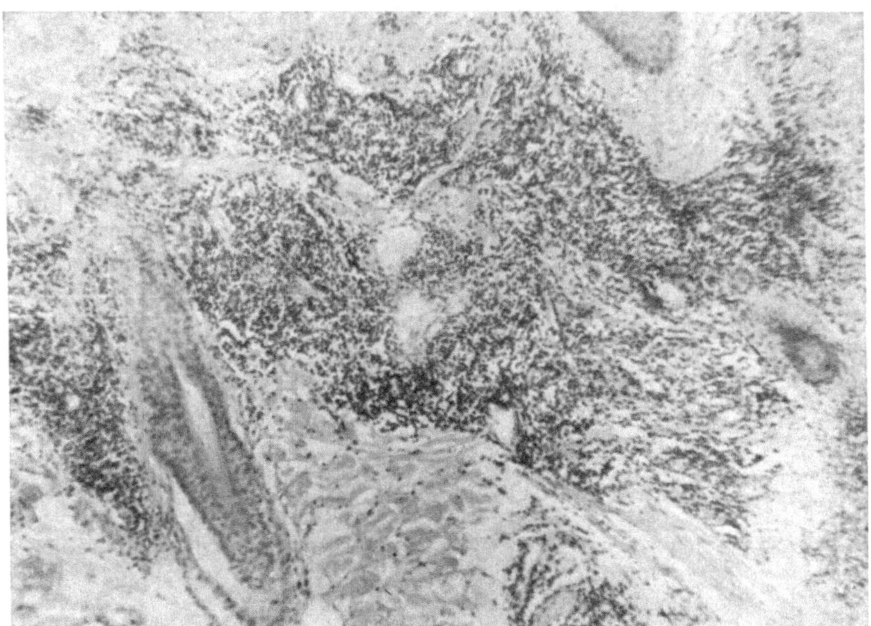

Fig. 40-16. Jessner–Kanoff lymphocytic infiltration in the corium around the hair follicles and capillaries, consisting mainly of lymphocytes. ×20 (Courtesy of Professor L. Szodoray, Debrecen)

keratosis and atrophy are absent, the symptoms are not photodependent, their development is rhapsodic or cyclic, three or four recurrences may occur on the same site within a year, antimalarial drugs are ineffective, there is no epidermal change in the histological pattern, the most striking feature is an intense lymphocytic infiltration in the dermis, which is predominantly perivascular and periadnexal (Fig. 40-16). Basophilic degeneration of the elastic tissue in the superficial dermis is a usual finding. It has been suggested that this condition might be a variant of lymphocytoma cutis [383].

VITILIGO

This skin disease may associate with diseases in which autoantibodies are present, e.g. anaemia perniciosa, hyposideraemia, hyperthyroidism, Hashimoto's thyroiditis, primary non-tuberculous Addison's disease, idiopathic hypoparathyroidism, etc. [166*a*]. Moreover, antibodies to gastric parietal cells, intrinsic factor, thyroid cytoplasm, thyroglobulin, microsome, adrenal gland, smooth muscle, and to nuclear substance (4–32 per cent) have been demonstrated in patients with vitiligo, without any associated disease [70, 135, 236, 434]. In five patients of the same family, a selective IgA deficiency was demonstrated [206]. Chronic atrophic gastritis was shown histologically in 38 per cent of patients with vitiligo. Supposedly, anti-intrinsic factor autoantibodies play a decisive role in the development of pernicious anaemia from chronic atrophic gastritis [473]. All these findings support the view that a global increase of immunological abnormalities is in the background of vitiligo. However, the pathological importance of the presence of different, often multiple, anti-organ antibodies is to be clarified. Vitiligo has been attributed to humoral anti-melanocyte-stimulating-hormone or anti-melanocyte antibodies [61, 135, 356, 385, 434], though negative cases have also been reported [156]. There is no convincing evidence for the presence of antibodies against melanin itself. Attempts to produce antibodies against melanoprotein in rabbits have failed [607]. It is suggested that the demonstration of antibodies in serum obtained from rabbits after injection of a melanoma homogenate (which contained cell debris) may be due to antibodies against unmelanized or incompletely melanized melanosomes [607].

Some indirect evidence supports the view that there might be an occasional connection, on an autoimmune basis, between the development of neoplasms in patients with vitiligo and *vice versa* [358]. Vitiligo seems to develop in patients with melanoma more often than expected by chance [197, 313]. Anti-melanocyte antibodies have been found in the serum of patients with malignant melanoma [374] and of those with multiple halo naevi [373]. Vitiligo developed in patients suffering from subacute virus encephalitis [428]; supposedly both processes might be due to a virus interfering with an enzyme common to both melanocytes and neurons. A case with a peripheral nerve tumour and loss of pigmentation has been described [331].

Several types of vitiligo are known: (*i*) vitiligo without any other pathological phenomenon; (*ii*) hereditary, probably inherited as an autosomal dominant trait [166*a*], closely associated with achlorhydria and organ-specific autoimmune disease [279]; genetic disposition is supported by familial cumulation and female excess [88]; (*iii*) vitiligo in which a neurogenic factor is involved [166*a*] and a cytotoxic agent is released close to or within the melanocyte, thus destroying the cell.

At present, there is no evidence for a primarily responsible anti-melanocyte antibody. It can be concluded that the aetiopathogenesis of vitiligo is still unclear. The evidence available is insufficient to prove that vitiligo is a genetically determined autoimmune disease. To suppress the assumed immune process, triamcinolone is injected below the vitiligous focus, a process which is mostly successful [90].

ALOPECIA AREATA

The primary patch, usually on the scalp, is circumscribed, rounded or oval in shape. The skin is smooth, soft and ivory-white and totally devoid of hair. Around the margin of the patch, exclamation-mark hairs may be present. The course is extremely variable. Further patches may develop whilst the earlier ones are regrowing, or gradual extension may lead to total alopecia.

Reflex irritation in connection with tonsillar, dental or ocular endogenous infectious foci has been incriminated, but this could only be proved in a few cases. Similarly, the role of endocrine influence on the course of alopecia areata and the pathogenetic role of emotional factors have only been clear in rare cases. (For connections with vasculitis, see Chapter 62, Vol. 6.)

Recent immunological investigations have suggested that the inherited defect (in 10–20 per cent of cases) may involve an increased propensity to form certain organ-specific autoantibodies. Patients with alopecia areata have a statistically increased incidence of three associated autoimmune diseases (Hashimoto's thyroiditis, Addison's disease, and pernicious anaemia). In males, thyroid antibodies were demonstrated in about 23 per cent, and adrenal antibodies in 7 per cent; in females, gastric parietal cell antibodies occurred in 9 per cent [313*a*]. The frequency of these antibodies did not correlate with the severity of alopecia. The presence of humoral antibodies directed against a specific tissue presumably reflects a disease of that tissue, although the state may be subclinical and non-progressive. Supposing that an antibody is formed against matrix cells, attempts have been made to produce alopecia areata experimentally in guinea pigs [576*a*, *b*]. Demonstration of humoral antibodies directed against any organ-specific hair antigen in the sera of patients with alopecia areata has failed [313*a*].

The association with autoimmune disease, the histological changes (lymphocytic inflammatory reaction resembling those in all the proven or suspected autoimmune diseases) and the temporary response to corticosteroids, all suggest that an immunological mechanism may be responsible for the partial inhibition of follicular activity.

LICHEN PLANUS

An immunohistological technique (Adams's DAMB nitrite reaction for tryptophan) resulted in demonstrating fibrin deposits in the subepidermal infiltrate [165*a*]. In accordance with this, fibrin deposits were revealed in a band-like pattern at the dermoepidermal junction also with glutaraldehyde (Avrameas), using a peroxidase enzyme–anti-human fibrinogen serum conjugate [165*b*]. The direct immunofluorescent technique with labelled antihuman fibrin(ogen) showed a fluorescing band along the dilated capillaries in the apex of the papillae [27, 124, 165*b*]; furthermore, there were irregularly shaped inhomogeneous fluorescence [27], or globular or cytoid fluorescent bodies [523] (Fig. 40-17*a*, *b*).

Location of immunoglobulins in the epidermal basement zone has been reported [22*b*], but not confirmed [27]. Intra- and pericapillar fluorescing homogeneous bodies corresponding to 'hyaline' or 'colloid' bodies with H-E staining were also

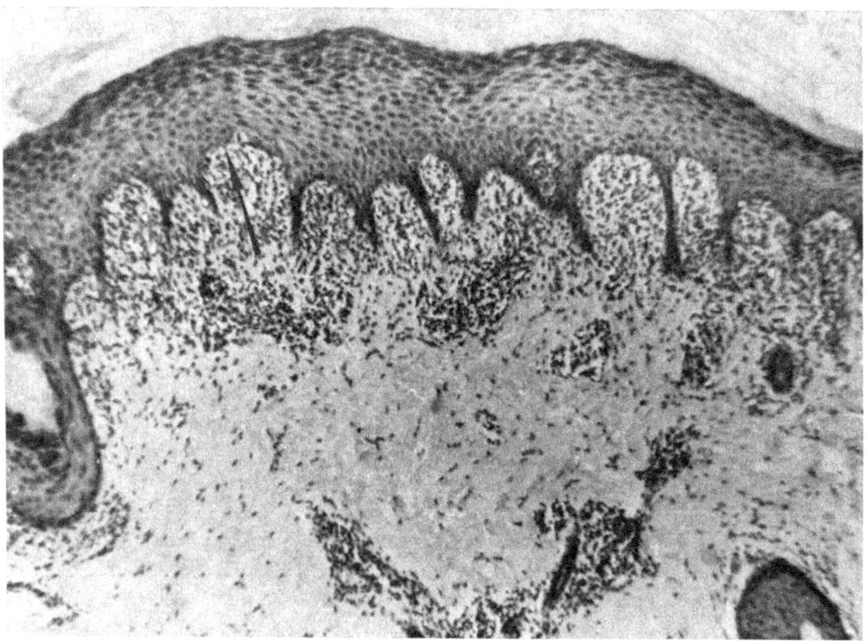

Fig. 40-17*a*. Lichen planus. Hyperkeratotic stratum corneum and widened stratum granulosum. The dome-shaped connective tissue papillae are filled with lymphocytic infiltrate. The basal cell layer is, at places, unrecognizable (arrow) ×20. (Courtesy of Professor L. Szodoray, Debrecen)

described [27]. These colloid bodies contain immunoglobulins including β_1C glod ulin, albumin and fibrinogen, whose deposition seems to be a secondary phen om enon [27, 165*a*, 589*a*]. Furthermore, the presence of IgM and β_1C/β_1A in the epidermal basement zone has been reported in several cases of lichen planus [124]. In the papillary dermis, near the epidermodermal junction, strongly fluorescent bodies of γ-globulin, IgG, IgM, and IgA specificity were seen in over 95 per cent of patients [603] and those specific for C occurred occasionally [407, 603]. These bodies, consisting of a complex of DNA, RNA and immunoglobulins, are not disease-specific, being present in SLE, dermatomyositis, and poikilodermia of unknown origin, too. They are absent in lichen sclerosus et atrophicus, and in lichen nitidus [603]. The only finding common to both lichen nitidus and lichen planus is the presence of fibrinogen at the BM zone, but this is a non-specific phenomenon [603], being independent of either the presence of dermal inflammation or the hydropic degeneration of the basal layer. Electron-microscopically, extracellular fibrillar masses of high density and a banding of approximately 140 Å were seen [165*a*].

In bullous lichen planus, a linear deposit of IgG and C4/C3 has been found [22*b*] in the epidermal basement zone of peribullous areas. In several cases an affinity for the human epidermal basement zone has been detected [22*b*]. Recent findings

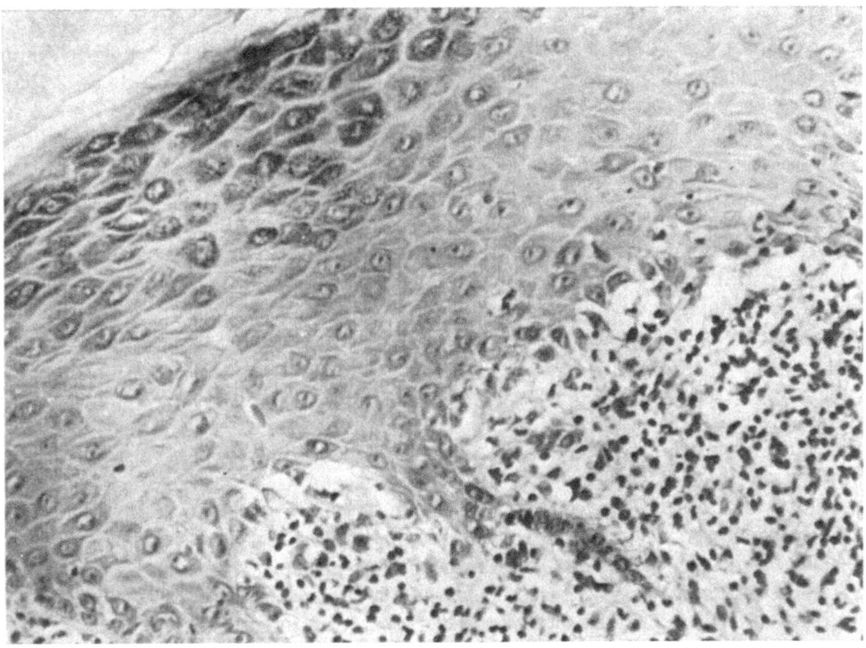

Fig. 40-17*b*. Lichen planus. Acanthosis, widened stratum granulosum. The stratum basale is unrecognizable. The epidermis is, at places, separated from the corium. The subepidermal infiltrate contains mainly lymphocytes. × 60 (Courtesy of Professor L. Szodoray, Debrecen)

[23] have been: (*i*) the occurrence of fibrin or related substances and of IgM in the upper part of the dermis; (*ii*) different amounts of various C components and fragments located in the epidermal basement zone and in the colloid bodies; (*iii*) IgE, IgM, IgA and fibrin in the colloid bodies, sometimes together with albumin.

Lichen planus seems to be of variable pathogenesis. The lymphocyte transformation test with skin homogenate from a lesion of the patient's own skin as mitogen gave a positive result in 2 of 6 cases. When proliferation of mononuclear cells infiltrating the dermis was investigated by incubation with ^{3}H-thymidine and radioautography, the labelling index was found relatively high [348]; it is supposed that the proliferating cells are lymphoblasts. This is compatible with the hypothetic autoimmune nature of lichen planus [519]. It is nevertheless possible that the immunoglobulins in lichen planus represent secondary non-specific binding due to an altered physical status of the damaged epidermal cells [603].

The earliest pathological sign is the appearance in the upper dermis of pigment-containing macrophages [23]. Deposition of fibrin appears to be another early phenomenon, as it occurred in areas without an inflammatory infiltrate [23]. Recent studies have indicated that in lichen planus the epidermis is damaged by the primary aetiological factor(s). Electron-microscopic studies have shown in the basal epidermal cells a fibrillar transformation resulting in formation of colloid bodies [164]. The concomitant occurrence of immunoglobulins and C may indicate that the former have played a part in the activation process. Their presence might be explained by pathologically enhanced capillary permeability, nevertheless it is more likely that their presence in and around the colloid bodies indicates that C has been activated via the classical pathway [359*a*]. It is also possible that immunoglobulins are involved in the genesis of colloid bodies either as antibodies or as non-antigen-induced aggregates [23]; furthermore, a secondary (auto)immune mechanism might be directed against antigenic debris of degenerated basal cells. C may have been activated by non-immunological mechanism, such as enzymes produced during coagulation and fibrinolysis [359*a*]. Whether C activation is the cause or result of the epidermal pathology remains unknown.

The antigenicity of the skin might originate in the skin itself or by absorption of low molecular weight compounds, e.g. drugs. Alternatively, it might result from bacterial or viral products. Demonstration of globular deposits of immunoglobulins and C at the dermoepidermal junction is helpful in the diagnosis, though not disease-specific [603].

In patients with *lichen sclerosus* when compared with control subjects a significantly increased prevalence of autoantibodies against thyroid cytoplasm (40 per cent) and gastric parietal cells (44 per cent) has been found [225*a*]. The presence or absence of these antibodies was not related to the severity or duration of the disease, suggesting that these autoantibodies did not arise as a consequence of lichen sclerosus. The increased prevalence of autoantibodies suggests that the condition may be related to or caused by an autoimmune process.

ULCUS CRURIS CHRONICUM

Ulcus cruris of venous origin is, in a quarter of the cases, surrounded by allergic dermatitis or eczema, which has a secondary aggravating role [75]. Leg ulcers developing on the basis of a systemic disease of the arteries, such as vasculitis necrotisans and arteritis obliterans, have been dealt with in Chapter 62 (Vol. 6). Infectious origin has been supposed in 12.5 per cent of the different phlebitides [179]. Leg ulcers have been observed in systemic autoimmune diseases including SLE, polyarteritis nodosa, progressive systemic sclerosis and ulcerating rheumatic nodules, in dysglobulinaemia (cryoglobulinaemia) and macroglobulinaemia (plasmacytoma, Waldenström's disease). In each of these diseases the role of neurodystrophy and of biologically active substances released as a consequence of anoxia has been assumed. Autograft failure was observed in patients with chronic leg ulcers having serum antibodies to skin, furthermore, immunization with freeze-dried autologous skin was followed by the appearance of skin autoantibodies and autograft failure [111]. In ulcus cruris an autoimmune origin may be assumed [76] if (*i*) ulcers are refractory to all therapeutic investigations and the course is protracted without any apparent cause, (*ii*) skin autografts are rejected, (*iii*) autoantibodies to leukocytes, DNA, skin connective tissue and/or blood vessels are detectable in the circulating blood, (*iv*) the auto-antibodies decline or disappear and autografts survive, if corticosteroid therapy is applied, and (*v*) the ulcer heals as a result of corticosteroid and/or immunosuppressive treatment supplemented with vasoactive drugs in the second phase of the therapy [75].

PROBLEMS OF THERAPY

The therapy of diseases of possible autoimmune origin presents a difficult problem. At present the complete suppression of the immune response to autologous antigens seems to be impracticable [357]. Prevention of the production of committed lymphocytes would be promising. For this purpose large dose corticosteroid therapy combined with antibiotics and a careful dosage of immunosuppressive drugs (azathioprine, 6-mercaptopurine, methotrexate or an alternate therapy) might be given. Methotrexate should be administered for several years in the lowest effective dose. Owing to the toxicity of the drug, methotrexate therapy cannot be standardized. Its main advantage is that the dosage of the corticosteroids can be reduced. The efficiency of the combined therapy is reflected by the objective clinical remission and the gradual disappearance of symptoms. The biological tests of inflammation and the titres of pathological antibodies do not parallel the clinical course.

DIVERSE SKIN DISORDERS HAVING SOME IMMUNOPATHOLOGIC RELATIONS

CUTANEOUS AMYLOIDOSIS

Amyloidosis is a disorder characterized by the accumulation in the connective tissue of a unique extracellular filamentous glycoprotein rich in tryptophan and devoid of hydroxyproline [116*a*, 163]. The deposition of amyloid may be widespread with involvement of major organs, leading to serious clinical consequences (amyloidosis systematisata and amyloidosis generalisata secundaria) or it may be rather limited in extent with little effect on health (amyloidosis localisata) [494]. The primary (familial or sporadic) form of amyloidosis is unrelated to any demonstrable predisposing disease, its secondary form follows certain chronic infections, inflammatory disorders or neoplasms. Amyloidosis is prone to occur as a concomitant of multiple myeloma. There is no basic difference between the systemic and localized forms, although data tend to suggest the existence of subtle biochemical and immunological differences between amyloid fibrils [317]. Electron-microscopically [631], all types of amyloid examined consist chiefly of fine fibrils 70 to 100 Å in diameter, each being composed of two filaments approximately 25 Å in diameter. The filaments are twisted to form a double helix in tissue section. The minor component, so-called doughnut, consists of disc-like pentagonal structures with a hollow centre; it was suggested to be an α-globulin different in its amino acid composition from the fibril protein; it does not bind Congo red.

The true nature of amyloid has been controversial, especially since Glenner et al. [221] revived the old concept that amyloid is related to immunoglobulin. It has been proved by sequence analysis that the amyloid fibril protein is, irrespective of its origin, homologous to immunoglobulin light chains [194, 219]. By chemical and immunological methods its $\varkappa$ and λ types could be differentiated; the latter seems to occur more frequently [220]. The N-terminal fragments of the amyloid fibrils appear to be similar to those of the light chains physico-chemically [222]. In a few cases the important role of light chains has been confirmed by immunological examination of the precursors of the amyloid substance [222]. The amino acid sequence of an amyloid fibril protein derived from systemic [221] or localized [443] amyloidosis was very similar to that of the variable portion of several species of Bence–Jones protein and fibres fully characteristic of amyloid fibrils have been prepared from Bence–Jones proteins by proteolysis [219]. Glenner et al. [219] have concluded that the amyloid fibrils arise from the light chains of circulating immunoglobulins. The amyloid fibrils have a constant portion and another one varying individually. However, an analysis of the major low molecular weight component of two human amyloid fibrils [193] showed that purified fibrils from secondary amyloidosis consist of a homogeneous protein whose partial amino acid sequence does not resemble that of any known immunoglobulin. The non-immunoglobulin nature of some amyloid fibrils has been supported by further studies [282, 456, 474].

Since any organ may be involved, the clinical manifestations of amyloidosis are extremely variable. Infiltration of amyloid along peripheral nerves as well as in the skin, tongue, smooth and cross-striated muscles, joints and the heart are particularly common in primary amyloidosis, whereas in the secondary form, the liver, spleen and kidneys are the sites of predilection. Amyloid can be distinguished from hyalin by (*i*) its ability to stain with crystal violet, fluorochrome dye, thioflavine T and Congo red; (*ii*) its extracellular deposition, (*iii*) a characteristic birefringence and (*iv*) a fibrillary ultrastructure to be shown by polarization microscopy or electron microscopy. Elevated or reduced serum IgG, IgA and IgM levels are frequently encountered in patients with secondary amyloidosis as well as in those suffering from idiopathic disease and multiple myeloma [96].

Cutaneous amyloidosis may represent a localized disorder or may be part of a multisystemic disease [72]. The thighs, shins, arms, upper back, breasts, and buttocks may be involved. The lesions are moderately pruritic, symmetrically distributed, brown in colour, and lichenoid, macular or tumefactive in type. Islands of amyloid extending to the dermoepidermal junction were found in the papillary dermis. Many of these aggregates were surrounded by fibroblasts [72]. Electron-microscopically, amyloid appeared to be in close relation with fibroblasts in the papillary dermis [250] and amyloid fibrils were demonstrated within the cytoplasm of fibroblasts and within the epidermis [253]. The hyalin bodies and amyloid deposits within the dermal papillae are in a close apposition to the basal layer [52]; it may, therefore, be stated that the epidermis plays an important role in the histogenesis of cutaneous amyloidosis [72].

Freudenthal's lichen amyloidosus only affects the skin, and mainly of old subjects. It runs a chronic course; histologically, the amyloid is of pericapillary location and surrounding the capillaries in a construction resembling an onion. It is generally accepted that epidermal hyperplasia is the only sign differentiating the clinical form of primary amyloidosis from macular amyloidosis [72, 558]. By immunofluorescent test γ-globulin was detected in the horny layer of the skin in lichen amyloidosus [589*b*]. Other investigators found an intense IgG fluorescence in the intercellular space, and weaker IgM and IgA fluorescence at the same sites [435]. The formation of amyloid in the skin is attributed to local factors, first of all, the reduced blood supply in the connective tissue. Supposedly, the local metabolism disturbed by the hypoxidosis leads to amyloid production [599]. It is not quite clear whether amyloid is a pathological protein or a normal constituent of the connective tissue. In the latter case amyloidosis should be considered to be a disbalance of the fibrous constituents of the connective tissue.

Amyloidosis can be readily induced experimentally in many animal species with a number of chemically unrelated agents [86, 194]. Animal experiments have led to the hypothesis that the amyloid substance may result from an immunological mechanism. This is supported by the structural relationship between amyloid fibrils and immunoglobulins [194]. Antisera raised with water-soluble human amyloid fibres [192] react optimally with the very same preparation used for raising the antiserum but not with all fibril preparations. The pentagonal structure appears to have specific antigenic determinants not shared by the fibrils [86]. This hypothesis has been further supported by immunohistochemical demonstration of γ-globulin and C3 in amyloid lesions [598]. Gamma-globulin deposits have been detected in amyloid substance by the immunofluorescent technique as well, both in man and in experimental animals [404]. Demonstration of C [366, 525], β_1C globulin (C3 factor) and 7S γ-globulin [349] in visceral lesions of human amyloidosis has also been reported. It has been suggested that amyloid is a local product of cells belonging to the RES [116*b*]; accordingly, secondary amyloidosis would results from a chronic stimulation of the RES by various factors some of which might be immunogenic [5]. Increased or abnormal synthesis of polypeptides in plasma cells and polymerization of light (or heavy?) chains to build a fibrous helical protein instead of normal immunoglobulin molecules have also been proposed [317]. However, recent chemical and immunological investigations [85, 87, 95, 553] have been inconsistent with this view. It has been suggested [277] that the presence of γ-globulin might be attributed to a transudation from the serum where the γ-globulin level is raised. Incubation with antisera raised to IgG, IgA, IgM and C3 did not evoke specific immunofluorescence at amyloid deposits demonstrable by fluorochrome thioflavine T [558]. According to these results, the immunopathogenesis should be ruled out, at least in the case of lichen amyloidosus. Although the unstimulated and absolute PHA lymphocyte response was found to be decreased in patients with amyloidosis [67], their PHA-stimulation indices were normal. In nearly half of the cases tested, a positive response to PPD as stimulating antigen has been observed. The delayed sensitivity to unrelated antigens, e.g. diphtheria toxoid and mumps virus has been considered normal in amyloidosis diseases [67]. Ultrastructurally, amyloid differs from γ-globulin in its particle size; it is also different from the antigen–antibody complexes, resembling α-globulin more closely [51, 117]. Considering that the amyloid fibrils are ultrastructurally similar to tropocollagen, it has been proposed [558] that the amyloid substance in the skin might be due to an abnormal secretory activity of histiocytes and fibroblasts; in the cytoplasms of these cells fine amyloid fibrils have been found. To the epidermis, a modulating role has been attributed [72]. The purely cutaneous form of amyloid is a local abnormality and is most likely produced by fibroblasts under the influence of epidermis or epithelial tumours [251].

Furthermore, infiltrates of lymphocytes and plasmocytes are practically nonexistent in the dermis of patients with amyloidosis [558]. It may, therefore, be concluded that the formation of amyloid is not necessarily based on an immunological mechanism, at least not in all clinical forms.

Rabbits and mice were given s.c. human γ-globulin, bovine serum albumin or immune complexes of these antigens in Freund's adjuvant for a long period of time [590*a*]. During the immune complex treatment deposition of amyloid was observed in lymph nodes, in the liver and in the kidneys. The same was a rare finding when antigen or Freund's adjuvant was administered alone. The typical reaction was a generalized hyalin thickening of the media corresponding to acellular vasculitis in the arterioles of each animal. In the surroundings of these, lympho-plasmacellular infiltration occurred (so-called immune dissociation). Utsuki et al. [590*a*] attribute the acellular vasculitis, the amyloidosis as well as the immune dissociation to a common cause: a disturbance in the immune mechanism due to the tissue toxicity of the immune complexes.

An appropriate treatment of the underlying infectious or chronic inflammatory disease may be beneficial in secondary amyloidosis, but the primary forms remain untreatable [494]. The use of cytotoxic agents is under study.

CUTANEOUS MUCINOSES

In these diseases, deposition in the connective tissue of mucoproteins, viz. proteins, hyaluronic acid and chondroitin sulphate (natural constituents of the skin), is the basic pathological process. In mucin deposition the role of the hypophysis and the thyroid gland, the organs influencing the degree of polymerization has been known for a long time. Supposedly, the histiotropic factor of the thyrotropic hormone stimulates the fibroblasts and mast cells, which in turn may have a role in the deposition of mucin. Mucinosis may be associated with hypothyroidism (diffuse myxoedema) or hyperthyroidism (myxoedema circumscriptum praetibiale symmetricum), but may occur in euthyroidism (mucinosis papulosa or lichen myxoedematosus and scleromyxoedema) as well. From the immunological point of view, myxoedema circumscriptum praetibiale symmetricum and mucinosis papulosa may be discussed in detail.

Myxoedema circumscriptum praetibiale symmetricum (MCPS)

This clinical picture develops almost exclusively in hyperthyreotic patients, accompanied by exophthalmus. The majority of the patients have been suffering from hyperthyroidism and have undergone drug-mediated (propylthiouracil) or surgical thyroidectomy or received radioactive iodine; as a result, the hyperthyroidism has ceased, but the exophthalmus has remained practically unchanged, with periophthalmic oedema. The possibility has arisen that an over-correction of struma might serve as a pathogenetic basis of the disease. Clinically, the disease is characterized by a pretibial, usually symmetrical oedema and a thick infiltrate. The affected skin is painless, cold to the touch, hypertrichosis may be present. In the histological picture a moderate hyperkeratosis, thickened cutis, fragmentation of connective tissue fibres and metachromasic masses of mucin separating the fibres from one another are the characteristic features. The follicles, and the sweat and sebaceous glands are, as a rule, atrophic.

It has been supposed that MCPS might represent a side-phenomenon of Graves' disease, a multisystem disease of unknown aetiology. Long-acting thyroid stimulator (LATS) is encountered in significant amounts only in these diseases. Since LATS is considered an autoantibody [461] of the IgG class, MCPS has been believed to be an immunological disease. LATS is inhomogeneous in its composition. It resembles TSH in its biological effect,but it is produced by the lymphoplasmocellular apparatus. After thyroidectomy its consumption decreases, it is therefore understandable that the highest serum levels are encountered in MCPS. Nevertheless, the responsibility of LATS in MCPS is questionable, for there is no clear-cut correlation between the serum levels of LATS and the severity of the skin lesions [30].

MCPS in itself is rarely serious. Topical application of glucocorticoids, if applied properly, is effective.

Papular mucinosis of Dalton–Seidell (PM)

The following synonyms are used: lichen myxoedematosus Dubreuilh, lichen paramyloidosus Marks-Shuster. The skin phenomena develop independently of the thyroid function.

Reddish-yellow elastic or compact nodules, the size of a pinhead or somewhat larger appear close to one another, mainly on the arms, trunk and thighs; they tend to regress spontaneously. The following morphological variants are known: generalized lichenoid; discrete papular, localized lichenoid plaque; nodular lesions; and urticarial forms. Scleromyxoedema of Arndt–Gottron might be considered a generalized form of PM [284, 522]. In the histological picture, accumulation of acid mucopolysaccharides in superficial parts of the corium, oedema and histiocytes are seen. Perivascular infiltration of lymphoid, eosinophil and mast cells often separate the collagenous fibres from each other. In the pathological skin neutral glycoproteins, hyaluronic acid and chondroitin sulphates were found to be present in increased amounts and the presence of heparin and keratane sulphates was demonstrated [351]. Pretreatment of sections with hyaluronidase renders the positive Hale reaction and the metachromatic staining with toluidine blue negative [522]. The acid mucopolysaccharides of the interstitial substance incubated in colloidal ferric hydroxide can be visualized in the electron microscope [522]. Occasionally elevated γ-globulin, serum mucoid and hexose levels were demonstrated and the liver parenchyma was found damaged. However, any pathogenetic role of the liver damage could not be proved.

The aetiopathogenesis of PM is still unclear. Occasionally the immunoelectrophoretic pattern showed an increase in the IgA or in the IgG. Immunohistologically

[499], sometimes IgG, more often IgM was detectable between collagenous fibres. The mucicarmin-positive substance separating the collagenous fibres from one another appeared fibrillar or felt-like and reacted with anti-human renal connective tissue antiserum. However, the majority of the authors failed to demonstrate either immunoglobulin deposits or immunoglobulin synthesizing cells [351]. Indirect immunofluorescence revealed no abnormalities. Serum protein studies revealed in several cases [146, 190, 198, 292, 406, 440, 469, 499, 522] the presence of an unusually basic cationic myeloma-type IgG (subclass γ_1), a monoclonal protein with a light chain of the λ [610] or, exceptionally, $\varkappa$ type [351]. IgA and IgM paraproteins have also been reported [59, 190, 444]. These proteins have a strong affinity to bind to constituents of the normal dermis, most probably to acid mucopolysaccharides. Thus, the myeloma-type protein appears to have the property of an autoantibody reactive with components of the dermis. Antisera against the γ chains of normal IgG reacted in a considerable percentage with the $F(ab')_2$ fragments of the PM proteins; their specificities may have been directed to different substances or to different determinants on an acid skin substance [610]. Others [351] failed to demonstrate immunofluorescent antibodies against the connective tissues ground substance or other skin constituents in patients' sera. Cultures from bone marrow cells showed monoclonal IgG synthesis [351]. Cultured cells from a biopsy specimen obtained from diseased skin yielded low-speed IgG. It was concluded that the bone marrow and the pathological skin synthesized a paraprotein closely resembling that present in the serum. The lymphoid cells which synthesize the monoclonal immunoglobulins in the skin are thought to have originated from lymphoid organs and migrated to the skin via the blood stream. Since PM has been found occasionally associated with Waldenström's macroglobulinaemia [59, 284] it has been suggested that the paraproteinaemia might be the primary disease and the cutaneous phenomena in PM might represent its cutaneous manifestation; the paraproteinaemic reticulosis might have remained in a latent form for years. However, the benign clinical course of PM is quite different from multiple myeloma with cutaneous involvement.

As to the role of the paraproteins in PM a hypothesis has been proposed [351]. Accordingly, the paraprotein having an antibody activity against an unknown antigen, specific for PM may play a role in a homeostatic mechanism and in this way control the progress of the disease. The assumption that the paraprotein plays no pathogenetic role in PM might be inconsistent with its synthesis in the skin. Further investigations should elucidate these problems.

The therapy of PM is not satisfactory. Favourable results on the skin lesions have been reported with cytostatics such as Alkeran [146] and Chlorambucil [284].

HERPES GESTATIONIS

This is a rare, irregularly recurrent, polymorphous skin disease of unknown aetiology occurring in the second and third trimesters of pregnancy and in the postpartum period. The eruption is pruritis, consisting of grouped papules, vesicles or bullae on an erythematous base. Systemic manifestations are usually minimal, the maternal prognosis is good, but the incidence of foetal abnormalities is high. Leukocytosis and, mainly, eosinophilia are frequent laboratory findings. Serum IgA may be raised. The histological picture shows subepidermal bullae which may contain eosinophils and a few lymphocytes and, less regularly, multilocular intraepidermal vesicles. A dermal infiltrate of eosinophils, sometimes accompanied by lymphocytes and histiocytes, is particularly prominent around blood vessels and appendages.

As aetiopathogenetical features, hypersensitivity reactions, infectious agents, toxic and immunogenic effects of placental and foetal tissues, impaired renal and hepatic function and endocrine disturbances have been observed [526]. The role of infections, renal or hepatic causes have not been substantiated [526]. The increased incidence of foetal abnormalities and history of spontaneous abortions in diseased women have suggested a causal relationship in terms of autosensitization to abnormal foetal products or chorionic antigens [133, 214]. Antibodies to maternal hormones or their metabolites have also been suggested. The finding of elevated serum and urine gonadotropin levels and the repeated observations that exogenous oestrogens may worsen the course of the disease while progesterone may be of beneficial effect, have suggested an endocrine relationship. However, there are contradictions in this respect [382]. It has been observed recently that anticoncipients of the ovulation-inhibitor type (megoestrol acetate + ethinyl oestradiol) induced a generalized relapse in women who had suffered from herpes gestationis [226, 412]. Herpes gestationis should be distinguished from progesterone dermatitis [586]. It has been observed in a nonpregnant patient suffering from choriocarcinoma [586]. The incompatibility has also been considered a possible factor [99]. In a patient the serum IgA and IgM levels were significantly lower than in normal pregnant women in association with steatorrhoea [338]. This might be suggestive of an immunological dysfunction, but as an alternative explanation of the reduced IgM level an increased IgM consumption owing to the formation of the intestinal immune complex deposit may be considered.

Opinions vary as to whether HG is a single disease entity or whether it may be related with bullous pemphigoid or dermatitis herpetiformis. In some cases direct immunofluorescence did not show fixation of circulating antibodies to BM zone *in vivo* [300], while in others such a fixation could be demonstrated [82*c*]. Thus the relation with bullous pemphigoid could not be clarified. IgA deposition in seemingly intact skin areas of patients was demonstrated by means of direct immunofluorescence, suggesting a relationship to dermatitis herpetiformis [225*a*]. Other investigators found C (mainly C3) in the BM zone [92*b*], while C1q and immunoglobulins were absent [476*a*]. Others succeeded in confirming these findings and also demonstrated C4. On this basis, HG was regarded as a separate disease entity [289*e*]. Deposition of IgG, C1q, C3 and properdin was shown by others, implicating both classical and alternate C pathway activation [82*c*].

Corticosteroids in adequate doses are the drugs of choice if there is no contraindication [526]. Favourable responses have been reported to sulphapyridine, progesterone and pyridoxine. Antibiotics given topically or systemically may be necessary to control secondary infection.

PRURIGO GESTATIONIS

This is a dermopathy of immunological interest. It occurs in pregnant women at term as a form of intensely itching dermatosis characterized by an intense erythema which rapidly extends to almost the entire body surface. The IgG in the fluid of provoked bullae was found to be active both on lyophilized placenta and lyophilized skin preparations [414]. In the fluid of spontaneous bullae, it was not possible to detect anti-placental or anti-skin IgG, these had probably been absorbed by cutaneous antigens. The results of radial immunodiffusion tests in agar gel suggest that prurigo gestationis represents a disease connected with the presence of anti-ovular maternal serum antibodies of the IgG class, cross-reacting with some skin antigen [414]. Human chorionic gonadotropin therapy resulted in a complete remission of the itching symptoms and the almost total disappearance of the cutaneous manifestations.

PORPHYRIA CUTANEA HEPATICA (PCH)

The patients are as a rule over 35 years of age; the disease is characterized by bullae on exposed skin, increased skin fragility and occasional photosensitivity. Excess copro- and uroporphyrin are present in the urine and variable porphyrins in the faeces. The porphyrin content of the erythrocytes is at the normal level. The Watson–Schwartz test for urinary porphobilinogen as well as the UV microscopy for porphyrin fluorescence in erythrocytes are negative. The disease is nearly always associated with some, usually alcoholic, intoxication and with chronic liver dysfunction. In its development mitochondrial damage of endogenous and exogenous origin plays an important role [294, 609]. Considering that the δ-aminolaevulinic acid synthetase production and the last steps of the porphyrin and haem synthesis take place in the mitochondria, even mild mitochondrial damage may be of great pathogenetic significance.

Characteristic changes common to the porphyrias include deposition of PAS-positive diastase-resistant mucopolysaccharides and immunoglobulins in and around the superficial dermal blood vessels. Reduplication of the vascular basal lamina and an extensive perivascular deposition of a fine fibrillar material were found as the most prominent electron-microscopic findings [170]. The vascular abnormality seems to be due to structural alterations as well as to deposition of substances from circulation. Direct immunofluorescent studies [22*a*, 24, 170, 411] have shown a remarkable pattern of mainly homogeneous fluorescence in, and adjacent to, the upper and mid dermis blood vessels and, to a somewhat lesser degree, at the dermoepidermal IgG deposits. The fluorescence was in correlation with the severity of the bullous eruption. The deposition of IgG was more intense in erythropoietic porphyria than in PCH [170]. IgM deposits were noted in vessels and at the dermoepidermal junction irregularly [170]. Occasionally fibrinogen was found in vessels [577]. It has been emphasized [563] that an intensive fluorescence in itself may indicate plasmapheresis due to membrane damage or proliferation of reticular fibres. Indirect immunofluorescent studies have yielded negative results [170]; this finding speaks against the presence of autoantibodies to cutaneous antigens, though, errors of the methods used cannot be excluded. It is not quite clear whether the deposits in the BM zone represent only an indicator of an inflammation-mediated alteration caused by damage to the vessel walls by light [577], i.e. a non-disease-specific consequence of the reactions owing to porphyrin derivatives and sunlight [565*b*], or the IgG deposits have an autoimmune function playing a part in the provocation of bullae. It seems to be a reasonable hypothesis [565*b*] that sometimes immunopathogenesis might contribute to the progression of the porphyric liver lesion manifesting itself in fibrosis.

Though to a variable degree, phenomena suggestive of an enhanced immunoreactivity have been observed in PCH. Immunodiffusion studies [541] have shown reduced haemopexin and prealbumin plasma levels and a raised fibrinogen level. It has been supposed that porphyrin might form a conjugated antigen with haemopexin as carrier [97]. The C-activating effect of the fibre proliferation demonstrated at the dermoepidermal junction and along the vessel walls has been proved using an anti-human C-conjugate [578]. In 14 of 20 cases indirect immunofluorescence tests have shown low-titre autoantibodies, mainly of the IgG type, to epithelial cell cytoplasm and sometimes to nuclear substance, and also to mesenchymal cells; in three cases similar, mono-organospecific antibodies were demonstrable [563]. In four of the same group of patients, direct immunofluorescent examination of liver biopsy material showed a pattern corresponding to autoimmune hepatitis of varying severity. Migration inhibition was demonstrated with sera from 90 per cent of patients with PCH, using embryonic rat liver mitochondria as antigen [538, 540]. This finding suggests that the primary toxic liver injury after porphyrin disposition may progress secondarily on an immunological basis. In part of the patients direct immunofluorescence showed immunoglobulin binding around liver sinuses, bile canaliculi and hepatocytes [565*b*]. Immunoglobulin bound to tissues could not be demonstrated mainly because toxic (alcohol, drug) membrane injury is followed by plasmapheresis; in addition, the evaluation is disturbed by an enhanced autofluorescence of the proliferating fibres [563, 564]. In rats treated with hexachlorobenzol the characteristic red cytoplasmic fluorescence of the hepatic macrophages was the first sign of the enhanced porphyrin production [563, 564]; in animals showing severe symptoms of hepatic porphyria, the same phenomenon was observed in the periadventitial macrophages of the skin as well. Antibodies reacting with vascular fibres and different structural elements of parenchymal organs were demonstrable in one third of the experimental animals from the third week of the intoxication on [563, 564].

Using adequate optical systems, a basic difference has been demonstrated between the skin phenomena accompanying diseases based on an autoimmune pathogenesis and those in PCH [129, 130]. At the dermoepidermal junction as well as at the secretory portion and the luminal surface of the sweat glands, human C and fibrinogen were present in two-thirds of the patients in correlation with the clinical symptoms and the degree of exposure to light; at the same sites monovalent immunoglobulin conjugate was not bound. As to the occurrence of C, the findings are inconsistent [129, 130, 170], suggesting that immune complexes play no considerable role in PCH [170]. Autotransplantation studies failed to confirm an autoimmune pathomechanism of PCH [130, 577].

Simultaneous occurrence of lupus erythematosus has been described [265]. If optimal immunofluorescence technique is applied, the immunofluorescence patterns of sun-exposed skin in PCH cannot be mistaken for lupus erythematosus

[577]. None of the exchange autografts of sun-exposed skin with covered skin were rejected in contrast to chronic lupus erythematosus and normal skin, suggesting that the operating mechanism in PCH and lupus erythematosus are different [577].

It may be concluded that *(i)* the liver disease manifesting itself in an enhanced porphyrin production and thus leading to PCH may progress on an immunopathological basis [563, 565*a*]; *(ii)* the primary injury of skin occurs in the superficial dermal blood vessels, owing to the presence of porphyrin molecules and sunlight energy [170]; an additional damage has been found at the dermoepidermal zone, which may be responsible for the unique fragility of the sun-exposed skin.

EPIDERMOLYSIS BULLOSA ACQUISITA (EBA)

EBA has no hereditary pattern. It occurs in adult life and presents the clinical picture of epidermolysis bullosa dystrophica. The majority of the cases are associated with systemic disorders, such as amyloidosis, chronic ulcerative colitis, regional enteritis, multiple myeloma and diabetes mellitus.

Although the pathogenesis of EBA is still obscure, the cutaneous fragility seems to be related to an abnormal synthesis of collagen. Histochemical studies suggest abnormalities in the connective tissue with increased mucopolysaccharide levels in the upper half of the dermis [517]. The PAS-positive BM was found to be divided between the roof and floor of the bulla, with a decrease [520] or increase [517] in dermal elastic tissue. Pearson [457] detected by electron microscopy connective tissue degeneration. The first immunofluorescent studies yielded negative results [43, 496]. Recent investigations have demonstrated the presence of localized IgG and C3 at the BM zone [347]. Indirect immunofluorescence with sera and blister fluid yielded negative results. There is no satisfactory explanation for the pathogenesis of EBA. The histochemical and immunological findings are suggestive of primary and secondary features in this disease. It is of interest to speculate on the interrelationship between cutaneous and systemic lesions and on the role of the immunoglobulin in the BM zone.

RECURRENT APHTHOUS ORAL ULCERATION OF MIKULICZ AND KÜMMEL (RAOU)

This disease is characterized by well-defined painful, recurrent single or multiple shallow erosions with discrete erythematous margins on the oral (most frequently labial and buccal) mucosa. It should be differentiated from gingivostomatitis herpetica [512]. The aetiology of RAOU is unknown. Recurrences appeared to have been precipitated by trauma, drug effects, hormonal, nutritional, psychogenic (emotional stress), genetic and local factors, especially microbes persisting in the oral cavity [6, 511, 537]. Streptococci [230], first of all L forms of group A streptococci have been implicated. *S. sanguinis* strain 2A [26, 537] was isolated from 94 per cent of the cases tested; streptococci were demonstrated in histological lesions; laboratory animals inoculated with *S. sanguinis* or its cell wall material developed oral lesions and delayed hypersensitivity; the latter was also found in human patients suffering from RAOU. It has been proposed that during remissions the L form of *S. sanguinis* might be present. Cell-mediated immunity was demonstrated by the leukocyte migration test [160]. Recently viral agents, first of all herpes simplex virus, have been suggested as possible causes. The intraoral introduction of herpes simplex virus may cause recurrent vesicles and erosions [232].

As to the pathogenesis of RAOU the possible role of humoral 'anti-mucosa' antibodies [362*a*, *d*] (mast cells, present in large numbers in the early lesions [69]) and cell-mediated immunity has been considered. The occurrence of humoral antibodies to adult human oral epithelium and an increase in titres—as compared with controls—was shown using a double-layer immunofluorescence staining method [159*e*]. It has been supposed that the anti-mucosa antibody would bind to the cytoplasm of prickle cells [362*b*] in an early phase of the disease. However, the serum level of this antibody did not parallel the course of the disease. In immune absorption studies, antigens obtained from different human sources (mucosa, colon, skin) showed cross-reactivity and no species specificity. The bulk of the anti-mucosa antibody was mainly found in the IgM fraction, less frequently in the IgG fraction [362*d*]. Using gingival epithelial cells as target cells in tissue culture [159*a*], adding a serum from patients with RAOU caused no change, but the survival time of the cells was significantly reduced when peripheral blood lymphocytes from patients were added [496*a*]. The lymphocytotoxicity was blocked by preincubation of RAOU lymphocytes with rabbit antihuman lymphocyte serum [109*b*]. Lymphocytes from active RAOU elicited a higher lymphocytotoxicity than those from inactive RAOU. Stimulation of lymphocyte transformation by tissue homogenates (using a saline extract of foetal oral mucosa as mitogen) was positive in 43 per cent of RAOU patients during the period of ulceration [362*c*]. The histological picture of the aphtha supports a substantial role of lymphocytes in the development of the ulcer; it is characterized by subepithelial infiltration of mononuclear cells covered by necrotic epithelium [159, 406]. In the mononuclear cells, cytoplasmic phagosome-like bodies have been demonstrated [363]; these might be forerunners of delayed hypersensitivity damage to antigen-bearing epithelial cells. Lehner [362*f*] demonstrated binding of IgG, IgM and IgA as well as C3 in the cytoplasm of oral mucosal specimens obtained from RAOU patients. Occasionally, cell-mediated immunity appeared to be impaired; five patients were attempted to be sensitized with DNCB, but two of them developed no delayed-type hypersensitivity [599]. To restore cutaneous delayed hypersensitivity reactions, Levamisol was administered to nine patients [599]; of these 6 remained free of symptoms for 25 months.

It is generally thought [512] that the Mikulicz–Kümmel aphtha as well as Sutton's aphtha, differing from the former in its larger size, are autoimmune diseases, whereas the herpetiform ulceration, in which virus-like bodies have been found [363], might be due to a virus infection. In the last years the connection between viruses and the immune system has come into prominence. Adenovirus type 1 [345] and herpes simplex virus hominis [509*a*] have been isolated from recurrent aphthous oral ulcerations. However, these viruses may occur even in the normal nasopharyngeal cavity and the patients' sera did not show elevated antibody titres to the isolated viruses. For this reason, transformation tests were performed with the patients' lymphocytes, using heat-inactivated type 1 adenovirus and herpes simplex virus hominis as antigen. The lymphocytes from patients suffering from recurrent aphtha showed a higher transformation rate than those obtained from control subjects [139]. Owing to the possible carcinogenic effect of these viruses, skin tests were not made. Direct immunofluorescent tests were carried out with antisera to the viruses mentioned above [510]. In the majority of the cases, herpes simplex virus or adenovirus antigens were detected in 1–2 per cent of the lymphocyte population, viz. IF with anti-adenovirus or anti-herpes antiserum alone was demonstrated in 52.5 per cent and 3.3 per cent, respectively, and both sera gave positive results in 11.6 per cent. In the control group only 4.6 per cent of the subjects proved to be positive for either of the antigens [139]. Based on these studies, the possible pathogenetic role of circulating virus–antigen-carrying lymphocytes may be presumed.

It has been known for a long time that aphthae in the oral mucosa may be induced by mechanical trauma. Superficial excoriation of the inner surface of the lower lip of aphthous patients is followed by development of an ulcer of inflamed margin by the 6th day; the ulcer heals spontaneously within another six-day period [509*b*]. In non-aphthous patients healing is complete in 2 days. Provocation of aphtha as a positive Köbner's isomorphous phenomenon cannot be excluded, but alternatively it may be an organ-specific symptom due to autoimmunity [512]. There has been no evidence to support the hypothesis that aphthous ulceration is primarily caused by hypersensitivity to food antigens. The incidence of serum antibodies to food-proteins was found significantly higher in aphthous patients than in a control group [584]. The existence of the ulceration on the other hand might contribute to the absorption of antigenic food molecules from the mouth.

Eradication of the corresponding chronic infectious agent and influencing of the cell-mediated immunity may be employed in the therapy of RAOU [599].

PYODERMA GANGRAENOSUM (PG)

Synonyms: *phagédénisme géométrique*, essential dermatitis ulcerosa, pyodermia phagedenica, pyodermia ulcerosa serpiginosa, pyodermia chronica vegetans. PG is a rare chronic disease of unknown aetiopathogenesis with recurrent deep ulcer or ulceration of the skin. The borders are purple, tender, boggy and undermined. It frequently appears at sites of trauma initially as papules, nodules or areas resembling folliculitis. It ulcerates progressively or may coalesce into large ulceration, acute and chronic inflammation and thrombosis of the superficial blood vessels are the characteristic changes. Scarring occurs frequently. Iodides and bromides may aggravate or even generalize the lesions.

The microorganisms isolated from PG lesions (*Streptococcus pyogenes* group A, *Staphylococcus pyogenes*) are probably not the primary aetiological agents; they should be considered secondary invaders. It has nevertheless happened [149] that a streptococcal antigen (streptokinase, streptodornase) provoked large ulcers at the sites of injection, accompanied by a constant rise in the antistreptolysin O titre. This finding might be explained by two alternative hypotheses [149]; (*i*) PG might be a 'post-streptococcal skin disease' like the vasculitis of Levene; or (*ii*) PG might be a 'Köbner-like phenomenon' (Piérard), a concomitant phenomenon unrelated to the pathogenesis of PG. A dermonecrotic factor has been found in patients' sera [149], but this γ-globulin is not specific for any disease, it occurs in low amounts in normal individuals as well. In rabbits PG has been produced by typhoid vaccine in carriers of *E. coli* or some other Gram-negative bacteria [291]; the symptoms thus induced healed readily as a result of diiodoquine or Enterovioform therapy, supposedly through the effect of these drugs on the intestinal flora. Reportedly, even viruses have been isolated from PG lesions, besides bacteria [209].

Various diseases have been reported in association with PG, including ulcerative colitis (40 per cent), less frequently regional ileitis, intestinal polyps, duodenal and gastric ulcer, perforation of the bowel, rheumatoid arthritis (30 per cent), focal sepsis, viral infections, diabetes, etc.

Immunoelectrophoresis showed normal or slightly increased levels of IgG, IgA and IgM [359]. Attention has been called to association with various immunological alterations, such as hypo- and dysgammaglobulinaemia, paraproteinaemia and monoclonal or polyclonal gammopathies [147, 158, 161, 255, 291, 379, 545] and to possible disturbances of humoral and cell-mediated immunity. Patients immunized with group D or H Salmonella bacteria responded with normal humoral antibody production. Similarly, three-fourths of the immunized patients developed protective levels of tetanus antitoxin [359]. The idea that PG might represent an immune complex disease or Shwartzman phenomenon [417] has also arisen; primary vasculitis has rarely been found [545]. Direct and indirect immunofluorescent tests [149] failed to yield abnormal results. As to the possible role of cell-mediated immunity, first of all the cutaneous anergy should be mentioned. Negative responses have been observed to skin tests with various antigens including PPD, streptokinase-streptodornase, mumps virus, trichophytin and Candida antigens [149, 359]. Sensitization of the skin with DNCB [359] or DNFB [149] has failed. In three-fourths of patients with PG the lymphocyte transformation test with PHA was normal, similarly the incorporation of ^{3}H-thymidine into, and the blastogenic response to streptokinase-streptodornase; lymphocytes from half of the patients gave a normal response to PPD [359]. All these suggest that there is no defect in the production of lymphocyte-mitogenic factor. In contrast, the production of the macrophage migration inhibition factor was found negative *in vitro* in response to PPD and streptokinase-streptodornase [359]. Further investigations are needed to show whether this defect might play any part in the pathogenesis of PG. Normal thymic function is necessary for the manifestation of delayed hypersensitivity *in vivo* and for the production of migration inhibition factor by lymphocytes [492]. Rejection of autografts is delayed by corticosteroids, but intracutaneous injection of autologous lymphocytes failed to evoke any reaction [149]. The rejection of autografts might result from an enhanced inflammatory response and not from a specific cellular reaction. The non-disease-specific dermonecrotic factor may be present in the serum [149]. Lack of cytotoxicity of lymphocytes has also been reported [149].

PG appears to be a polypathogenetic syndrome in which immunological disturbances play the main role. Initially humoral immunity was incriminated, supposing some unknown relationship between the PG lesions and monoclonal gammopathies. Recently attention has been called to an, at least partial, defect of cell-mediated immunity including lack of normal thymic function. However, similar immunological defects occur in chronic mucocutaneous candidiasis, sarcoidosis and Hodgkin's disease, too. There is no convincing evidence for an autoimmune pathogenesis. Cross-reactivity between lipopolysaccharides of *E. coli* or other Gram-negative bacteria on the one hand, and colon antigens, on the other, in some cases has been suggested [291].

An efficient therapy of PG needs systemic administration of high doses of corticosteroids, supplemented with local injections if necessary. Antibiotic therapy is not essential.

KAPOSI'S ANGIORETICULOSIS

This is a benign tumour developing from pluripotential endothelial and perithelial cells in tissues proliferating with angiopoiesis. It occurs as small and larger bluish-grayish-brown painful compact nodules on the feet and hands, less frequently on mucous membranes and in viscera. The pigmentation of the nodules is due to haemosiderin.

The cause of Kaposi's angioreticulosis is still unknown. It has been suggested that it is (*i*) a neoplasm (vascular, neural or reticuloendothelial); (*ii*) an infectious granuloma with neoplastic potential; (*iii*) a systemic vascular disease; or (*iv*) a reticuloendothelial hyperplasia. Factors such as the presence of inflammatory cells, the histological picture, which may resemble a granulomatous process, and the irregular geographic distribution have suggested the role of an infectious agent. Bacteria, fungi and viruses have been incriminated, but their role has not been confirmed. Maintenance of tumour cells in tissue culture has generally failed.

Herpes-type particles were observed under the electron microscope [217]. Comparative immunological studies showed high serum titres to soluble antigen of human cytomegalovirus and low titres to Epstein-Barr virus [217].

As regards immunological disorders, some clinical and histological features suggest that the clinical manifestations and progression of the disease may be influenced by host immunity (spontaneous remissions; infiltration of the tumour by lymphocytes and plasma cells). Antibody responses to *E. coli* Vi antigen and immunoglobulin levels were found normal, but an impairment in the delayed-type response to DNCB was observed in patients with the malignant type of tumour [396]. In 39 per cent of Ugandan patients, the PHA stimulation index for cultured lymphocytes was decreased [570]. The serum immunoglobulins were examined in 6 cases of histologically confirmed Kaposi's angioreticulosis; the γ-globulin level was reduced in 3 cases as tested by agar gel electrophoresis. IgG and IgA paraprotein was demonstrated by immunoelectrophoresis in 2 and 1 cases, respectively. IgM deficiency was found in one case [157], and the PHA stimulation index was below the normal level in 2 cases. The results are suggestive of a damaged humoral and/or cell-mediated immunity in a varying number of cases.

COMMON HUMAN WARTS (CHW)

CHW are caused by the human papilloma virus, a DNA virus of the Papovavirus group. They are benign epidermal tumours ready to regress (Fig. 40-18). The role of immunity has arisen in connection with the spontaneous resolution of CHW [500]. There are observations suggesting that their persistence or regression may relate to host immunity; these are as follows: (*i*) warts mainly occur in children; (*ii*) they may proliferate in an uncontrolled fashion in immunosuppressed patients; (*iii*) regression frequently follows trauma to a single lesion. Immune response may be directed toward structural proteins of the virion and/or virus-induced cellular antigens. The serum of some patients contains IgG to human papilloma virus, and this may explain the regression. Twenty-one per cent of the tested patients had precipitating serum antibodies of the IgG class to purified virions or virion components; IgM antibodies were demonstrable in 3 per

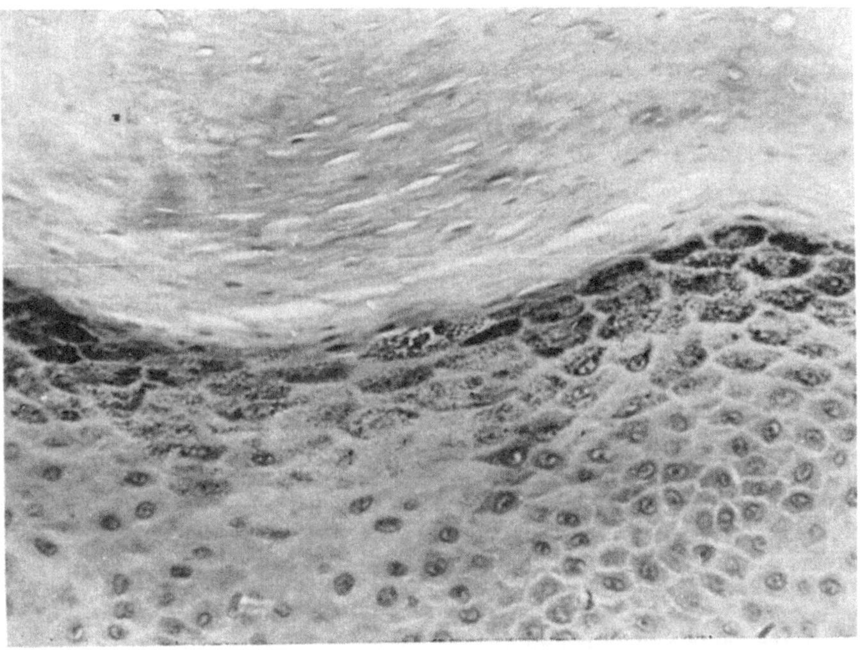

Fig. 40-18. Verruca vulgaris. Some cells in the stratum granulosum are vacuolated. ×60 (Courtesy of Professor L. Szodoray, Debrecen)

cent [452]. The precipitating antibodies were directed to the major structural protein of the viral capsid C-fixing antibodies [212*b*]. Others [68] found C-fixing antibodies in only 12 per cent of patients with CHW in regression. However, it is not clear whether the virus-specific IgG is a cause or a consequence of regression. Sera of patients with regressing warts contained virus-specific IgM (100 per cent), IgG (97 per cent) and IgA (80 per cent) [398], and IgM against wart-virus-infected cells in 46 per cent, and wart-virion-specific IgM in 12 per cent. The role of cell-mediated immunity has been examined by the leukocyte migration inhibition test [415]. Cell-mediated immunity increased at the time of resolution of the infection, suggesting that it is involved in the elimination of infection or, alternatively, the change in the immune status may be a result of the elimination of infection. This may be of practical importance, namely, a successful cryotherapy like excision may completely separate the antigen from the host, preventing any change in the immune status.

Regressing wart lesions all contained virus, but non-regressing lesions often did not. However, histologically no evidence of lymphocyte infiltration has been demonstrated [68]. The inconsistence of the immunological results might be attributed to differences in technique and in the selection of the material.

Recently [453] two soluble antigens of human wart tissue have been isolated from whole-tissue homogenates by elution from antibody-Sepharose immuno-adsorbents: the one is a nuclear antigen which appears diffusely throughout the nucleus of epidermal cells, the other is a cell-surface antigen, either a component of the cell membrane or localized within the intercellular space. Neither of them is a structural protein of the virion. The antigens, occurring in rapidly growing and dividing cells, were detected by immunofluorescence in warts, squamous cell carcinomas, foetal skin and psoriatic epidermis, but neither in normal skin nor in basal cell carcinomas. However, extracts from large sheets of normal epidermis reacted in immunodiffusion with antisera to the wart-associated antigens. A possible explanation for the apparent discrepancy between the two techniques might be that warts may be much richer in the antigens, which appear to be organ-specific, than normal skin or, alternatively, the antigens may reside in cryptic sites in normal cells. In rabbits immunized with human wart tissue, antibodies were formed that reacted with the surface of epidermal cells, and an immunofluorescent reaction was demonstrable in the intercellular area of the wart tissue [144]. Antisera to crude wart homogenates, absorbed with pooled human sera and liver extract, showed positive immunofluorescent reaction [451*a*] in the nuclei and cell surfaces in warts and epidermal squamous cell tumours. The same reaction was negative in the normal epidermis and in basal cell tumours. In agarose gel diffusion test an aqueous extract of wart tissue showed a single precipitation band [451*b*].

Human plantar warts were studied by immunofluorescence [212*a*], using crude homogenates from selected plantar warts as antigen and rabbit and guinea pig antisera. Specific intranuclear fluorescence was demonstrated corresponding to the basophil inclusion body. The fluorescence was more intensive in the direct than in the indirect immunofluorescence test.

Contact dermatitis induced by DNCB at the site of warts led to disappearance of the warts 10 to 14 days after challenge [231], supposedly due to delayed hypersensitivity mechanisms. The host response to DNCB with destruction of the warts may have been secondary to a non-specific lymphocyte or macrophage stimulation or, alternatively, DNCB as hapten might have conjugated with wart-virus. In another series [371*a*] of the 77 refractory warts patients only 7 failed to respond to topical immunotherapy with DNCB. Three patients already sensitive to nickel or formalin responded adequately to application of their respective sensitizers in epicutaneous testing concentrations. Therapeutic use of DNCB requires thorough consideration. In a series of 23 cases of recalcitrant verrucae, severe systemic reaction to DNCB occurred in one case and severe pain due to the development of bullae at the site of treated verrucae was noted in 4 cases [92*a*].

CHRONIC ACRAL DERMATITIS ASSOCIATED WITH EXTREME ELEVATION OF IgE

This clinical picture was described by Winkelmann and Gleich [624] in 1973. It appears as a chronic, pruritic papulovesicular and hyperkeratotic dermatitis, particularly involving the acral areas (extensor surface of the extremities) associated with markedly, more than 100-fold, raised serum IgE levels. The chronicity of the disease is reflected by de- and hyperpigmentation. Nail dystrophy has been observed. There was no personal or family history of atrophic disease. A variety of immunological, physiological and pharmacological studies of the skin yielded normal results. Mast cells were observed in large numbers in the dermis, and even in the epidermis. The illness lasts many years and is resistant to all treatments except corticosteroid therapy.

The elevation of IgE and the prominence of mast cells in the inflammatory exudate suggest the involvement of certain immunological mechanisms in the pathogenesis. IgE binds to mast cells and when combined with antigen can trigger release of the mediators of type I hypersensitivity reaction, which may play an important role in the development of the cutaneous lesions.

WISKOTT-ALDRICH SYNDROME (WAS)

According to present knowledge, WAS is sex-linked, inherited in an X-linked recessive manner. Its clinical characteristics are as follows; eczema, thrombocytopenia, haemorrhage, predisposition to infections and autoimmune disorders, isohaemagglutinin deficiency, dysgammaglobulinaemia and an increased frequency of malignancies [207]. The eczema usually begins on the scalp, face, flexures or buttocks during the second or third months of life and may suggest seborrhoeic or atopic dermatitis. Bleeding often begins in the first six months. Gastrointestinal bleeding, petechiae, certain forms of thrombocytopenia causing intracranial bleeding and epitaxis are often observed. Recurrent infections also begin early in life. Bacterial infections (otitis media, pneumonia, meningitis, septicaemia) tend to persist, and resist therapy [399]. The defence mechanisms against both bacterial and some viral (e. g. herpes simplex, cytomegalovirus) infections are seriously impaired. Among the clinical laboratory findings thrombocytopenia, mild anaemia, lymphopenia and eosinophilia may be mentioned. Pathological findings include the absence of characteristic or consistent features of thymus involvement, though the thymus may be atrophic or fibrotic. The lymphoid tissue of the thymus and of the spleen may become enlarged. Among the immunological abnormalities it is noted that serum IgM is often reduced and the IgA level raised; occasionally [604], but not consistently [399], very high levels of IgE have been observed. The high levels might reflect chronic non-specific stimulation of immunoglobulin synthesizing cells by residual antigens. In older children the isohaemagglutinin titres may rise to the low normal range [399].

The pathogenesis of WAS is still practically unknown. The thrombocytopenia is caused by an unknown cellular defect leading to shortened survival times. The patient's own platelets, labelled with ^{51}Cr and reinfused, showed markedly shortened survival times [25]. There is a failure to regulate the oxidative phosphorylation residing in cell granules [346]. The reduced IgM antibody response to some (e.g. polysaccharide) antigens is related to a disorder of antigen processing and/or recognition [53]. Cell-mediated immunity is also impaired, perhaps again due to deficient antigen recognition. Delayed hypersensitivity response to common skin test antigens (as PPD, streptokinase-streptodornase, *C. albicans*, trichophytin, mumps vaccine) and experimental DNCB sensitization was found to be reduced or absent [53*a*, 439]. There was fairly good correlation between the cutaneous PHA response and several measures of cellular immunity including delayed and contact type hypersensitivity [53*a*]. Lymphocyte transformation test resulted in selective failure of response to pneumococcal polysaccharides and a less than normal response to streptolysin O, diphtheria and tetanus toxoid and isologous leukocytes. Impaired cellular resistance to herpes simplex virus has been reported [556]. Normal response to optimal concentration of PHA *in vitro* after 5 days of culture to produce lymphotoxin and MIF has been reported [53*a*].

Aimed bactericidal antibiotic therapy has been recommended to prevent infectious complications. Severe bleedings can be managed by platelet transfusion if necessary; however, platelets may induce an autoantibody response [399]. The immunohaemolytic anaemia responded well to corticosteroids and the antibody disappeared after a year of treatment [399]. Splenectomy is not recommended because of an excessive risk of pneumococcus septicaemia. After the administration of transfer factor, clinical improvement was reported and the development of delayed hypersensitivity to antigens to which the patient had been sensitized [370].

Unfortunately, it has happened [25*a*] that transfer factor therapy, by restoring cell-mediated immunity, enabled responding to antigens to which the patient had been unresponsive. In this way a humoral autoimmune response was evoked with consequent Coombs-positive haemolytic anaemia.

CHRONIC GRANULOMATOUS DISEASE (CGD)

CGD is characterized by a defect in neutrophil bacterial activity and an eczematoid dermatitis associated with haematological abnormalities [37, 93, 354]. Before the first year of life usually dermatitis (scaly, seborrhoeic, dry, weeping or eczematoid lesions, sometimes pustular, usually around the head) or suppurative lymphadenitis occur; during early childhood major infections occur (perirectal, abdominal, chest wall abscess, osteomyelitis, pyarthrosis, empyema, peritonitis, meningitis, otitis media, hepatic abscess and, as terminal event, septicaemia). Recurrent and chronic pneumonitis progresses to widespread consolidation and abscess formation. Hepatosplenomegaly is a common phenomenon. Clinical laboratory findings include leukocytosis, anaemia and increased erythrocyte sedimentation rate. The myelogram shows myeloid hyperplasia with neutrophil leukocytosis. The most frequent bacteriological finding is isolation of *Staphylococcus aureus* from the site of infection. Gram-negative organisms come into prominence after repeated antibiotic treatment. Fungal infections are less common. Granuloma formation and a picture of chronic infection characterized by lymphocytes, macrophages and plasma cells are the usual pathological findings. The significance of pigmented-lipid histiocytes is not clear. Diagnostic laboratory features are: elevation of serum immunoglobulin levels progressively with the recurrence of the bacterial infection. Immunoglobulin response to antigenic stimulation is normal. To establish the diagnosis it must first be demonstrated that there is no other cause for the recurrent bacterial infections [399]; neutrophils must respond appropriately to infectious challenge (usually with *Staph. aureus* strain 502/A) [479], and chemotaxis must be evident from the suppurative nature of the lesions. Next, the functional capacity of the neutrophils should be studied [399]. In the neutrophils in which no activation of the hexose monophosphate shunt pathway occurs during phagocytosis, there is no precipitated dye after incubation with latex particles and nitroblue tetrazolium [622]. To make bactericidal assay more specific, antibiotics or lysostaphin [569] were added to kill bacteria outside neutrophils. Other anomalies such as the lack of normal increase in respiration, glucose oxidation and hydrogen peroxide production have been demonstrated in cells of patients during phagocytosis [270]. The pattern of genetic transmission of CGD is X-linked recessive. Defective bactericidal function and the typical metabolic abnormalities exist as autosomal recessive form [478]. It may be concluded [399] that all of the manifestations can clearly be linked to an intracellular defect of neutrophil bactericidal activity. The specific abnormality causing the defective cell function is not yet known. The relationship of the eczema associated with this blood cell defect to the rest of the disease pattern has not been defined.

Therapy is so difficult and the control of bacterial infections is so imperfect that early death is common [399]. Bactericidal antibiotics must be given for prolonged periods and in right dosage. Surgical drainage should be applied to remove pus.

PSORIASIS AS SYSTEMIC DISEASE

Psoriasis cannot be regarded as an isolated disease of the skin, but as an oligo- or plurisystemic disease [268]. The participation of the osseous system has been proved by clinical, radiological, histological and electron-microscopic studies; the participation of joints (arthritis psoriatica) has been evidenced by a scintigraphic method. The latter ranges between 1 per cent and 15 per cent in different countries [275*b*]. Myopathia psoriatica is characterized by clinical, histological, electron-microscopic, electromyographic and enzymatic changes; in the connective tissue the biosynthesis of glycosaminoglycans and collagen is enhanced. Enteropathia psoriatica (with pathological xylose loading test, steatorrhoea) has been observed in 43 per cent of patients; in the mucous membrane of the small intestine light- and electron-microscopic alterations have been found. The functional disturbance of the spleen is indicated by a protracted clearance of heat-injured erythrocytes from the blood and the highly reduced sequestration index. Anaemia has also been demonstrated. In widespread scaling psoriasis the iron loss may cause iron deficiency. The pentose-sulphate cycle in the erythrocytes is raised, whereas the dehydroepiandrosterone content is low [268]. The participation of the pancreas is suggested by hyperinsulinism and limited glucose tolerance. The hepatic lesion, though evidenced histologically and enzymologically, is of unknown nature. Gout and amyloidosis occur as secondary phenomena. The humoral parameters, viz. the elevated 'collagen-like' protein level in the serum, hyperuricaemia, dehydroepiandrosterone deficiency and high androstendiol content in the plasma, the enhanced mucopolysaccharide and hydroxyproline and decreased dehydroepiandrosterone excretion with the urine, suggest [268] that systemic psoriasis is a disease of genetic origin probably with an autosomal dominant pattern [315], due, probably, to a structural protein abnormality. The proliferative processes and hyperplasias, including an increased epidermopoiesis with consecutive acanthosis, capillary hyperplasia, an increase in nerval elements in the corium, and the enhanced glycosaminoglycan and collagen biosynthesis in the connective tissue, all suggest that organs other than the skin are also involved [275*a*, 315].

As to the pathogenesis of psoriasis two models are investigated at present; both are based on a presumed genetically determined predisposition; the clinical manifestation of the disease would then need provocative mechanisms like endogenous crises, infection and/or immunological events [178*a*]. Further endogenous and/or exogenous stimuli would exaggerate the clinical picture. One of the models presumes a defect in the adenylcyclase-cyclic AMP cascade in the psoriatic epidermis. The second model is based on a latent dehydroepiandrosterone deficiency; the latter has been supported by biochemical studies [268].

Immunopathological factors have also been considered. However, the existence of neither antibodies to a special antigen, nor immune complexes and immunological defects has been unequivocally demonstrated. The pathogenetic roles of bacteria (firstly *Streptococcus pyogenes* and secondly *Staphylococcus aureus* and *E. coli*) and less frequently fungi (*Candida albicans*) have been studied. Helminths have also been incriminated. However, the immunological hypothesis has been neither confirmed nor refuted [119, 235, 263, 324, 332, 333, 429]. The pathogenetic role of the primary and secondary immune response has been supposed first of all in the development and recurrence of the eruptive-exanthematic form of the punctate-guttate type, for in this clinical form the history of infections, strong cutaneous sensitivity to bacterial antigens and high antibody levels are more common than in the chronic static forms. Relatively quicker and more lasting improvement may be expected from properly chosen antibiotic therapy and/or extirpation of the infective focus [365].

On this basis it has been proposed that dermal capillaropathy can develop not only on the effect of toxic bacterial products, but also as a result of allergic reactions [119]. As to the immunoglobulins a rise in IgA level in the serum and in the saliva [240], in correlation with the extent and duration of the psoriasis, is a common finding [195, 392, 597]; elevated IgG levels have also been reported; other immunoglobulins behave variably; the C3 level is normal. There is no characteristic immunological pattern [384*b*]. The immunoglobulin changes might be concomitant phenomena to the non-specific hepatic lesion. Immunofluorescent studies [267] of lesions and uninvolved skin from patients did nor reveal *in vivo*-bound immunoglobulin, fibrinogen or C, neither could circulating skin antibody be demonstrated. In contrast to this, IgG and IgM were detected around the dermo-epidermal junction and above the dermal papillae [343*b*]. Anti-immunoglobulin activity was detected by the mixed agglutination technique in epidermal lesions of psoriatic patients. The anti-immunoglobulin factors could be eluted from the sections by acid buffer [343*b*]. Recently anti-IgG activities of lymphocytes and IgM have been revealed [488], suggesting that firmly bound antigen–antibody complexes appear in psoriatic lesions and the anti-IgG in the serum may combine with the Fc portion of the IgG in these complexes. The existence of other antigens that would be suitable for the demonstration of mainly humoral autoantibodies (antibodies of the anaphylactic type, skin-sensitizing against psoriatic skin homogenates demonstrable by PCA in the guinea pig skin; specific haemagglutinin) has not been confirmed [306*b*]. Demonstration of the anti-nuclear factor has often failed [268]. The double diffusion precipitation (Oakley–Fulthorpe) test with normal human or autologous apparently intact skin as antigen was found positive in 10 per cent, the leukoagglomeration test of Fleck in 30–46 per cent, and the intracutaneous test with autoantiserum in 59 per cent [471]. With body tissues and metabolites as antigen, the C consumption test was positive more frequently than in healthy controls [329], but there was no demonstrable relationship to the severity and period of the disease. The presence of cytophilic heterophil antibodies has also been demonstrated. The apparent existence of such side-antibodies does not indicate a causal relationship. They may be even consequences of the pathological process [384*b*]. Recently [44*a*], direct immunofluorescent tests of psoriatic lesions revealed the presence of *in vivo* bound IgG as well as of other immunoglobulins and C in the stratum corneum. By means of a double immunofluorescent staining technique the concomitant occurrence of IgG and C could be demonstrated suggesting the presence of immune complexes on the membranes of polymorphous leukocytes [126*a*].

The possible role of cell-mediated immunity has been investigated from several aspects. The results of the i.c. test have been discussed most thoroughly. As antigens microbial (Streptococcus, Candida) [488] inhalative [261*b*] antigens and homogenates of psoriatic and normal epidermis [406] have been used. Slight or no difference was observed (partial defect of cell-mediated immunity) as compared to the reaction of control subjects. Thus the results of these tests cannot be considered diagnostically conclusive [353, 544]. Up to now the existence of a specific psoriasis antigen [189*a*] has not been satisfactorily demonstrated nor has a specifically altered cutaneous reactivity been proved. The PHA transformation index for the lymphocytes was normal [276*b*, 488], that for autologous or homologous epidermis extracts was slightly raised [186]. According to others [276*b*] the lymphocyte transformation was significantly stimulated only by plaque epidermis in one case of 11 psoriatics. The leukocyte migration inhibition test with streptolysin O was positive in 55 per cent [151]. The autologous leukocyte migration indices with extracts from psoriatic skin and scales was the same as that of the normal controls [276*b*]. A protracted latency after epicutaneous sensitization with DNCB was suggested, but could not be confirmed [113, 488]. The rheumatoid rosette test based upon the immunocyte-adherence phenomenon has been suggested to detect the rheumatoid factor on peripheral blood lymphocytes. The biological significance of this test is different from that of the Waaler–Rose test, which only demonstrates agglutinating antibodies of the IgM class. Rheumatoid rosettes were described in some cases of psoriatic arthritis [533]. Recently [487*b*] this test has been found positive (>6 rosettes per 1,000 lymphocytes) in 40 per cent of patients with complicated (generalized, erythrodermic, arthritic) or uncomplicated psoriasis, the reaction was positive in 4 per cent of control subjects and in none of patients suffering from eczema. This finding has raised the possible significance of anti-IgG activity, suggesting that psoriasis might be a cell-mediated immunological disorder. Indirect immunofluorescent studies [239] showed the presence of an anti-IgG factor in 46 per cent of Waaler–Rose-negative patients, but the correlation with the results of the rheumatoid rosette test was not convincing (42 per cent positivity). The hypothesis has been proposed [487] that the decrease in cyclic AMP activity in the psoriatic epidermis would involve immunological disorders either directly by blocking the β-adrenergic receptors, which have an immunological adjuvant effect, or act indirectly by modifying skin antigenicity.

As to the behaviour of psoriatic and normal skin transplants, it was believed that the psoriatic autograft would retain its characteristics in the normal skin, but the normal skin transplant would become psoriatic. However, according to recent investigations [245] autografts in psoriatics lose their psoriatic features. Perhaps the fate of the transplant is essentially influenced by the actual activity of the disease before the transplant is innervated [245]. From the aspect of transplant immunity it seems to be of importance that 80 per cent of the skin autografts to psoriatic skin (psoriatic plaque to psoriatic plaque) are rejected, especially if they first set. Perhaps the high O_2 requirement of the psoriatic epidermis plays a part in this phenomenon. Successive autografts are partially (2nd set) or totally (3rd and 4th set) accepted, suggesting the possibility of a desensitizing effect [261*a*]. Grafting was generally followed by clinical improvement [261*a*].

Some defect of the immune system has also been searched for [77]. Familial cumulation seems to support the role of some genetic factor [391*a*]. However, the fact that not all monozygotic twin pairs are concordant concerning the occurrence of psoriasis indicates that also environmental factors are of importance [122*a*]. Multifactorial mode of inheritance for psoriasis implies a polygenic mechanism. If an individual has the necessary quantity of genetic factors, he is prone to develop psoriasis. Once this liability is present, environmental factors will determine the manifestation of the disease. Of the histocompatibility antigens HL-A13 and W17 have been found predominating in psoriatics. It seems therefore reasonable to conclude that there is no convincing evidence for the immunopathological genesis of psoriasis vulgaris [391*b*].

Nevertheless, it has repeatedly been proposed [134, 384*a*] that complicated forms of psoriasis, e. g. arthritis psoriatica, pustular psoriasis, erythroderma psoriaticum, may arise on an immunological basis. Psoriasis vulgaris is characterized by a mild myopathic tissue syndrome, while in arthritis psoriatica, the so-called mesenchymal maximal variant of psoriasis [275*a*], especially in severe cases, the lymphocytic-histiocytic reaction extends and thus damages the muscle fibres secondarily. Consequently, the cross-striation changes or disappears, the sarcolemma becomes hyperplasic, the fibres hyalinize or even undergo atrophy. Thus, the histological and electron-microscopic picture (thickening of the BM and muscle-fibre changes in muscle capillaries) is consistent with the electro-myographic findings and the presence of anti-muscle antibodies demonstrable by the anti-human globulin consumption test [550*a*]. Since high-titre anti-nuclear factor was not found by specific immunofluorescent techniques [550*a*] it has been concluded that, in addition to the anti-nuclear factor, other components co-operate in the positivity of the loose-body test and the anti-human globulin consumption test.

The rheumatoid factor is absent in the serum of patients with arthritis psoriatica. A reduced IgM level was found in 11 per cent of cases with arthritis psoriatica by Mancini's radial immunodiffusion test [576]. High anti-IgG levels were demonstrated in the serum of some patients with psoriatic arthritis [278] as compared to the moderate serum levels in patients with uncomplicated psoriasis. Subcutaneous immunization with a brucella antigen induced much higher antibody titres in patients with arthritis psoriatica than in normal subjects or in patients with psoriasis vulgaris [550*a*]. A statistical analysis of the curve for the anti-human globulin consumption test of Steffens has been suggestive of the presence of anti-skin autoantibodies in arthritis psoriatica, but not in psoriasis vulgaris [550*a*]. In arthritis psoriatica 10–25 per cent spontaneous transformation was observed in the lymphocyte transformation test [550*a*]. The immunoadherence test is positive (the rosette formation indicating an anti-IgG activity of lymphocytes) [487*a*, 533], but the pathogenetical importance of this finding is doubtful. According to Hénocq [261*a*], the human arthritis psoriatica disease has common features (inflammatory lesions in joints and periarticular tissues) with experimental adjuvant arthritis in rats (chronic lesions induced by injection of Freund's complete adjuvant without added antigen). The majority of the authors consider arthritis psoriatica and the concomitant immune processes essentially independent phenomena, but their interaction cannot be excluded.

ORAL LEUKOPLAKIA

On the oral mucosa, there may be small to extensive, well-defined, white patches like drops of candle-wax. In the histological picture hyperorthokeratosis or hyperparakeratosis and occasionally acanthosis are characteristic findings. In about 15 per cent of the cases epithelial atypia was observed. The incidence of malignant change was 4–6 per cent.

Leukoplakia may be regarded [468*a*] as a somewhat variable and non-specific response of the oral mucosa to external stimuli (e.g. tobacco smoking, snuff, hot or spiced foods, mechanical irritation, *Candida albicans* invasion) but it is often influenced by the pre-existing state of the mucosa and its underlying connective tissue stroma.

Recently 5 out of 11 patients with oral leukoplakia showed inhibition of migration with leukoplakial tissue and one showed inhibition with normal mucosa [494*a*]. It is assumed that oral leukoplakia is associated with a state of tissue-specific cell-mediated immunity against antigenic components of the leukoplakial tissue.

SUBSEPSIS ALLERGICA OF WISSLER–FANCONI IN ADULTS

Clinical characteristics of this disease are intermittent fever, transient, mainly polymorphic exanthems, morbilli-, scarlatini- and urticariform phenomena, polycyclic annular nodose erythemas, purpurae, migrating arthralgias, slightly swollen painful joints, subcutaneous nodules with swelling of the surrounding tissues, and neutrophil leukocytosis, occasionally leukaemoid in character [403*a*]. It is often associated with eosinophilia. The aetiology of the disease is unknown. Its first or recurrent appearance may be preceded by infection (most frequently staphylococcus, meningococcus or pneumococcus), but the haemoculture is negative and the course of the illness resists antibiotic therapy.

The disease seems to be of allergic origin [403*a*], but the antigen is unknown and no antibody or autoantibody could be made responsible. Occasionally, it turns into rheumatoid arthritis and in its therapy corticosteroids are the drugs of choice. The symptoms are partly of infective-septic character (in most cases leukocytosis with a shift to the left, accelerated erythrocyte sedimentation, and splenomegalia), partly allergic (transient chameleon exanthems, eosinophilia, raised γ and α_2 globulin levels). It has been proposed to classify the disease into the group of non-differentiated autoimmune diseases [454*a*]; occasionally the latex T, the Waaler–Rose test, the L agglutination, the anti-human globulin consumption test, the loose body test and the LE cell phenomenon may be positive.

HERPES SIMPLEX VIRUS INFECTION

Herpes simplex virus (*Herpesvirus hominis*; HVH) has two serotypes, viz. type 1, the common causative agent of labial herpes, gingivostomatitis and kerato-conjunctivitis herpetica, and type 2 which causes vulvovaginitis, cervicitis and gluteal and preputial herpes. The clinical manifestation is determined by the site of entry of the virus and the actual immune status of the host. The primary infection occurs in 99 per cent in the first five years of the life, usually soon after the protection provided by maternal immunity has become unsatisfactory. Occasionally, in about 1 per cent the primary infection is accompanied by heavy viraemia and fever. HVH type 1 antibodies could be demonstrated in a population study in Atalanta in 30–50 per cent among the groups of population with higher living standards and in 80–100 per cent among those living in less favourable conditions [426*a*]. For type 2 the frequency was 10 per cent vs 20–60 per cent for type 1. About one-third of the world population is supposed to be infected with type 1 virus.

The primary infection is followed by an antibody response. From the diagnostic point of view the neutralizing and the C-fixing antibodies are of importance. C-fixing antibodies are formed to both virion-fixed (V) and soluble (S) antigens. The anti-V titre is usually more persistent than the anti-S titre [377*b*]. HVH type 2 antibody was demonstrated in the serum of genital herpes cases of less than 5 days' standing in 44 per cent using C-fixation and in 57 per cent using immunofluorescent antibody technique [363*a*].

HVH, being able to spread in the organism from cell to cell may persist despite the presence of neutralizing antibodies in the serum. This has been proved recently by isolating HVH types 1 and 2 from trigeminal [175*b*] and sacral ganglia and even from unselected cadavers [25*a*].

Recurrences, due to the persistent virus, occur in predisposed subjects as more or less circumscribed phenomena. The mechanism of the recurrences is still unclear. Considering the severe manifestations in immunosuppressed patients, predisposing factors of immunological nature must be assumed. It has been suggested [377*b*] that a decline in the anti-S C-fixation titre of the serum may be a forerunner of recurrence. On the other hand, comparative studies (lymphocyte transformation test, C-fixation and skin tests) with sera from patients suffering from, and those without history of, chronic recurrent herpes simplex have shown that the lack or deficiency of cell-mediated immunity cannot be an essential predisposing factor [503*c*].

Recurrent genital herpes seems to be of special importance in women, for HVH antigens have been demonstrated by immunofluorescent techniques in exfoliated cells of cervical carcinoma [498*a*]. Attempts to prove a correlation between HVH type 2 seropositivity and cancer of the uterine cervix and vulva led to equivocal results [94*a*, 483*a*, 503*e*]. Hamster fibroblasts exposed *in vitro* to HVH partially inactivated with UV irradiation developed transformed foci. Cells from these foci proved to be oncogenic in newborn hamsters [160*b*]. Experimental infection of rats with consequent tumour formation has also been reported.

HVH-infected cells are susceptible to the immune cytotoxic effect of human anti-HVH sera [627*a*] as demonstrated by the loss of ability of HVH-infected cells to attach to plastic cell-culture plates after reaction in suspension with anti-HVH serum in the presence of C. Human serum without neutralizing antibody to HVH showed no cytotoxic effect against HVH-infected cells.

Local virostatic drugs such as 5-iodo-2'-deoxyuridine (IdU) adamantinamine derivatives (tromantadine) and cytosine arabinoside [184*a*] are used for therapy [175*a*]. Application of IdU in ointment on skin lesions failed to yield uniform results, but in a controlled trial in which small paintbrushes were used for the local application of a 5 per cent solution of IdU, the duration of the IdU-treated recurrences was significantly reduced [382*a*]. To stimulate the defence mechanism of the organism, HVH antigen was administered in a form of inactivated virus vaccine. After repeated vaccinations the interval between recurrences has prolonged and, later on, only a forme fruste developed; a few patients became free of recurrences. The reduction in recurrences was 77 per cent [175*b*].

HERPES ZOSTER INFECTION

Epidemiological and clinical experience has suggested and virological experiments have proved that varicella and herpes zoster are caused by the same virus, i.e. the varicella-zoster (VZ virus) (*herpes-virus varicellae*). The primary infection occurs in most subjects in the first 8 to 10 years of the life, probably through the respiratory and/or alimentary tract. About 30 per cent of the primary infections are subclinical.

The infection is followed by a long-lasting immunity while the virus may persist in a latent form. During latency the virus may be reactivated when the immunity falls below a threshold level. This may occur in old age or during an intercurrent illness, e.g. various fevers, tumour, leukaemia, or owing to cytostatic or corticosteroid therapy. Reactivation of virus may manifest itself in clinical herpes zoster. Thus, herpes zoster is an immunologically modified varicella. This is supported by the course of the different clinical pictures and the dynamics of the C-fixing and platelet agglutinating antibody titres to VZ virus antigens [549*b*, *c*]. In patients with herpes zoster both of these titres were found to be at high or moderate levels [443*a*]. Those suffering from uncomplicated varicella developed C-fixing antibodies, but no demonstrable antibodies aggregating platelets. In post-varicella encephalitis antibodies were produced that were detectable by both tests. Of serum samples collected from healthy medical students 15 to 31 per cent reacted in the platelet aggregation test and only 4 per cent in the C-fixation test. If the residual immunity is sufficiently high, herpes zoster remains localized and its course is usually mild. In such cases the antibody titres rise, sometimes very rapidly, the infection does not generalize and further recurrences are extremely rare [276a]. In contrast, in patients with insufficient antibody response and poor non-specific defence herpes zoster may generalize and take a gangrenous form [396a]. The protective effect of the immunity is supported by a case of unilateral trigeminal zoster in which necrosis with axon and myelin destruction was found in both Gasser ganglia [191a].

Cell-mediated immunity to VZ antigen was assessed by lymphocyte transformation test in patients with acute HZ infection [503d]. There was a significant diminution in cell-mediated immunity to this antigen, but no definite difference in the response to PHA and PPD.

Painting with 5-iodo-2'-deoxyuridine is applied as local therapy. Systemic administration of antineuritic drugs and/or interferonogenic virus preparations may shorten the course of the disease. Gamma-globulin is ineffective when vesicles are already present. Corticosteroid therapy should be limited to the treatment of post-zoster neuralgia. Even the presence of aberrate vesicles contraindicates corticosteroid therapy. Dihydroergotamine, X-irradiation of the ganglia or ganglion blockade may be considered.

In malignancy or immune deficiency, convalescent zoster plasma or zoster immune globulin should be given within 72 h after exposure to VZ virus. This may be supplemented with cytosine arabinoside infusion for several days [418a].

SKIN TUMOUR IMMUNITY IN MAN

Tumour immunity has been reviewed in detail recently in numerous excellent papers [24a, 115, 228, 241, 256a, 259b, 320, 321, 322, 426b, 549, 559, 585]. In this chapter only some important concepts will be outlined.

Cells may acquire new antigens (neoantigens) during neoplastic transformation. These may be localized in the tumour cell nucleus, cytoplasm or cell membrane. Tumour-associated antigen (TAA) is a broad term comprising all neoantigens present in or on the neoplastic cell. Surface-membrane antigens are of importance for growth control as they may elicit transplantation immune responses in genetically compatible (isogeneic) hosts, ultimately leading to rejection. Cell-surface TAAs are, therefore, called tumour-associated transplantation antigens (TATA). The presence of TATA has been demonstrated in a large number of animal tumours induced by viral or chemical carcinogens as well as in spontaneously occurring tumours. Different tumours induced by the same virus show antigenic uniformity or extensive cross-reactivity, whereas the TATA of chemically induced and spontaneous tumours usually do not cross-react, they are individually distinctive. Apart from this type of TATA, many tumours bear some foetal antigens. The classic concept of the 'autonomous tumour cell' is slowly being replaced by the theory of a dynamic host–tumour interaction.

Since tumours are foreign to the organism, they elicit an immunological response in the host. An immunological basis is supported by clinical observations, such as (*i*) the spontaneous regression, either of the primary tumour or of metastases after removal of the former; (*ii*) the survival of patients despite circulating tumour cells at the time of surgery; (*iii*) survival for prolonged periods in spite of incomplete removal of the primary tumour; (*iv*) an increased incidence of neoplasia in immunosuppressed and immunodeficient patients; (*v*) the presence of tumour at autopsy in patients without any clinical evidence of tumour; (*vi*) the wide individual variation within the same type of tumour.

Many experimental data suggest that immune T lymphocytes (killer cells) are of primary importance in the defence mechanism against tumours. B lymphocytes concerned with the production of humoral antibodies are cytotoxic in the presence of C and thus may play a role in the rejection of some malignant tumours. The demonstration of cell-mediated immunity against tumour antigens is based on tissue culture systems such as cytotoxicity and colony-inhibition tests whereas C fixation, gel diffusion, immunofluorescence and mixed-cell agglutination tests serve for the demonstration of serum antibodies. The sensitive serological techniques have at least three implications: (*i*) they may give aetiological clues or (*ii*) facilitate the establishing of an immunological diagnosis and (*iii*) immunological approaches to tumour therapy. In general, high antibody titres correlate to remission of the disease while low or no titres have been found in relapses. Skin reactions to autologous tumour extracts were found positive when the tumour was localized or when a remission had been induced, whereas they were found negative when the tumour was widespread or recurrent. Indirect membrane immunofluorescent tests with live tumour cells in suspension, e.g. cells treated with mouse antibody to surface antigens and subsequently with conjugated anti-mouse globulin serum, resulted in a dotted or ring-shaped membrane fluorescence. In some tumours, e.g. testicular seminomas, a positive correlation has been found between the prognosis and the degree of lymphocyte infiltration in the tumour tissue. There is little doubt that immunosuppression may sometimes facilitate the growth of malignant tumours. In such cases interruption of therapy resulted in disappearance of the tumour. An increase in neoplasia may be due to lack of immunological surveillance.

Although humoral mechanisms may play some part in tumour destruction, most evidence suggests that tumours are killed primarily via the cell-mediated immunity. However, the reason why tumours grow in face of cell-mediated immune reaction is strongly disputed. The current hypotheses suggest (*i*) specific immunological tolerance to the TATA; (*ii*) 'immunological enhancement', i.e. the cytotoxic effect of immune lymphocytes is blocked by humoral antibodies, leading to an enhanced tumour growth. The blocking factors involved in the enhancement behave like IgG gel filtration and there is some evidence that they represent antigen–antibody complexes. Certain sera contain an 'unblocking' factor capable of counteracting the blocking serum activity. Such sera have been shown to have an anti-tumour therapeutic effect *in vivo*. (*iii*) 'Sneaking through' refers to the hypothesis that a tumour may grow so fast that it reaches a size preventing cytotoxic reactions until an adequate response has developed. (*iv*) Tumours may be protected by substances, e.g. sialomucins, α-2-globulins, which non-specifically coat the tumour cells. (*v*) A tumour cell population may be subject to immunoselection so that only the least antigenic cells are allowed growing (antigenic deletion). (*vi*) Contrary to this, according to an immunostimulation theory, an immune reaction may at times produce more intensive tumour growth than would occur in the total absence of immune responsiveness.

The demonstration of humoral antibodies in cell-mediated immunity may have some prognostic value, but is of little importance as regards the diagnosis, and at present highly inferior to conventional diagnostic procedures.

Many facts indicate that the development of some cutaneous malignant tumours is modified by immune responses [175]. Spontaneous regression might have an immunological basis, especially in patients who received an incomplete or insufficient treatment [322]. The fate of patients may be essentially influenced by their immune responses [322]. In many, if not all, of the major human tumours the early relapses may be due to the outgrowth of immunoresistant cell variants, insensitive to, or protected by, antibody. Biopsied tumour cells derived from early relapses are frequently coated by IgG, demonstrable by direct immunofluorescence [322]. Late relapses may be due to new induction events or to regrowth of the long-dormant tumour cell clone, owing to a temporary and/or local weakening of host defence [322].

The existence of immunological surveillance on tumours is supported by the increased incidence of lymphomas in patients with hypogammaglobulinaemia [409], the development of malignancies and dysplastic cells in many tissues following prolonged immunosuppressive treatment [181], the association of autoimmune haemolytic anaemia and lymphoma in man [409] and NZB mice, and the behaviour of malignant cells unwittingly transferred with renal homografts [620].

The pathogenesis of skin tumours is not discussed in this chapter, but the principles of a possible immunotherapy are outlined. The practical problems of immunological intervention are related to the complexities of the tumour–host relation [547]. Unfortunately, the factors playing a role in these complex relations are poorly understood. Immunotherapy of tumours may require both the enhancement of a specific response and a means of making tumour cells accessible as early as possible [518*b*]. The major role of immunotherapy seems to reduce the possibility of recurrences and metastases rather than the eradication of large numbers of tumour cells [322].

The afferent lymphatics and regional lymph nodes, although important for early recognition of tumour-specific transplantation antigens, are not necessary for the eventual development of tumour-specific immunity [137*a*]. The removal of the local lymphatics once a tumour has reached a clinically detectable size would not adversely affect the host's ability to mount an immune response to the tumour since a systemic tumour-specific sensitization has already ensued.

The term immunotherapy of human malignancies refers to initiation or augmentation of an immunological reaction against tumour antigens [448]. Four types of interventions are used [24*a*]: (*i*) Adjuvant immunotherapy. Non-specific stimulation of the reticuloendothelial system by injection of foreign materials has been shown to enhance immune responsiveness in patients, and has caused increased immunological resistance to transplanted animal tumours. Remissions in malignant diseases have been associated with intercurrent bacterial infections. (*ii*) Active immunotherapy. The most promising results in the prevention and treatment of animal tumours come from studies in which active immunotherapy has been induced to tumour cells or viruses. (*iii*) Adoptive immunotherapy. Exogenous immunologically competent cells have in the case of animal tumours largely been shown to retard rather than prevent growth of tumours. This is, therefore, a less successful tool than active or adjuvant therapy. (*iv*) Passive immunotherapy. Immunotherapy with passively transferred antisera has met with variable success in different systems but, in general, has been successful only in preventing the take of a small inoculum of cells.

Patients to be treated are sensitized by local application to normal skin of BCG vaccine or other non-specific immunological stimulant (primary phase) and 'challenged' (secondary phase) by administration of the antigen directly to the malignant lesion or its vicinity. The non-specific stimulation potentiates the cytotoxicity of lymphocytes that are specifically immunoactive against tumour cells. The more intense the reaction at the tumour site as compared to normal skin, the greater is the likelihood of successful therapy. If the patient is unable to develop cell-mediated immunity to BCG vaccine, a battery of other antigens, e.g. diphtheria toxoid, *Candida albicans*, PPD, vaccinia virus, mumps vaccine, trichophytin, streptokinase-streptodornase, *Corynebacterium parvum*, can be used in the hope that, singly or in combination, they would activate the dormant immune 'memory' of lymphocytes sensitized by a previous exposure. It should be noted [53*b*] that, (*i*) owing to the great variability of the techniques used for skin testing, the interpretation of the skin responses is uncertain; (*ii*) sensitization may carry some risk for the patients, for cross-reactivity may develop to chemically related substances; (*iii*) a decreased responsiveness over 50 years of age might be attributed to an alteration of the permeability or other physicochemical properties of the skin.

Initial indications were that immunostimulant therapy was relatively free of side-effects, but with increasing experience major and minor problems have been encountered with BCG. Many patients have fever, which may be high and associated with rigors, lassitude, nausea, and anorexia [166*d*, 551*a*]. Other toxic effects (rash, lymphopenia, leukopenia) have been reported even when a clinically significant BCG infection could not be identified [427]. Usually these symptoms are short-lived, but they may persist and confine the patient to bed. Injections of tumour cells and BCG can cause severe and persistent local skin necrosis, ulceration with a continuing purulent discharge which contains living mycobacteria [229*a*]. Major problems are presented by granulomatous hepatitis [58*a*], mycobacterial pneumonia [229*a*], disseminated lung granulomas [166*d*], and splenomegaly. These granulomatous lesions are not just hypersensitivity reactions; they result from spread of BCG organisms through the blood stream. In case of intracutaneous administration development of blocking serum activity is thought to be possible [62], but this can be avoided by using the nodule-scarification method. Though such dissemination of organisms may provide an excellent stimulant to the immune system, granulomatous disease can give rise to severe liver and lung dysfunction, and patients receiving BCG must be watched closely for these. Fortunately the lesions respond well to conventional antituberculous therapy, which should be applied promptly.

With the aim of inducing localized hypersensitivity reactions at the site of skin tumours Eva Klein and her group [260*a*, 319*c*, *d*, *e*, 320*a*] have applied topical chemical sensitizers, usually DNCB, to skin tumour sites. Challenging doses caused more intense reaction in cutaneous neoplasms than in adjacent normal skin and daily topical application often caused tumours to regress completely. Regressions of accessible lesions vary from partial to complete and last from several months to more than 5 years. Combination of immunotherapy with other treatment modalities resulted in augmentation of antitumour effects. Antitumour activities of challenge reactions are selective for tumour cells and appear to be independent of the types of antigens used or the types of malignant neoplasms. Non-cellular mediators derived from lymphocytes and monocytes induce antitumour activities that may be significant in the regressions of neoplasms induced by cell-mediated challenge reactions.

In the current enthusiasm for non-specific immune stimulants, other approaches, such as administration of transfer factor, of immune RNA, or of chemotherapeutic agents bound to tumour-directed antibodies, should not be forgotten [212*c*].

Nevertheless these investigations and other similar ones listed by the International Registry of Tumor Immunochemotherapy were of short duration, and confirmation of the efficacy of immunochemotherapy must await longer follow-up [288*a*]. According to Baker and Taub [24*a*], the clinical trials of immunotherapy have yielded limited information on tumour antigens and host responses but there has been little success in causing regression of malignant disease. It has been limited to prolongation of duration of remissions but these studies have generally suffered from lack of controls.

KERATO-ACANTHOMA (KA)

This rapidly evolving benign tumour is mainly situated on exposed areas of the skin (Fig. 40-19); it is composed of keratinizing squamous cells originating in pilosebaceous follicles and resolving spontaneously within 6 to 12 months even

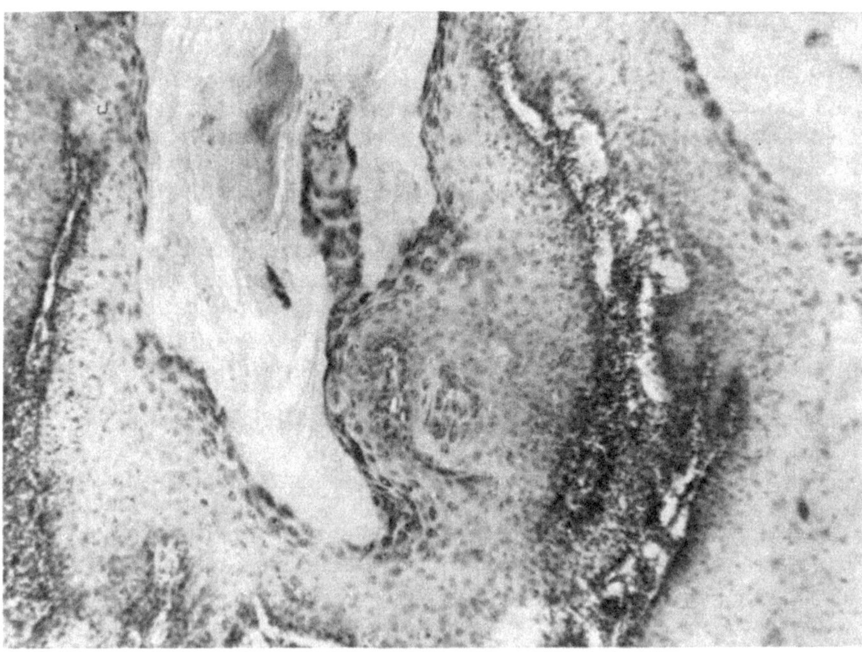

Fig. 40-19. Kerato-acanthoma. Proliferating epidermis surrounding the central horny cone; on the right, inflammatory reaction in the corium. Initial stage. $\times 20$ (Courtesy of Professor L. Szodoray, Debrecen)

if untreated. The patients display delayed-type skin hypersensitivity to antigens prepared from ground KA tumour [430]. Using antigens prepared by Behçetin's method [389], the skin reaction of patients with an extensive KA lesion positively correlates with the extent of the KA lesion. The reaction is mainly of delayed type. The positive skin test is useful in differentiating KA from basal cell epithelioma.

By immunofluorescent techniques, *in vivo* fixation of IgG, IgM and C3 was demonstrable in areas of tumour adjacent to the dermis or in necrotizing tumour tissue [71]. In some areas, immunoglobulin and C were deposited in intercellular spaces of tumour tissue. Fibrinogen-fibrin deposits were also present, but did not correspond to the immunoglobulin and C deposits. The characteristics of immunoglobulin and C fixation in KA suggest that immunologically mediated mechanisms might participate in the spontaneous resolution of the disease. Association of multiple KA with deficiency of cell-mediated immunity (as shown by the intracutaneous test, artificial sensitization with DNFB and LTT) has been reported [582]. Differentiating between KA and squamous cell carcinoma is sometimes difficult [229]. In KA eosinophils are common, micro-abscess may occur and glycogen is prominent in cells. All these are usually negative in squamous cell carcinoma.

SQUAMOUS CELL CARCINOMA

In this disease an 'epidermal cell-surface antigen' is demonstrable by immunofluorescence [303]. Using the indirect method in malignant and benign tumours with PV or BP sera as markers to locate the antigens, a reduced fluorescence was shown and the degree of reduction depended on the type of the antigen and the degree and duration of the infiltration [464]. Supposedly, the antigen is definitely lost as the cells become involved or, as an alternative explanation, the antigen undergoes a change sufficient to become unrecognizable by the antibody. It is possible that the loss of the 'pemphigus antigen' reported in squamous cell carcinoma may reflect a decreased cellular cohesion and hence increased capacity for tissue invasion [420].

In a study of skin carcinomas, complete regression of lesions was noted in 9–25 per cent of cases with BCG adjuvant therapy [243*a*]. The response of squamous cell carcinomas of the head and neck to a combination of BCG plus methotrexate and isoniazid appeared to be superior to the results achieved with methotrexate alone [159*d*]. Fifty patients with superficial basal cell carcinomas and squamous cell carcinomas in situ were treated with DNCB sensitization and followed up for 5 years without recurrence [319*e*]. Others [557*a*] also confirmed the success of DNCB treatment in basal cell carcinoma, granuloma fungoides, lymphoma metastatic to the skin and carcinoma of the breast metastatic to the skin as well. On the effect of allergic delayed-type inflammation, the tumour (e.g. basal cell carcinoma) decomposes, and the lesion heals with cicatrices [470]. This therapy is recommended with multiple lesions as well as with marginal recurrences after surgical and X-ray therapy. Recurrences have ben reported. Topical application of DNCB on basal cell carcinomas caused complete regression in 32 per cent and partial regression in 29 per cent, but croton oil, a primary irritant that induces inflammation without evidence of cell-mediated immunity also caused complete regression in 23 per cent of the tumours treated [377*a*].

As regards its rise, extension, regression and therapeutic possibilities MM is now in the focus of the interest of immunologists. This, usually malignant, tumour develops from pigment-producing melanocytes, often from pigmented naevi or pigmented moles [518*a*]. It may be variable in course and independent of sex, age, location, extent, histological picture and the pigmentation of the primary tumour. It has been suggested that MM might occur as a secondary deposit in regional lymph nodes where the primary tumour has regressed [141, 375, 442]. Occasionally MM regresses partially or completely, without any specific treatment [173]. In this case spontaneous regression does not mean complete recovery. Its occasional regression has raised the possibility that MM might be controlled by an immune mechanism.

Owing to the high percentage of false negative (50 per cent) and false positive (20 per cent) results [441], the available immunological methods are of little value in the diagnostics of MM. Most information may be derived from following the dynamics of the patient's immunological status. In the therapy of MM, on the other hand, an exploitation of the immunological possibility is promising.

Melanoma (M) antigen. In serum samples from MM patients antibodies against two large groups of tissue type-specific antigens of MM cells have been detected: (*i*) a group of cell membrane antigens of the transplantation type, apparently corresponding to the tumour-associated transplantation antigens (TATA) [323, 413, 416, 463*b*]. According to indirect immunofluorescent studies, the existence of a common and of an individually variable tumour antigen may be assumed [49]. The patient-specific antibody directed against the individual cell-membrane antigen can be determined by cross-absorption, immunofluorescence and immunodiffusion techniques in which different cell suspensions and their autologous positive sera are used [376]. (*ii*) A group of cytoplasmic antigens, present in the cytoplasm of snapfrozen M cell smear preparations and short-term cultures of M cells. These antigens appear to be more constant than the membrane antigens [63]. The antibodies to the cytoplasmic antigens are disease- and partly individual-specific [426*b*]; cross-reaction has only been observed with pathological cells from patients with the halo naevus syndrome [372*c*]. The cytoplasmic M antigens are able to elicit both humoral and cell-mediated responses. Further research is necessary to reveal their exact nature.

Immediate-type antibody-mediated reactivity in MM. The immediate-type reaction of patients with MM has been studied sporadically by injecting autologous MM material intracutaneously [137]. Positive results have been reported in the majority of the cases. If a tumour polysaccharide complex was injected together with the autologous serum, positive reaction was obtained in all the non-metastatic patients, in 60 per cent of those with metastasis and in 12 per cent of control subjects.

Circulating humoral antibodies have been found in the sera of some patients against their own tumour cells [463*a*, 465], even in the far exhausted stages of the disease [285*a*]. Immune response can be induced by human MM in rabbits [189, 225, 539]. The antibodies thus produced react with an antigen common to most human cases. However, in a few experiments the anti-M-cell rabbit antibodies failed to give the indirect immunofluorescence reaction with MM cells [539].

In other cases fluorescence appeared on the cell membrane in the absence, and in the cytoplasm in the presence, of C [189]. In the course of further experiments [225] antisera absorbed with a variety of normal tissues reacted strongly in immunofluorescent tests with most of the M cells tested in tissue sections. All antisera reacted with cells of four pigment-producing cultured M cell lines [225]. Absorption with whole M cells completely removed the activity against M cells [225]. The reaction was unrelated to melanin and was negative against benign mole and the other tumour cells tested. It should be noted that the same antiserum was not cytotoxic for the four cultured M-cell lines.

It is questionable whether patients' sera exert any influence on the growth of human or animal MM tissue cultures [410].

The cytotoxicity of serum M antibodies was examined in slide cultures of tumour cells by phase-contrast microscopy in comparison with the vitality of the tumour cells as examined by the trypan blue exclusion test. In one-third of the cases there was an agreement between the cytotoxicity, the result of the immunofluorescence test and the C dependent inhibition of the RNA synthesis [374]. The C dependent cytotoxicity test is frequently applied [153, 372*a*, 477] when the integrity of tumour cells is to be examined [100].

A variety of immunodiffusion and immunoelectrophoretic methods have been used for demonstrating humoral antibodies [325*a*, 377], but the results are inconsistent [410].

A decrease in the serum C level in the course of the illness is considered a sign of progression. This is not the result of a non-specific immunodepression, but reminds of an absorption of the continuously produced antibodies by the extending tumour ('sponge effect' of Klein).

The first immunofluorescent studies yielded negative results. Attempts to demonstrate antibodies on M cells by the direct method have failed [330]. The indirect test was also negative with autologous serum [330]. Other investigators [175] observed M cell membrane and cytoplasmic fluorescence in one-third of the non-metastatic MM cases. The indirect membrane fluorescence with autologous serum was positive in 100 per cent, with allogeneic sera in 80 per cent [150]. Bickhardt and Kunze [49] observed membrane fluorescence with the indirect test using sera from patients with MM and cultured M cells. Forty-seven per cent of the sera reacted with at least one cell line. To exclude intravital antibody deposition in the tissue, Oettgen et al. [433] applied M cells obtained from suspended cultures. They observed specifically absorbable membrane or ring-shaped fluorescence in 61 per cent of the MM sera tested. Lewis et al. [374] found individual-specific antibodies in 80 per cent of non-metastatic MM patients. Cytoplasmic fluorescence was obtained with homologous serum in fixed preparations. Bourgoin et al. [64], using an indirect immunofluorescent technique and autologous serum, succeeded in demonstrating immunoglobulins on the surface of human M cells at the stage of metastatic dissemination. These antibodies were not observed on tumour cells during local and regional invasion. This technique has been used by most of the authors examining humoral immunity in MM [63, 374, 416, 422, 465].

The radioimmunoassay [286] is suitable for measuring M antibodies and a simultaneous identification of their immunoglobulin class and, also for demonstrating circulating antibodies [83, 84].

Tumour-specific humoral immunity was demonstrable by at least one serological method in about the half of the patients tested [532]. The antibodies considerably influence the localization and rate of growth of metastases. Humoral tumour-specific antibodies have been detected by blocking and absorption studies only in patients with early or localized tumour [372*a*, 374, 375, 465]. In the case of localized MM, or MM with little tendency to spread, the cytotoxic antibodies, owing to their IgM nature, are able to inhibit the haematogenic spread of the tumour, but they do not influence the growth of solid tumours and the dissemination via the lymphatics. The disappearance of the immunoglobulins of antibodies with anti-M activity in the course of the disease is considered a consequence of some change in the tumour antigenicity or in the responsiveness of the patient. The loss of antibodies is associated with tumour spread via the blood stream [372*b*]. The basic properties of the anti-human-MM antibodies are still uncertain [410]. The individual specificity of the cell membrane antibodies does not exclude cross-reactions. Their immunological profile is unknown and it is questionable whether they are able to form immune complexes.

Delayed-type reactivity in MM. The possibility of immune reactions by patients against their MM has been raised as early as in 1907, when Handly described round-cell infiltrates around melanomas. The cellular stromal reaction in MM has been investigated by enzyme-cytochemical techniques [80]. The stromal cellular reaction in the tumour zone has been found variable in consistence and intensity. Parallel with the progression of the tumour depth, the lymphocytic-plasmacytic infiltration decreased in thickness. There are no plasma cells and lymphocytes in the cutaneous metastases. During the spontaneous regression of MM there is a correlation between the immunological findings and the histomorphological picture [285*c*]. The stages of regression and progression are reflected by the numbers of cytotoxic small lymphocytes, plasmacytes and macrophages, in accordance with the presence or disappearance of the cytotoxic antibodies in the serum. The intracutaneous test performed with autologous extracts of MM cells was found to be positive during spontaneous regression of the localized tumour, suggesting that the active cell-mediated immunity may lead to regression [178]. Patients with suppressed delayed hypersensitivity have developed increased number of spontaneous tumours and transplanted tumours have grown in immunosuppressed recipients [207]. The so-called general delayed-type reactivity has been examined by DNCB sensitization and intracutaneous and contact challenge. Both this and the lymphocyte transformation test were positive in each of the following groups: (*i*) patients with non-metastatic long-persisting MM; (*ii*) primary tumour of short history with metastasis; (*iii*) metastasizing MM without demonstrable primary tumour [628]. Others [54, 166*c*] succeeded in sensitizing with DNCB 95–98 per cent of tumour-free patients, but only 60–76 per cent of patients with MM. In a further study 62 per cent of the patients with MM could not be sensitized [296]. The delayed-type reactivity to bacterial and fungal antigens remained positive in the tested patients [610].

Some authors [178] failed to obtain positive delayed-type cutaneous reaction with autologous M materials in patients with metastatic MM. Others [55] reported 11 positive and 5 negative reactions, but 6 of 9 positive cases gave positive reaction to the extract of the autologous intact skin as well. Further authors [467], working with autologous tumour-cell extracts, obtained positive cutaneous delayed-type reaction in 16 per cent of tumour-bearing patients.

The mixed lymphocyte tumour cell culture (MLTC) test performed with autologous tumour cells was found negative at the time of the extirpation but it yielded positive results during chemo- or radiotherapeutic periods [426]. Before surgical removal of the MM all patients showed considerable cell-mediated immunity [386]. In the immediate postoperative period all such activity was lost, but returned in most of the patients between the 4th and 22nd postoperative days. The possible mediators of the depression of cell-mediated immunity might be an increased output of adrenal steroids in response to the stress of surgery or to the anaesthetic agents used (e.g. halothane).

As to the cellular microtoxicity assay, a specific lethal effect of peripheral lymphocytes was found in 7 of 12 MM cases when tested with autologous M cells and in 14 of 19 tests performed with allogeneic combinations [150].

Using the colony inhibition technique in dilute agar gel [260], cytotoxicity was observed, which was, however, independent of the clinical status and not individual specific.

In short-term mixed cultures of autologous M cells and lymphocytes [568] damages were only observed if the ratio of lymphocytes to M cells was over 300 : 1. Only 3 of 22 patients in the 2nd or 3rd clinical stage of MM had cytotoxic lymphocytes, i.e. in these cases more than half of the M cells died as evidenced electron-optically [136].

Cell- (and antibody-) mediated immunity was also studied by labelling tumour cells with ^{51}Cr [73]. The trypan-blue exclusion test, too, indicated immunocyte-mediated tumour immunity [178].

Inhibition of M cell viability with lymphocytes from normal donors as compared with growth in medium alone was found in 46 per cent; in 13 per cent stimulation was observed [262]. The results were independent of the ABO blood-group system. The inhibition was more pronounced when the microcytotoxicity test was applied. The viability of M cells was inhibited by lymphocytes from MM patients in 79 per cent. In this respect there was no difference whether the tumour was local, regional or had remote metastases. Similarly, the test failed to differentiate clinically active cases from inactive ones.

When PHA, tuberculin or $HgCl_2$ was used as mitogen in the lymphocyte transformation test, the transformation rate for the lymphocytes from MM patients showed no difference from the control value [611]. When autologous or homologous M cells were used as mitogen, the transformation index was found to correlate with the time that had elapsed from the onset of the disease [295]. However, a reduced stimulation index (29 vs 60) for the lymphocytes of patients with MM has also been reported [49]. The decrease became more prominent with the progression of the disease.

The production of migration inhibition factor by lymphocytes exposed to autologous tumour extracts has been studied in patients with MM [113*a*, 531*a*]. Some specificity of tumour antigenicity has been demonstrated but correlation with clinical data has not yet been presented. Lymphocyte transformation and migration inhibition tests *in vitro* showed some correlation with delayed-type skin hypersensitivity but *in vivo* this relation was not consistently demonstrable [240].

The spontaneous rosette test with T lymphocytes [49] showed a downward tendency parallel with the decrease in T lymphocytes during metastatic dissemination.

A new system for heterotransplantation which appears to augment tumour cell membrane antigenicity may be an important tool of further immunological studies [419*a*]. The observation that the HL-A5 sublocus is deleted in MM patients may provide a genetic marker in this tumour system.

A significant decrease was demonstrated in the serum lysozyme level in patients and an enhanced sensitivity of their lymphocytes to ALS produced in dogs, rats or mice [90]. On the other hand, there were no considerable differences as regards the percentage of phagocytic leukocytes, the serum C level and intraleukocytal lysozyme [90].

Immune phagocytosis of human immunoglobulin-coated M cells has been investigated *in vivo* [64]. The eluted immunoglobulin reacted with cultured M cells and induced phagocytosis in heterologous macrophages. The role of macrophages in the anti-tumour defence is disputed.

The studies on delayed-type immunity as a whole has proved the active role of immunocytes in the immunologic surveillance in MM. The degree of lymphocyte-mediated tumour immunity is higher in patients with little or no residual tumour than in those with large tumour loads [257]. In patients who showed no cell-mediated immunity (about one-third of the patients), the disease progressed until death [532]. However, in patients with MM care should be taken in the evaluation of diagnostic tests from the clinical-oncological aspect [410]. The humoral and cell-mediated immune responses should be followed parallel and in their dynamics: for instance, the ability of the patients' blood lymphocytes to destroy cultivated allogeneic or autochthonous M cells and the ability of their sera to block such a destruction [257]. Combination of specific and non-specific defence reactions should also be reckoned with.

Impairment of the immunologic surveillance in MM. Several ways of escaping immunological surveillance may be speculated on owing to such reasons as [410]: (*i*) Disturbances in the immune apparatus. The corresponding observations have been inconsistent, therefore the role of such a disturbance in MM growth seems to be unlikely. (*ii*) Immunosuppression due to the effect of oncogenic viruses which impair the function of the immune system. (*iii*) Congenital or acquired immune defects. (*iv*) Loss of tumour-specific antigenicity. Theoretically, blocking of antigenic determinants *in vivo* by substances like sialomucin is possible. (*v*) Immunological paradoxon owing to enhancement by blocking antibodies. The phenomenon of immunological enhancement has been described above. This may play a substantial role in the MM growth. The enhancing factor can be transferred passively with the serum. It is thought to consist of antigen–antibody complexes rather than of either antigen or antibody alone. The enhancement phenomenon seems to be due to an unfavourable immune response [410]. Blocking serum activity (blocking of the cytotoxic lymphocyte effect) could be detected in 30 per cent of cases with local MM, in 89 per cent of those with regional and in 80 per cent of those with far metastatic MM. As a rule, it cannot be demonstrated in patients who have become free of symptoms [256*c*, 257, 258]. In two subsequent studies blocking serum activity was demonstrated in 43 per cent and 23 per cent of the clinically inactive cases and 71 per cent and 34 per cent of the clinically active cases, respectively [262, 532]. In spite of the small differences, tests for blocking serum activity may be of practical value. It has remained obscure why blocking factors appear as late as in the 2nd and 3rd stages of the disease [410]. Encouraging attempts have been made to separate blocking factors or antigen–antibody complexes (deblocking) even *in vivo* [260]. According to Nairn [426*b*], blocking factors in serum may not operate *in vivo,* still less the serum unlocking factor. If blocking factors act on the target cells, they are unlikely to be significant in the body because of the inaccessibility of the cells of solid tumours but this would not be the case if they act centrally on the lymphoid tissues. For therapeutic purposes cell-mediated immunity should be intensified without increasing blocking serum activity [257]. (*vi*) Immunological paradoxon due to induction of tolerance. Transient or persistent specific unresponsiveness to tumour antigens or groups of antigens has been investigated in MM. Induction of high-zone tolerance by releasing large masses of MM antigen followed by a transient increase and a subsequent exponential fall in specific cytotoxic antibodies [224, 254]. (*vii*) Immunological paradoxon owing to an imbalance between the growth of MM and the defence mechanism is also possible theoretically.

Immunotherapy. Based on encouraging results of active immunization of experimental animals with MM antigens and systemic treatment of animals with non-specific (M-antigen-free) adjuvants as well as passive transfer of immunocytes or antibodies, the immunotherapy has been introduced into the treatment of MM. The recommendations of the WHO [310] seem to be competent in this respect. Effective immunological adjuvant therapy [454] has been applied by numerous authors [264, 285*a*, 410] as follows:

1. Active non-specific immunostimulation. This is aimed at a non-specific intensification of an already existing antitumour immunity or inducing of a non-specific reactivity. BCG vaccine has been shown to increase host resistance against transplantable animal tumours [437]. Clinical trials in MM have been encouraging, e.g. Bluming et al. [56] prolonged the duration of remissions (relapses did not occur for 50–59 weeks) after resection in five of six patients to whom BCG vaccine (Institut Pasteur, Paris) had been administered by dermal scarification. Intracutaneous injection of BCG (Glaxo) was much less efficient; relapses occurred from the 30th week on. The cellular reactivity was potentiated in both groups. Gutterman et al. [242] also used the scarification method and found the lyophilized vaccine (Tice) to be more effective than the fresh liquid BCG Pasteur. After resection of recurrent advanced MMs in 28 patients, these investigators immunized 19 patients with BCG Pasteur and 9 with BCG Tice. There was a significant decrease in the relapse rate and an improvement in the survival of patients treated with the latter. Patients receiving higher doses of the lyophilized BCG vaccine showed a pronounced rise in skin reactivity to a battery of antigens, thus suggesting the superiority of this as immunosuppressant. During BCG treatment 7 out of 10 negative Mantoux skin tests became positive. Immunoglobulin levels increased in 5 patients, leukocyte migration continued to be inhibited by tumour-derived materials in patients with advanced disease, and cytotoxic lymphocytes lethal to melanoma cells developed in 2 patients [229*a*]. A patient of Levy et al. [371] had lymphocytes which were highly toxic for autogeneic tumour cells; autogeneic serum did not block the cytotoxicity. Then BCG was injected into a small tumour nodule and three weeks later, in association with clinical deterioration, the lymphocytes of the patient were still cytotoxic, but his serum could block the tumour-specific lymphocyte reactivity completely. Nathanson's [427] 9 pa-

tients with intradermal metastates were treated with BCG intralesionally. Two and 5 showed complete and local regression, respectively. Conversion to positive reaction to PPD after BCG treatment was noted only in patients who had responded to the treatment. Ikonopisov [285*b*] compared the results obtained from postoperative immunotherapy with irradiated M cells with those of postoperative BCG therapy and the result obtained after the combination of both therapies. He found the continuous BCG therapy the most efficient. Patients with a single metastasis survived the radical operation and the subsequent immunization period. The patients with generalized metastases died, irrespective of immunotherapy. When MM nodules were directly injected with BCG, approximately 90 per cent of the nodules regressed [415*a*]. Moreover, 20 per cent of the uninjected nodules of these patients also regressed. Several patients were without recurrence even after 5 years. Another team [535*a*] tried a four-stage BCG therapy, consisting of intracutaneous injection of 0.1 ml, injection of the same volume directly into the tumour nodules, injection of neuraminidase-treated autochthonous tumour cells and subcutaneous injection of tumour cells plus BCG. The patients thus treated developed both cellular and humoral immune responses against both the common and the specific tumour-associated antigens. Following live BCG scarification immunotherapy, all relapse patients failed to develop delayed hypersensitivity or primary antibody response to the primary antigen keyhole limpet haemocyanin [241*b*]. In contrast, remission patients all developed delayed-type hypersensitivity and the majority developed primary antibody response to mitogens and antigens and quantitative immunoglobulin levels did not change significantly during BCG therapy and were similar in remission and relapse patients. According to other authors [175*a*], inhibition of migration was observed following oral BCG therapy when the tumour membrane antigens were derived from histologically similar tumours but not with those from unrelated tumours. Autologous serum produced complete abrogation of the response, but decreased inhibition of migration was also noted when allogeneic serum was added to the culture medium. No alteration in the reactivity of these patients' leukocytes to tumour membrane antigens was noted during the course of the disease. Baker and Taub surveyed the 82 BCG-treated cases reported in the literature and found that objective improvement occurred in 32 of these [24*a*]. Previous treatment of mice with BCG protects them against i.m. challenge with S91 melanoma, and *in vitro* BCG immune lymphocytes are cytotoxic to target cells [175*c*].

Immunotherapy with vaccinia virus has also been attempted [495*a*]. This kind of immunotherapy may activate specific immune mechanisms or may induce a non-specific cytotoxic inflammatory reaction. It seems likely that vaccinia virus may activate the production of cell-mediated cytotoxic immunity against M cells. This cytotoxic immunity could be passively transferred with transfer factor to other patients with metastatic MM. Vaccinia was injected into localized melanotic nodules with some success; there was regression of the injected nodules but only limited regression of uninjected nodules and no success with visceral metastases.

Delayed hypersensitivity was induced in or adjacent to accessible tumour deposite e.g. by DNCB injected directly into the lesions [415*b*] or by applying DNCB to the skin over primary or secondary tumour deposits [390*a*]. Application of DNCB before surgical excision has given promising results. The treatment could be beneficial especially in cases of MM with intradermal localization. The efficacy of the treatment in advanced stages of the disease with subcutaneous and visceral metastases is questionable. Histological examination of treated lesions suggests that involution of the tumour during DNCB treatment is mediated by a delayed hypersensitivity reaction [390*a*].

The strategies of immunostimulant therapy and of chemotherapy with its concomitant immunosuppressive effects are quite different and may, at first sight, seem incompatible [166*d*]. Despite this, attempts are being made to combine BCG therapy and chemotherapy, the separate agents being given in alternating courses. Initial results of BCG and DTIC (dimethyltriazenoimidazole carboxamide) treatment in disseminated MM are promising. The response-rate was 55 per cent in 89 patients compared to 18 per cent in 111 patients treated with DTIC alone [241*a*].

According to a *Lancet* Editorial [166*d*] at present the situation is as follows. With each of the immunostimulant techniques some clinical benefit has been observed, but the frequency, degree, and duration of treatment responses suggest that existing immunological stimulants *per se* will do no more than slightly increase the survival of patients with metastatic disease. The real value of immunostimulant therapy cannot yet be assessed.

2. Active specific immunization. A more specific approach has been to inject irradiated or enzyme-treated autologous or homologous M cells (with or without immunological adjuvants) [286]. This type of treatment can certainly induce or increase detectable tumour-directed antibodies and lymphoid cells cytotoxic to M cells *in vitro* [136]. The antibody production depended on the number of the injected tumour cells; the duration of the antibody production depended on the 'little residual disease'. High antibody levels were achieved with tumour antigens coupled with xenogeneic immunogens. Vaccines were supplemented [280] with subcellular corpuscular or cell-fixed fractions including microsomes and mitochondria; the aim of these supplementations was to stimulate the delayed-type reactivity passively and to avoid the risk represented by soluble antigens which may cause immunoparalysis. Of the 64 cases described in the literature objective clinical improvement occurred in only 8 [24*a*]. To reinforce immune mechanisms, autotransplantation of MM has also been attempted [143]. The combination of active immunization with adjuvants is most promising [24*a*].

3. Passive transfer of immunocytes (adoptive immunotherapy). Peripheral leukocytes from remission patients resulted in a complete regression of metastases, lasting several months [425]. Successful experiments with the transfer of plasma leukocyte concentrates and allo- and xenogeneic lymphocytes (cross-transfusion of leukocytes in patient pairs) have also been reported, but in this case GVH reaction cannot be excluded, especially during immunosuppressive therapy. A more indirect approach is exposing immunologically competent cells to an antigenic stimulus (e.g. irradiated tumour cells or PHA activation) *in vitro* and reinfusing the cells into the patient; with this technique less success (or no effect) has been achieved than with direct method. Cross-implantation technique (injections of M cells from the patient's daughter or transplantation of tumour) raises ethical problems. Successful transfer of transfer factor has also been reported. Of the 146 MM cases described in the literature who were given adoptive therapy 20 responded clinically but there were only 9 remissions [24*a*].

4. Passive transfer of antibodies. Immunotherapy with sera from patients in regression has yielded negative results [560].

It should be taken into consideration when assessing the results of immunotherapy that MM is notoriously unpredictable. Ten-year tumour-free survival has been observed in 45 per cent of patients with pathologically positive lymph nodes [121*a*] and more than 5-year survival has been reported for 17 per cent of patients with metastatic disease, without evidence of any recurrences [121*b*]. Further experiments are necessary to establish the real value of this procedure. Effective immunotherapy seems to be possible, but first of all the immune mechanism active against MM should be identified and followed by laboratory methods. If the tumour mass can be radically removed once or repeatedly and the immune apparatus is intact, active immunization with tumour antigens and systemic adjuvants requires consideration, for one should reckon with induction of an immune response to normal tissue antigens, especially of blocking antibodies and autoantibodies. Passive transfer of immunocytes also encounters difficulties. At present it seems impossible to propose an immunotherapy schedule which would be valid for every case and at all stages of the disease [63]. A technique for the selection of patients should be developed [63].

Recently some authors [123, 171, 399*a*] have pointed to an association of halo naevus with cutaneous MM or its removal. Humoral antibodies to the cytoplasm of MM cells have been found not only in patients with primary cutaneous MM without metastases, but also in resolving halo naevi. The antibodies disappear as the resolution of the naevus has been excised. It was concluded that halo naevus may represent an accelerated and successful rejection phase of a pigmented mole developing malignant change. Since halo naevus may not be associated with malignancy, it has been proposed [612] to name the demonstrated humoral antibody 'halo naevus cell cytoplasmic humoral antibody'.

Strong cell-mediated immunity to M antigens has been revealed in patients' lymphocytes [171]. The positive skin tests with common antigens are suggestive of intact cell-mediated immunity. Part of the patients with halo naevus do not react with M antigen in all available tests (lymphocyte transformation, MIF production, cytotoxicity and rosette formation). It has been suggested [612] that the common factor in cutaneous MM and halo naevus are not malignancy, but 'involution', not the neoplastic proliferation of pigment cells, but their proneness to death. The absence of lymphocytic infiltration in the region of the halo has suggested that the response might be mediated rather by humoral antibodies. The lymphocytes are quite sharply confined to the part of the dermis where naevus cells are present; the melanocytes concerned lie above the BM.

REFERENCES

1*a*. Ablin, J. R.: *Lancet* **ii,** 1397 (1968).
1*b*. id., *J. invest. Derm.* **53,** 463 (1969).
1*c*. id., *Z. Immun.-Forsch.* **146,** 8 (1973).
2*a*. Ablin, R. J. and Beutner, E. H.: *Int. Arch. Allergy* **33,** 227 (1968).
2*b*. id., *J. dent. Res.* **47,** suppl., 105 (1968).
2*c*. id., *Experientia* (*Basel*) **24,** 1055 (1968).
2*d*. id., *Clin. exp. Immunol.* **4,** 283 (1969).
3. Ablin, R. J., Bronson, P. and Beutner, E. H.: *J. Hyg. Epidemiol. Microbiol. Immunol.* (*Prague*) **13,** 321 (1969).
3*a*. Ablin, R. J., Holder, I. A.: *Arch. Derm.* (*Chicago*) **109,** 887 (1974).

3*b*. Ackermann Schopf, C., Ackermann, R., Terasaki, P. I. and Levy, J.: *J. Immunol.* **112,** 2063 (1974).
4. Albin, R. J. and Newman, G., jr.: *J. invest. Derm.* **52,** 388 (1969).
5. Abruzzo, J. L.: *Arthr. and Rheum.* **14,** 451 (1971).
6. Achard, H. O.: In *Dermatology in General Medicine.* Ed. by Fitzpatrick, Th. B., Arndt, K. A., Clark, W. H., jr., Eisen, A. Z., Van Scott, E. J. and Vaughan, J. H. McGraw-Hill, New York 1971, p. 821.
7. Akopyan, A. T., Pozdnyakov, O. L., Avakyan, A. A. and Kharitonova, A. M.: *Vestn. Derm. Vener.* (*Moscow*) **46**/10, 15 (1972).
8. Alexander, J. W., Bossert, J. E., McClellan, M. A. and Altemeier, W. A.: *Arch. Surg.* **103,** 167 (1971).
9. Alexander, J. W., Fisher, M. W. and MacMillan, B. G.: *Arch. Surg.* **102,** 31 (1971).
10. Alexander, J. W. and Good, R. A.: *Immunobiology for Surgeons.* Saunders, Philadelphia 1970.
11. Alexander, J. W. and Moncrief, J. A.: *Arch. Surg.* **93,** 75 (1966).
12. Alexander, J. W., Windhorst, D. B. and Good, R. A.: *J. Lab. clin. Med.* **72,** 136 (1968).
13. Allison, A. C.: In *Clinical Immunobiology.* Vol. I. Ed. by Bach, F. H. and Good, R. A. Academic Press, New York 1972, p. 113.
14. Allison, A. C., Denman, A. P. and Barnes, R. D.: *Lancet* **ii,** 135 (1971).
15. Anderson, H. J., Newcomer, V. D., Landau, J. W. and Rosenthal, L. H.: *Arch. Derm.* (*Chicago*) **101,** 538 (1970).
16. Anderson, P. C.: *J. invest. Derm.* **39,** 383 (1962).
17. Antonova, T. N., Kiseleva, M. L. and Trofimova, L. Ya.: *Vestn. Derm. Vener.* (*Moscow*) **46**/4, 41 (1972).
18. Aoki, T.: *Hifu* (*Osaka*) **7,** 219 (1965).
19. Aoki, T., Fujita, M. and Toyoshima, K.: In *Abstr. VIIIth Int. Congr. Allergol., Tokyo 1973.* Ed. by Munro-Asham. D. and Pugh, D. L. Int. Congr. Series No. 300. Excerpta Medica Foundation, Amsterdam 1973, p. 3.
19*a*. Arbesman, C. E., Wypych, J. I., Reisman, R. E. and Beutner, E. H.: *Arch. Derm.* (*Chicago*) **110,** 378 (1974).
20. Arturson, G., Johansson, S. G. O., Hogman, C. and Killander, J.: *Lancet* **i,** 546 (1969).
21. Atherton, A., Merill, N. and McCarthy, M. D.: *Fed. Proc.* **19,** 195 (1960).
22*a*. Baart de la Faille-Kuyper, E. H.: Lupus Erythematosus. An Immunohistochemical and Clinical Study of 485 Patients. Thesis. University of Utrecht 1969.
22*b*. id., *Ned. T. Geneesk.* **117,** 473 (1972).
23. Baart de la Faille-Kuyper, E. H. and Baart de la Faille, H.: *Brit. J. Derm.* **90,** 365 (1974).
24. Baart de la Faille-Kuyper, E. H. and Cormane, R. H.: *Acta derm.-venereol.* **48,** 578 (1968).
24*a*. Baker, M. A. and Taub, R. N.: *Progr. Allergy* **17,** 227 (1973).
25. Baldini, M., Kim, B., Steiner, M., Kuramoto, A., Okuma, M. and Otridge, B. W.: *Pediatr. Res.* **3,** 377 (1969).
25*a*. Ballow, M., Dupont, B. and Good, R. A.: *Pediatrics* **83,** 772 (1973).
26. Barile, M. F., Graykowski, E. A., Driscoll, E. J. and Riggs, D. B.: *Oral. Surg.* **16,** 1395 (1963).
26*a*. Baringer, J. R.: *New Engl. J. Med.* **291,** 828 (1974).
26*b*. Barranco, V. P.: Read at the *6th South Central Derm. Congr. Tulsa 1974*; cit. *Derm. News* **7**/5, 3 (1974).
27. Barthelmes, H. and Haustein, U.-F.: *Derm. Mschr.* **156,** 85 (1970).
28. Batchelor, J. R. and Hacket, M.: *Lancet* **ii,** 581 (1970).
29. Baur, S., Koo, N. and Taylor, K. B.: *Immunology* **19,** 891 (1970).
30. Beall, G. N. and Solomon, D. H.: In *Immunological Diseases.* Vol. II. 2nd ed. Ed. by Samter, M. Little-Brown, Boston 1971, p. 1198.
31*a*. Bean, S. F.: *J. invest. Derm.* **53,** 187 (1969).
31*b*. id., *Acta derm.-venereol.* **50,** 95 (1970).
32. Bean, S. F., Good, R. A. and Windhorst, D. B.: *Arch. Derm.* (*Chicago*) **102,** 205 (1970).

33. Bean, S. F., Jordon, R. E., Winkelmann, R. K. and Good, R. A.: *Amer. J. Dis. Child.* **122,** 137 (1971).
34. Bean, S. F. and Lynch, F. W.: *Arch. Derm. (Chicago)* **101,** 642 (1970).
35. Bean, S. F., Waisman, M., Michel, B., Thomas, Ch. I., Knox, J. M. and Levine, M.: *Arch. Derm. (Chicago)* **106,** 195 (1972).
35*a*. Benda, R. and Dbaly, V.: *J. Hyg. Epidemiol. (Prague)* **17,** 237 (1973).
36. Bendixen, G.: *Clinical Hypersensitivity Disorders.* Thomas, Springfield 1971, p. 112.
37. Berendes, H., Bridges, R. A. and Good, R. A.: *Minn. Med.* **40,** 309 (1957).
38. Berger, H.: *Ann. intern. Med.* **42,** 205 (1955).
39. Berrens, L. and Young, E.: *Dermatologica (Basel)* **128,** 287 (1964).
40. Beutner, E. H.: *Brit. J. Derm.* **84,** 594 (1971).
41. Beutner, E. H., Chorzelski, T. P., Hale, W. L. and Petrusewicz, I.: *J. Amer. med. Ass.* **203,** 10 (1968).
42*a*. Beutner, E. H., Chorzelski, T. P., Jarzabek, M., Wood, G. W., Cid de Abreu, L. and Bier, O.: *Int. Arch. Allergy* **42,** 545 (1972).
42*b*. ibid., **42,** 556 (1972).
43. Beutner, E. H., Chorzelski, T. P. and Jordon, R. E.: *Autosensitization in Pemphigus and Bullous Pemphigoid.* Thomas, Springfield 1970.
44. Beutner, E. H., Chorzelski, T. P., Petzold, D., Cormane, R. H., Thivolet, J. and Jabłońska, S.: *Dermatologica (Basel)* **140,** 7 (1970).
44*a*. Beutner, E. H., Jabłońska, S., Jarzabek-Chorzelski, M., Marciejowska, E., Rzeska, G. and Chorzelski, T. P.: *Int. Arch. Allergy* **48,** 301 (1975).
45. Beutner, E. H. and Jordon, R. E.: *Proc. Soc. exp. Biol. (N. Y.)* **117,** 505 (1964).
46. Beutner, E. H., Lever, W. F., Witebsky, E., Jordon, R. and Chertock, B.: *J. Amer. med. Ass.* **192,** 682 (1965).
47. Beutner, E. H., Rhodes, E. L. and Holborow, E. J.: *Clin. exp. Immunol.* **2,** 141 (1967).
48. Beutner, E. H., Sporer, R. and Chorzelski, T. P.: *J. invest. Derm.* **62,** 342 (1974).
49. Bickhardt, R., and Kunze, J.: *Z. Hautkr.* **49,** 315 (1974).
50. Bierman, S. M.: *Arch. Derm. (Chicago)* **107,** 896 (1973).
51. Binette, J. P. and Calkins, E.: *Arthr. and Rheum.* **10,** 107 (1967).
52. Black, M. M. and Wilson, J. E.: *Brit. J. Derm.* **84,** 199 (1971).
53. Blaese, R. M., Strober, W., Brown, R. S. and Waldmann, T. A.: *Lancet* **i,** 1056 (1968).
53*a*. Blaese, R. M., Weiden, P., Oppenheim, J. J. and Waldmann, T. A.: *J. Lab. clin. Med.* **81,** 538 (1973).
53*b*. Bleumink, E., Nater, J. P., Schraffordt Koops, H. and Thé, T. H.: *Cancer* **33,** 911 (1974).
54. Bleumink, E., Nater, J. P. and Thé, T. H.: In *Abstr. VIIIth Int. Congr. Allergol., Tokyo 1973.* Ed. by Munro-Asham. D. and Pugh, D. L. Int. Congr. Series No. 300. Excerpta Medica Foundation, Amsterdam 1973, p. 29.
55. Bluming, A. Z., Vogel, Ch. L., Ziegler, J. L. and Kiryabwire, J. W. M.: *Nat. Cancer Inst.* **48,** 17 (1972).
56. Bluming, A. Z., Vogel, Ch. L., Ziegler, J. L., Mody, N. and Kamya, G.: *Ann. intern. Med.* **76,** 405 (1972).
57. Bockendahl, H. and Remy, W.: *Klin. Wschr.* **52,** 346 (1974).
58. Bockendahl, H., Remy, W. and Peters, T.: *Z. klin. Chem. klin. Biochem.* **10,** 329 (1972).
58*a*. Bodurtha, A., Kim, Y. H. and Laucins, J. F.: *Amer. J. clin. Path.* **61,** 747 (1974).
59. Bohnstedt, R. M. and Ehlers, G.: In *XIIIth Int. Congr. Derm., München 1967.* Vol. III. Ed. by Jadassohn, W. and Schirren, C. G., Springer, Berlin 1968, p. 142.
60*a*. Bolgert, M.: *Sem. Hôp. (Paris)* **49,** 3357 (1973).
60*b*. ibid., **49,** 3497 (1973).
61. Bor, S., Feiwell, M. and Chanarin, I.: *Brit. J. Derm.* **81,** 83 (1969).
62. Bornstein, R. S., Yarbro, I. W. and Prehu, R. T.: *Ann. intern. Med.* **76,** 499 (1972).
63. Bourgoin, J. J.: *Ann. Inst. Pasteur* **122,** 789 (1972).
64. Bourgoin, J. J., Dargent, M., Bertoglio, J. and Gerlier, D.: *C. R. Acad. Sci. Ser. D.* **275,** 2183 (1972).

65*a*. Braun-Falco, O., and Vogell, W.: *Arch. clin. exp. Derm.* **223,** 328 (1965).
65*b*. ibid., **223,** 533 (1965).
66. Bray, J. P., Estess, F. and Bass, J. A.: *Proc. Soc. exp. Biol.* (*N. Y.*) **132,** 394 (1969).
66*a*. Brehm, K., Paul, E. and Schmitt, H.: *Hautarzt* **25,** 379 (1974).
67. Briccetti, A. B., Cathcart, E. S. and Cohen, A. S.: *Int. Arch. Allergy* **44,** 349 (1973).
68. Brodersen, I. and Genner, J.: *Acta derm.-venereol.* **53,** 461 (1973).
69. Brody, H. A. and Silverman, S.: *Oral Surg.* **27,** 27 (1969).
70. Brostoff, J., Bor, S. and Feiwel, M.: *Lancet* **ii,** 177 (1969).
71. Brown, F. C. and Tan, E. M.: *Cancer Res.* **33,** 2030 (1973).
72. Brownstein, M. H. and Hashimoto, K.: *Arch. Derm.* (*Chicago*) **106,** 50 (1972).
73. Brunner, K. T., Manuel, J., Cerottini, J.-C. and Chapuis, B.: *Immunology* **14,** 181 (1968).
73*a*. Buchvald, J., Borecky, L. and Doskocil, J.: *Čsl. Derm.* **48,** 176 (1973).
74. Buck, A. and Kalkoff, K. W.: *Arch. derm. Forsch.* **243,** 392 (1972).
75. Bucur, G.: *Derm.-Vener.* (*Buc.*) **17,** 129 (1972).
76. Bucur, G. and Noaghea, G.: *Derm.-Vener.* (*Buc.*) **13,** 393 (1968).
77. Burch, P. R. J. and Rowell, N. R.: *Acta derm.-venereol.* **45,** 366 (1965).
78. Bureau, B.: *Sem. Hôp.* (*Paris*) **48,** 1209 (1972).
79. Bureau, Y.: *Bull. Soc. franç. Derm. Syph.* **78,** 443 (1971).
80. Burg, G. and Braun-Falco, O.: *Arch. derm. Forsch.* **245,** 318 (1972).
81. Burnham, Th. K. and Fine, G.: *Arch. Derm.* (*Chicago*) **105,** 52 (1972).
82*a*. Burnham, Th. K., Fine, G. and Nesblett, T. R.: *Ann. intern. Med.* **65,** 9 (1966).
82*b*. id., *Arch. Derm.* (*Chicago*) **102,** 42 (1970).
82*c*. Bushkell, L. L., Jordon, R. E. and Goltz, R. W.: *Arch. Derm.* (*Chicago*) **110,** 65 (1974).
83*a*. Bystryn, J.-C.: Lecture delivered at the Meeting Soc. Invest. Derm. and Europ. Soc. Derm. Research, Amsterdam 1972.
83*b*. Bystryn, J.-C. and Abel, E.: *Arch. Derm.* (*Chicago*) **110,** 857 (1974).
83*c*. Bystryn, J.-C., Abel, E. A. and Teo, C. de: *J. invest. Derm.* **62,** 543 (1974).
84. Bystryn, J.-C., Abel, E. and Weidman, A.: *Arch. Derm.* (*Chicago*) **108,** 241 (1973).
85. Cagli, V., Carbonara, A. and Mancini, G.: *Boll. Soc. ital. Biol. sper.* **38,** 353 (1962).
86. Calkins, E.: In *Immunological Diseases.* 2nd ed. Vol. II. Ed. by Samter, M. Little-Brown, Boston 1971, p. 1073.
87. Calkins, E., Cohen, A. S. and Gitlin, D.: *Fed. Proc.* **17,** 431 (1958).
88. Callender, S. T., Spray, G. H. and Wright, R.: *Brit. J. Haemat.* **14,** 161 (1968).
89. Cameron, J. S.: *Proc. roy. Soc. Med.* **62,** 49 (1969).
90. Candil, E.: *Dermatologica* (*Basel*) **140,** 195 (1970).
91. Caputo, R., Bellone, A. G. and Crosti, C.: *Arch. derm. Forsch.* **247,** 181 (1973).
92. Carraz, M., Bourgoin, J. J., Veysseyre, C. and Frobert, Y.: *Rev. Inst. Pasteur Lyon* **4,** 361 (1971).
92*a*. Carrel, J. M. and Davidson, D. M.: *J. Amer. pediat. Ass.* **63,** 293 (1973).
92*b*. Carruthers, J. A. and Black, M. M.: *Brit. J. Derm.* **93,** Suppl. 11 (1975).
93. Carson, M. J., Chadwick, D. L., Brudaker, C. A., Cleland, R. S. and Landing, B. H.: *Pediatrics* **35,** 405 (1965).
94. Casson, P. R., Gesner, B. M., Converse, J. M. and Rapaport, F. T.: *Surg. Forum* **19,** 509 (1968).
94*a*. Catalano, L. W. and Johnson, L. D.: *J. Amer. med. Ass.* **217,** 447 (1971).
95. Cathcart, E. S. and Cohen, A.: *J. Immunol.* **96,** 239 (1966).
96. Cathcart, E. S., Ritchie, R. F., Cohen, A. S. and Brandt, K.: *Amer. J. Med.* **52,** 93 (1972).
97. Cator, G. W.: *J. Lab. clin. Med.* **77,** 65 (1971).
98. Caufield, J. B. and Wilgram, G. F.: *J. invest. Derm.* **39,** 307 (1962).
99. Cawley, E. O., Wheeler, C. E. and Wilhite, P. A.: *Sth. med. J.* **45,** 827 (1952).
100. Celeda, F. and Rothman, B.: *Proc. nat. Acad. Sci.* (*Wash.*) **57,** 630 (1967).
101. Chambler, K. and Batchelor, J. R.: *Lancet* **i,** 16 (1969).
102. Chapel, H. M. and Batchelor, J. R.: *Brit. med. J.* **iv,** 385 (1973).
103. Charles, A.: *Brit. J. Derm.* **72,** 439 (1960).
104. Chorzelski, T. P., Beutner, E. H., Jabłońska, S., Blaszczyk, M. and Trifshauser, C.: *J. invest. Derm.* **56,** 373 (1971).

105. Chorzelski, T. P., Beutner, E. H. and Jarzabek, M.: *Int. Arch. Allergy* **39,** 106 (1970).
106*a*. Chorzelski, T. P. and Jabłońska, S.: *Derm. Wschr.* **153,** 558 (1967).
106*b*. id., *Hautarzt* **23,** 477 (1972).
107*a*. Chorzelski, T. P., Jabłońska, S. and Blaszczyk, M.: *Arch. belg. Derm.* **23,** 353 (1967).
107*b*. id., *Brit. J. Derm.* **80,** 211 (1968).
108*a*. Chorzelski, T. P., Jabłońska, S., Blaszczyk, M. and Jarzabek, M.: *Hautarzt* **18,** 521 (1967).
108*b*. id., *Dermatologica* (*Basel*) **136,** 325 (1968).
109. Chorzelski, T. P. and Jarzabek, M.: *Przegl. Derm.* (*Warsaw*) **54,** 22 (1969).
109*a*. Chorzelski, T. P., Maciejowski, E., Jabłońska, S., DeMento, F. J., Grover, R. W., Holubar, K. and Beutner, E. H.: *Arch. Derm.* (*Chicago*) **109,** 849 (1974).
110. Christophers, E.: *Hautarzt* **21,** 95 (1970).
111. Chytilová, B. and Kulhánek, V.: *Plast. Reconstr. Surg.* **26,** 109 (1960).
112. Clark, W. H., jr., Yip, S. Y. and Tolman, M. M.: *Fed. Proc.* **24,** 433 (1965).
113. Clendenning, W. E. and van Scott, E. J.: *J. invest. Derm.* **45,** 46 (1965).
113*a*. Cochran, A. J., Spilg, N. G. S., Mackie, R. M. and Thomas, C. E.: *Brit. med. J.* **iv,** 67 (1972).
114. Coe, J. E. and Salvin, S. B.: *J. Immunol.* **93,** 495 (1964).
115. Cohen, A. M., Burdick, J. F. and Ketcham, A. S.: *J. surg. Res.* **11,** 421 (1971).
116*a*. Cohen, A. S.: In *Metabolic Basis of Inherited Diseases*. 3rd ed. Ed. by Stanbury, J., Wyngaarden, J. B. and Fredrikson, D. S. Blakiston-McGraw Hill, New York 1972, p. 1273.
116*b*. id., *New Engl. J. Med.* **277,** 522 (1967).
117. Cohen, A. S. and Paul, W. F.: *Nature* **197,** 193 (1963).
118. Cohen, M. and Nelken, D.: *Clin. exp. Immunol.* **13,** 417 (1973).
119. Cohen Tervaert, W. C. and Esseveld, H.: *Dermatologica* (*Basel*) **140,** 282 (1970).
120. Comaish, S. and McVittie, E.: *Brit. J. Derm.* **89,** 127 (1973).
121*a*. Conrad, F. G.: *Arch. Surg.* **104,** 587 (1972).
121*b*. id., *Cancer* **30,** 144 (1972).
122. Coombs, R. R. A.: In *Progress in the Biological Sciences in Relation to Dermatology*. Ed. by Rook, A. Cambridge University Press, London 1960, p. 247.
123. Copeman, P. W. M., Lewis, M. G., Phillips, T. M. and Elliott, P. G.: *Brit. J. Derm.* **88,** 127 (1973).
124. Copeman, P. W. M., Schroeter, A. L. and Kierland, R. R.: *Brit. J. Derm.* **82,** 269 (1970).
125. Cormane, R. H. and Chorzelski, T. P.: *Dermatologica* (*Basel*) **134,** 463 (1967).
126. Cormane, R. H. and Gianetti, A.: *Brit. J. Derm.* **84,** 523 (1971).
126*a*. Cormane, R., Hunyadi, J. and Hamerlinck, F.: *J. invest. Derm.* **64,** 289 (1975).
127. Cormane, R. H. and Petzold, D.: *Dermatologica* (*Basel*) **140,** 1 (1970).
128. Cormane, R. H. and Szabó, É.: *Brit. J. Derm.* **83,** 435 (1970).
129. Cormane, R. H., Szabó, É. and Hauge, L. S.: *Brit. J. Derm.* **82,** Suppl. 5, 26 (1970).
130. Cormane, R. H., Szabó, É. and Thio, Th. H.: *Brit. J. Derm.* **85,** 531 (1971).
131. Cram, D. L. and Fukuyama, K.: *Arch. Derm.* (*Chicago*) **106,** 819 (1972).
132. Cram, D. L., Griffith, M. R. and Fukuyama, K.: *Arch. Derm.* (*Chicago*) **109,** 235 (1974).
133. Crawford, G. M. and Leeper, R. W.: *Arch. Derm.* (*Chicago*) **61,** 753 (1950).
134. Csákány, Gy., Bozsóky, S., Bakos, L. and Korossy, S.: *Acta radiol.* **57,** 121 (1962).
135. Cunliffe, W. J., Hall, R., Newell, D. J. and Stevenson, C. J.: *Brit. J. Derm.* **80,** 135 (1968).
136. Currie, G. A., Lejeune, F. and Fairley, G. H.: *Brit. med. J.* **ii,** 305 (1971).
137. Czajkowski, N. P., Rosenblatt, M., Cushing, F. R., Vazquez, J. and Wolf, P. L.: *Cancer* **19,** 739 (1966).
138. Dabelsteen, E., Ullman, S., Thomsen, K. and Rygaard, J.: *Acta derm.-venereol.* **54,** 189 (1974).
138*a*. Dahl, M. V., Katz, St. I., McNair Scott, R. and Binn, L. N.: *J. invest. Derm.* **62,** 96 (1974).

139. Dán, P., Kulcsár, G., Sallay, K. and Nász, I.: *Blut* **22,** 211 (1971).
140. Dantzig, P.: *Arch. Derm.* (*Chicago*) **108,** 264 (1973).
141. Das Gupta, T., Bowden, L. and Berg, J. W.: *Surg. Gynaec. Obst.* **117,** 341 (1963).
142*a*. David, J. R., Lawrence, H. S. and Thomas, L.: *J. Immunol.* **93,** 274 (1964).
142*b*. ibid., **93,** 279 (1964).
143. Day, E. D.: *The Immunochemistry of Cancer.* Thomas, Springfield 1965.
144. Decherd, J. W., Rubin, M. B., Goldschmidt, H. and Heiss, H. B.: *Acta derm.-venereol.* **52,** 116 (1972).
145. De Coteau, W. E., Gerrard, J. W. and Cunningham, T. H.: *Lancet* **ii,** 679 (1973).
146. Degos, R., Civatte, J., Clauvel, J. P. and Danon, F.: *Bull. Soc. franç. Derm. Syph.* **77,** 579 (1970).
147. Degos, R., Touraine, R., Danon, Mme, Lauret, P., Rigolet, D., Debat, M. and Zillerman, Mme J.: *Bull. Soc. franç. Derm. Syph.* **73,** 370 (1966).
148. De Gowin, R. L.: *Arch. intern. Med.* **120,** 242 (1967).
149. Delescluse, J., de Bast, Cl. and Achten, G.: *Brit. J. Derm.* **87,** 529 (1972).
150. Della Porta, G., Balzarini, G. P. and Canevari, S.: *Rev. Inst. Pasteur Lyon* **4,** 329 (1971).
151. Del Rey Calero, J. and Calbo Torrecillas, F.: *Rev. Diagn. Biol.* (*Madrid*) **20,** 541 (1971).
152. De Mento, F. J. and Grover, R. W.: *Arch. Derm.* (*Chicago*) **107,** 883 (1973).
153. De Vries, J. E., Van T Hoog, A. G. and Rumke, P.: *Rev. Inst. Pasteur Lyon* **4,** 369 (1971).
154. Dick, H. D., Frazer, N. G. and Murray, D.: *Brit. J. Derm.* **81,** 692 (1969).
155. Diem, E.: *Z. Hautkr.* **48,** 835 (1973).
156. Dobmeier, L. J. and Sams, W. M., jr.: *J. invest. Derm.* **56,** 410 (1971).
157. Dobozy, A., Husz, S., Hunyady, J., Berkó, Gy. and Simon, M.: *Lancet* **ii,** 625 (1973).
158. Dobrotina, N. A., Remizova, C. I. and Postnikova, G. A.: *Vestn. Derm. Vener.* **47**/11, 74 (1973).
159*a*. Dolby, A. E.: *Immunology* **17,** 709 (1969).
159*b*. id., *Clin. exp. Immunol.* **7,** 681 (1970).
159*c*. Domonkos, A. N.: *Arch. Derm.* (*Chicago*) **109,** 587 (1970).
159*d*. Donaldson, R. C.: *Amer. J. Surg.* **124,** 527 (1972).
160. Donatsky, O. and Bendixen, G.: *Acta allergol.* **27,** 137 (1972).
160*a*. Donatsky, O. and Dabelsteen, E.: *Acta allergol.* **29,** 308 (1974).
160*b*. Duff, R. and Rapp, F.: *Nature, New Biol.* **233,** 48 (1971).
161. Duperrat, B., Puissant, A., David, V. and Bernuau, Mme D.: *Bull. Soc. franç. Derm. Syph.* **79,** 615 (1972).
162. Dygin, V. P. and Kliachkin, L. M.: *Probl. Gemat.* (*Moscow*) **10,** 37 (1965).
163. Ebner, H., Ehringer, H. and Hausteiner, H.: *Z. Hautkr.* **48,** 779 (1973).
164. Ebner, H. and Gebhart,W.: *Arch. derm. Forsch.* **242,** 153 (1972).
165*a*. Ebner, H. and Kraft, D.: *Arch. derm. Forsch.* **243,** 305 (1972).
165*b*. id., *Dermatologica* (*Basel*) **146,** 101 (1973).
166*a*. Editorial: *Lancet* **ii,** 1298 (1971).
166*b*. ibid., **i,** 621 (1972).
166*c*. ibid., **ii,** 949 (1973).
166*d*. ibid., **ii,** 1119 (1974).
167*a*. Editorials: *J. Amer. med. Ass.* **223,** 554 (1973).
167*b*. ibid., **225,** 1242 (1973).
168. Eilber, F. R. and Morton, D. L.: *Cancer* **25,** 362 (1970).
169. El-Hefnawi, H., Abdel Gawad, Z. and El-Marsafy, M. K.: *Arch. klin. exp. Derm.* **218,** 422 (1964).
170. Epstein, J. H., Tuffanelli, D. L. and Epstein, W. L.: *Arch. Derm.* (*Chicago*) **107,** 689 (1973).
171. Epstein, W. L., Sagebeil, R., Spitler, L., Wybran, J., Reed, W. B. and Blois, S.: *J. Amer. med. Ass.* **225,** 373 (1973).
171*a*. Erenius, K. and Mortenstein, R. F.: *Int. Arch. Allergy* **40,** 707 (1971).
172. Escande, J. P.: *Presse méd.* **77,** 415 (1969).
173. Everson, T. C. and Cole, W. H.: *Spontaneous Regression of Cancer.* Saunders, Philadelphia 1966.

174. Faber, W. R. and van Joost, Th.: *Brit. J. Derm.* **89,** 519 (1973).
175. Fairley, G. H.: *Brit. med. J.* **ii,** 467 (1969).
175*a*. Falk, R. E., Mann, P. and Langer, B.: *Arch. Surg.* **107,** 261 (1973).
175*b*. Fanta, D., Kraft, D. and Söltz-Szöts, J.: *Z. Hautkr.* **49,** 597 (1974).
175*c*. Faraci, R. P. and Schour, L.: *Science* **185,** 68 (1974).
176. Farah, F. and Shbaklu, Z.: *J. Allergy clin. Immunol.* **48,** 357 (1971).
177. Farber, E. M., Nall, M. L. and Watson, W.: *Arch. Derm.* (*Chicago*) **109,** 207 (1974).
178. Fass, L., Herberman, R. B., Ziegler, J. L. and Kiryabwire, J. W. M.: *Lancet* **i,** 116 (1970).
179. Fayolle, R. and Rouhani, R.: *Bull. Soc. franç. Derm. Syph.* **70,** 560 (1963).
180. Fedorov, N. I.: *Vestn. Derm. Vener.* (*Moscow*) **46/4,** 44 (1972).
181. Feingold, M. L. and Koss, L. E.: *Arch. intern. Med.* **124,** 66 (1969).
182. Feller, I., Pierson, C. and Arbor, A.: *Arch. Surg.* **97,** 225 (1968).
183. Fellner, M. J., Fukuyama, K., Moshell, A. and Klaus, M. V.: *Brit. J. Derm.* **89,** 115 (1973).
184. Fellner, M. J., and Prutkin, L.: *J. invest. Derm.* **55,** 390 (1970).
184*a*. Fiala, M., Chow, A. W., Miyasaki, K. and Guze, L. B.: *J. infect. Dis.* **129,** 82 (1974).
185. Fincher, D. F., Dupree, E. and Bean, S. F.: *Arch. Derm.* (*Chicago*) **103,** 88 (1971).
186. Finzi, S. F.: *Rass. Derm. Sif.* **22,** 265 (1969).
187. Fisher, J. P.: *J. invest. Derm.* **44,** 43 (1965).
188. Fjellstrom, K. E. and Arturson, G.: *Acta path. microbiol. scand.* **59,** 257 (1963).
189. Forrester, J. A., Dumonde, D. C. and Ambrose, E. J.: *Immunology* **8,** 37 (1965).
189*a*. Forsey, R. R., Haberman, H. F. and Langman, L.: *Arch. Derm.* (*Chicago*) **91,** 512 (1965).
190. Fowlkes, R. W., Blaylock, W. K. and Mullinai, F.: *Arch. Derm.* (*Chicago*) **95,** 370 (1967).
191. Frank, H. and Beetz, H.-M.: *Hautarzt* **25,** 201 (1974).
191*a*. Frankl, J. and Sabján, V.: *Bőrgyógy. Vener. Szle.* (*Budap.*) **49,** 61 (1973).
192. Franklin, E. C. and Pras, M.: *J. exp. Med.* **130,** 797 (1969).
193. Franklin, E. C., Pras, M., Levine, M. and Frangione, B.: *FEBS Letters* **22,** 121 (1972).
194. Franklin, E. C. and Zucker-Franklin, D.: In *Advances in Immunology*. Vol. 15. Ed. by Dixon, F. J. and Kunkel, H. G. Academic Press, New York 1972.
195. Fraser, N. G., Dick, H. M. and Crichton, W. B.: *Brit. J. Derm.* **81,** 89 (1969).
196. Fraser, N. G., Kerr, N. W. and Donald, D.: *Brit. J. Derm.* **89,** 439 (1973).
197. Frenk, E.: *Dermatologica* (*Basel*) **139,** 84 (1969).
198. Fudenberg, H. H., James, K., Epstein, W. L. and Shuster, J.: *Clin. Res.* **14,** 267 (1966).
199. Fukuyama, K., Douglas, S. D., Tuffanelli, D. L. and Epstein, W. L.: *Amer. J. clin. Path.* **54,** 410 (1970).
200. Futrell, J. W. and Myers, G. H., jr.: *Ann. Surg.* **177,** 1 (1973).
201*a*. Fülöp, É. and Vajda, Mrs. T.: *Bőrgyógy. Vener. Szle.* (*Budap.*) **47,** 145 (1971).
201*b*. ibid., **49,** 17 (1973).
202. Fry, L. and Johnson, F. R.: *Brit. J. Derm.* **81,** 44 (1969).
203. Fry, L. and Seah, P. P.: *Brit. J. Derm.* **90,** 137 (1974).
204. Fry, L., Seah, P. P., McMinn, R. M. H. and Hoffbrand, A. V.: *Brit. med. J.* **iii,** 371 (1972).
205. Fry, L., Seah, P. P., Riches, D. J. and Hoffbrand, A. V.: *Lancet* **i,** 288 (1973).
206. Gatti, R. A.: *Lancet* **i,** 91 (1972).
207. Gatti, R. A. and Good, R. A.: *Cancer* **28,** 89 (1971).
208. Gauto, M. W., Beutner, E. H. and Chorzelski, T. P.: *J. invest. Derm.* **58,** 166 (1972).
209. Gay Prieto, J., Jaqueti, G., Rodriques-Pérez, A. P., Gancedo, A. G. and Alonso Puertas, M.-L.: *Hautarzt* **17,** 26 (1966).
210. Geber, H.: *Derm. Z.* **32,** 143 (1921).
211. Gebhard, R. L., Katz, S. I., Marks, J., Shuster, S., Trapani, R. J., Rogentine, G. N. and Strober, W.: *Lancet* **ii,** 760 (1973).
212*a*. Genner, J.: *Acta derm.-venereol.* **51,** 361 (1971).

212*b*. ibid., **51**, 365 (1971).
212*c*. Ghose, T., Norvell, S. T., Guclu, A., Cameron, D., Bodurtha, A. and MacDonald, A. S.: *Brit. med. J.* **iii**, 495 (1972).
213. Gianetti, A.: *Ann. Derm. Syph.* **100**, 288 (1973).
214. Gianotti, F. J.: *Zbl. Haut-Geschl. Kr.* **87**, 48 (1954).
215. Gillette, R. W., Cooper, S. and Lance, E. M.: *Immunology* **23**, 769 (1972).
216. Gingrich, R. E. and Fusaro, R. M.: *J. invest. Derm.* **43**, 235 (1964).
217. Giraldo, G., Beth, E. and Coeur, P.: *J. nat. Cancer Inst.* **49**, 1495 (1972).
218. Gjonea, E. and Nordöy, A.: *Brit. med. J.* **i**, 610 (1970).
219. Glenner, G. G.: *Acta path. microbiol. scand., Sect. A.* **233**, 114 (1972).
220. Glenner, G. G., Ein, D. and Terry, W. D.: *Amer. J. Med.* **52**, 141 (1972).
221. Glenner, G. G., Terry, W. D., Harada, M., Isersky, C. and Page, D.: *Science* **172**, 1150 (1971).
222. Glenner, G. G., Terry, W. D. and Isersky, C.: *Semin. Haematol.* **10**, 65 (1973).
223. Goldber, Ch. B. and Whitehouse, F. jr.: *Nature* **228**, 160 (1970).
224. Goldner, H., Girardi, A. J., Larson, V. M. and Hilleman, M. R.: *Proc. Soc. exp. Biol. Med.* **117**, 851 (1964).
225. Goodwin, D. P., Hornung, M. O., Leong, S. P. L. and Krementz, E. T.: *Surgery* **72**, 737 (1972).
225*a*. Goolamali, S. K., Barnes, E. W., Irvine, W. J. and Shuster, S.: *Brit. med. J.* **iv**, 78 (1974).
226. Gordon, B.: *Brit. med. J.* **i**, 51 (1967).
227. Graber, W., Laissue, J. and Krebs, A.: *Ther. Umsch.* **29**, 16 (1972).
228. Götz, H.: *Antigenität von Tumorproteinen.* W. de Gruyter, Berlin 1972.
229. Graham, J. H.: Lecture delivered at the *Meeting of North Amer. Clin. Dermat. Soc., San Diego 1973*, ref. in *Dermat. News* **6**/7, 4 (1973).
229*a*. Grant, R. M., Mackie, R., Cochrane, A. J., Murray, E. L., Hoyle, D. and Ross, C.: *Lancet* **ii**, 1096 (1974).
230. Graykowski, E. A., Barile, M. F., Lee, W. B. and Stanley, H. R.: *J. Amer. med. Ass.* **196**, 637 (1966).
231. Greenberg, J. H., Smith, T. L. and Katz, R. M.: *Arch. Derm.* (*Chicago*) **107**, 580 (1973).
232. Griffin, J. W.: *Oral Surg.* **19**, 209 (1965).
233. Griffith, M. R., Fukuyama, K., Tuffanelli, D. and Silverman, S., jr.: *Arch. Derm.* (*Chicago*) **109**, 195 (1974).
234*a*. Grob, P. J. and Inderbitzin, Th. M.: *J. invest. Derm.* **49**, 285 (1967).
234*b*. ibid., **49**, 637 (1967).
234*c*. ibid., **50**, 352 (1968).
234*d*. id., *Schweiz. med. Wschr.* **98**, 207 (1968).
234*e*. id., *Int. Arch. Allergy* **35**, 141 (1969).
235. Gróf, P.: *Bőrgyógy. Vener. Szle.* (*Budap.*) **49**, 136 (1973).
236. Grupper, Ch., Benacerraf, C., Roussel, G. and Eyquem, A.: *Bull. Soc. franç. Derm. Syph.* **77**, 852 (1970).
237. Guerra-Rodrigo, F.: *Brit. J. Derm.* **86**, 348 (1972).
238. Guerra-Rodrigo, F. and Morais Cardos, J. P.: *Arch. Derm.* (*Chicago*) **104**, 412 (1971).
239. Guilhou, J.-J., Meynadier, J. and Clot, J.: *Nouv. Presse méd.* **2**, 2750 (1973).
240. Guilhou, J.-J., Meynadier, J., Robinet-Levy, Mme M. and Bascoul, Mme S.: *Nouv. Presse méd.* **2**, 3047 (1973).
241. Guinan, P., Sadoughi, N., Bush, I. M., John, Th., Eghrari, F. and Ablin, R. J.: *Urology* **2**, 493 (1973).
241*a*. Gutterman, J. U., Mavligit, G., Gottlieb, J. A., Burgess, M. A., Mc Bride, C. E., Einhorn, L., Freireich, E. J. and Hersh, E. M.: *New Engl. J. Med.* **291**, 592 (1974).
241*b*. Gutterman, J. U., Mavligit, G. and Mc Bride, C. E.: *Cancer* **32**, 321 (1973).
242. Gutterman, J. U., Mavligit, G., Mc Bride, C., Frei III., E., Freireich, E. J. and Hersh, E. M.: *Lancet* **i**, 1208 (1973).
243. Guy, W. H., Jacobs, F. M. and Guy, W. B.: *Arch. Derm.* (*Chicago*) **63**, 377 (1951).
243*a*. Hadziev, S. and Kavaklieva-Dimitrova, J.: *Folia med. neerl.* **11**, 8 (1969).
244. Haferkamp, O.: *Med. Welt* **21**, 999 (1970).

244*a*. Hakim, A. A.: *Experientia (Basel)* **29,** 865 (1973).
245. Haneke, E.: *Derm. Mschr.* **158,** 227 (1973).
246. Hardy, K. M., Perry, H. O., Pingree, G. C. and Kirby, Th. J., jr.: *Arch. Derm. (Chicago)* **104,** 467 (1971).
247. Hashem, N. and Carr, D. H.: *Lancet* **ii,** 1030 (1963).
248. Hashem, N., Hirschhorn, K., Sedlis, E. and Holt, L. E., jr.: *Lancet* **ii,** 269 (1963).
249. Hashimoto, I.: *Tohoku J. exp. Med.* **89,** 45 (1966).
250. Hashimoto, K., Gross, B. G. and Lever, W. B.: *J. invest. Derm.* **45,** 204 (1965).
251. Hashimoto, K. and King, L. E., jr.: *J. invest. Derm.* **61,** 293 (1973).
251*a*. Hashimoto, K., King, L. E., jr., Yamanishi, Y., Beachey, E. H. and Maeyens, E.: *J. invest. Derm.* **62,** 423 (1974).
252. Hashimoto, K. and Lever, W. J.: *Arch. Derm. (Chicago)* **101,** 287 (1970).
253. Hashimoto, K. and Yoong Onn, L. L.: *Arch. Derm. (Chicago)* **104,** 648 (1971).
254. Hattler, B. and Amos, B.: *Monogr. surg. Sci.* **3,** 1 (1966).
255. Haufe, U., Berdau, W., Lubs, H., Rose, H.-J. and Stoff, K.: *Derm. Mschr.* **158,** 727 (1972).
255*a*. Heid, E., Maleville, J. and Basset, A.: *Bull. Soc. franç. Biol. Med.* **80,** 10 (1973).
256*a*. Hellström, I. and Hellström, K. E.: *J. Ret. End. Soc.* **10,** 131 (1971).
256*b*. id., *Nature* **240,** 471 (1972).
256*c*. id., *Fed. Proc.* **32,** 156 (1973).
257. Hellström, I., Warner, G. A., Hellström, K. E. and Sjögren, H. Ö.: *Int. J. Cancer* **11,** 280 (1973).
258. Hellström, K. E.: In *Immune Surveillance*. Ed. by Smith, R. T. and Landy, M. Academic Press, New York 1970, p. 261.
259*a*. Hellström, K. E. and Hellström, I.: *Advanc. Cancer Res.* **12,** 167 (1969).
259*b*. id., *Triangle* **11,** 23 (1972).
260. Hellström, K. E., Hellström, I., Sjögren, H. Ö. and Warner, G. A.: In *Progress in Immunology*. First Int. Congr. Immunol. Ed. by Amos, B. Academic Press, New York 1971, p. 939.
260*a*. Helm, F. and Klein, E.: *Arch. Derm. (Chicago)* **91,** 142 (1965).
261*a*. Hénocq, E.: *Abstr. Ann. Meeting Europ. Acad. Allergol. Clin. Immunol., Oslo 1972*, p. 19.
261*b*. id., *Acta allergol.* **29,** 152 (1974).
262. Heppner, G. H., Stolbach, L., Byrne, M., Cummings, F. J., McDonough, E. E. and Calabresi, P.: *Int. J. Cancer* **11,** 245 (1973).
263. Herbert, W. J. and Wilkinson, P. C.: *A Dictionary of Immunology*. Blackwell, Oxford 1971, p. 21.
264. Hersh, E. M., Gutterman, J. U. and Mavligit, G.: *Immunotherapy of Cancer in Man: Scientific Basis and Current Status*. Thomas, Springfield, Illinois 1973.
265. Hetherington, G. W., Jetton, R. L. and Knox, J. M.: *Brit. J. Derm.* **82,** 118 (1970).
266. Hewitt, J., Lessana-Leibowitch, M., Benveniste, M. and Saporta, L.: *Ann. Méd. interne (Paris)* **122,** 1003 (1971).
267. Heydenreich, G., From, E. and Diderichsen, H.: *Dermatologica (Basel)* **144,** 314 (1972).
268. Hoede, N., Morsches, B. and Holzman, H.: *Internist* **15,** 186 (1974).
269. Hoischen, W. and Steigleder, G. K.: *Dtsch. med. Wschr.* **91,** 398 (1966).
270. Holmes, B., Page, A. R. and Good, R. A.: *J. clin. Invest.* **46,** 1422 (1967).
271. Holubar, K. and Beutner, E. H.: *Arch. Derm. (Chicago)* **109,** 409 (1974).
272. Holubar, K., Chorzelski, T. P., Gauto, M. and Beutner, E. H.: *Int. Arch. Allergy* **44,** 631 (1973).
273. Holubar, K., Doralt, M. and Eggerth, G.: *Brit. J. Derm.* **85,** 505 (1971).
274. Holubar, K., Hönigsmann, H. and Wolff, K.: *Arch. Derm. (Chicago)* **108,** 50 (1973).
275*a*. Holzmann, H., Hoede, N. and Morsches, B.: *Dtsch. med. Wschr.* **98,** 1535 (1973).
275*b*. id., *Med. Welt* **24,** 523 (1973).
276. Honeyman, J. F., Honeyman, A., Lobitz, W. C., jr. and Storrs, F. J.: *Arch. Derm. (Chicago)* **106,** 22 (1972).
276*a*. Hope-Simpson, R. E.: *Proc. roy. Soc. Med.* **58,** 9 (1965).
276*b*. Hopsu-Havu, V. K. and Helander, I.: *Acta derm.-venereol.* **54,** 333 (1974).

277. Horowitz, R. E., Stuyvesant, V. W., Wigmore, W. and Tatter, D.: *Arch. Pathol.* **79,** 238 (1965).
278. Howell, F. A., Chamberlain, M. A., Perry, R. A., Torrigiani, G. and Poitt, I. M.: *Ann. rheum. Dis.* **31,** 129 (1972).
279. Howitz, J. and Schwartz, M.: *Lancet* **i,** 1331 (1971).
280. Hughes, L. E., Kearney, R. and Tully, M.: *Cancer* **26,** 269 (1970).
281. Hunter, J. A. A., Ryan, T. J. and Savin, J. A.: *Brit. med. J.* **i,** 283 (1974).
282. Husby, G., Steffen, K., Michaelsen, T. E. and Natvis, J. B.: *Nature* (*New Biol.*) **238,** 187 (1972).
283. Hutchinson, R., Patel, R. and MacArthur, J.: *Amer. J. Surg.* **122,** 520 (1971).
284. Huth, K., Ehlers, G., Knoth, W., Kunze, K., Löffler, H., Mähr, G. and Petzold, D.: *Dtsch. med. Wschr.* **97,** 152 (1972).
285*a*. Ikonopisov, R. L.: *Rev. Inst. Pasteur Lyon* **4,** 321 (1971).
285*b*. id., *Tumori* **58,** 121 (1972).
285*c*. id., *Derm.-Vener.* (*Sofia*) **11,** 15 (1972).
286. Ikonopisov, R. L., Lewis, M. G., Hunter-Craig, I. D., Bodenham, D. C., Phillips, T. M., Cooling, C. I., Proctor, J., Hamilton Fairley, G. and Alexander, P.: *Brit. med. J.* **ii,** 752 (1970).
287*a*. Inderbitzin, Th. M. and Grob, P. J.: *J. invest. Derm.* **49,** 642 (1967).
287*b*. id., *Int. Arch. Allergy* **33,** 576 (1968).
288. Inderbitzin, Th. M. and Katz, St. I.: In *Immunology and the Skin.* Ed. by Montagna, W. and Billingham, R. E. Appleton-Century-Croft, New York 1971, p. 267.
288*a*. International Registry of Tumor Immunotherapy: *Compendium of Tumor Immunotherapy Protocols*, No. 2. Nat. Inst. Health, Bethesda 1974.
289*a*. Jabłońska, S. and Chorzelski, T. P.: *Ital. Gen. Rev. Derm.* **10,** 11 (1970).
289*b*. id., *Ann. Derm. Syph.* **98,** 377 (1971).
289*c*. id., *Hautarzt* **23,** 431 (1972).
289*d*. id., *Brit. J. Derm.* **89,** Suppl. 9, 11 (1973).
289*e*. id., *Z. Hautkr.* **49,** 721 (1974).
290. Jabłońska, S., Chorzelski, T. P. and Lebioda, J.: *Hautarzt* **21,** 156 (1970).
291. Jabłońska, S., Stachow, A. and Dabrowska, H.: *Ann. Derm. Syph.* **94,** 121 (1967).
292. James, K., Fudenberg, H. H., Epstein, W. L. and Shuster, J.: *Clin. exp. Immunol.* **2,** 153 (1967).
293. Jasser, S. and Nasilowski, W.: *Pol. med. J.* (*Warsaw*) **8,** 110 (1969).
294. Jean, G., Lambertenghi, G. and Ranzi, T.: *J. clin. Path.* **21,** 501 (1968).
295. Jehn, U. W., Nathanson, L., Schwartz, R. S. and Skinner, M.: *New Engl. J. Med.* **283,** 329 (1970).
296. Johnson, M. W., Maibach, H. I. and Salmon, S. E.: *New Engl. J. Med.* **284,** 1255 (1971).
297. Jones, R. J.: *Brit. J. exp. Path.* **52,** 100 (1971).
298. Jones, W. N. and Gordon, V. H.: *Arch. Derm.* (*Chicago*) **99,** 57 (1969).
299. Jordon, R. E., Bean, S. F. Trifshauser, C. T. and Winkelmann, R. K.: *Arch. Derm.* (*Chicago*) **101,** 629 (1970).
300. Jordon, R. E., Beutner, E. H., Witebsky, E., Blumental, G., Hale, W. L. and Lever, W. F.: *J. Amer. med. Ass.* **200,** 751 (1967).
300*a*. Jordon, R. E., Day, N. K., Luckasen, J. R. and Good, R. A.: *Clin. exp. Immunol.* **15,** 53 (1973).
301*a*. Jordon, R. E., Sams, W. M., jr. and Beutner, E. H.: *J. Lab. clin. Med.* **74,** 548 (1969).
301*b*. id., *J. invest. Derm.* **56,** 249 (1971).
301*c*. id., *Int. Arch. Allergy* **39,** 107 (1970).
302. Jordon, R. E., Sams, W. M. jr., Diaz, G. and Beutner, E. H.: *J. invest. Derm.* **57,** 407 (1971).
302*a*. Jordon, R. E., Schroeter, A. L., Rogers III, R. S. and Perry, H. O.: *J. invest. Derm.* **63,** 256 (1974).
303. Jordon, R. E., Winkelmann, R. K. and De Moragas, J. M.: *J. invest. Derm.* **54,** 352 (1970).
304. Kandhari, K. C., Pasricha, J. S. and Sharma, N. K.: *Indian J. med. Res.* **58,** 1443 (1970).

305. Kano, K., Beutner, E. H. and Milgrom, F.: *Proc. Soc. exp. Biol. (N. Y.)* **127**, 355 (1968).
306*a*. Kano, K., Milgrom, F. and Rapaport, F. T.: *Proc. Soc. exp. Biol. (N. Y.)* **125**, 142 (1967).
306*b*. ibid., **128**, 1165 (1968).
307. Kano, K., Milgrom, G., Witebsky, E. and Rapaport, F. T.: *Proc. Soc. exp. Biol. (N. Y.)* **123**, 930 (1966).
308. Kapkaev, R. A.: *Vestn. Derm. Vener.* (*Moscow*) **43**/10, 26 (1969).
309. Kaplan, M. H.: *Lancet* **i**, 706 (1962).
310. Karrer, K. and Schneider, C. C.: *Öst. Z. Krebsforsch.* **25**, 152 (1970).
311. Katz, H. I., Dahl, M. V., Penneys, N., Trapani, R. J. and Rogentine, G. N.: *Arch. Derm.* (*Chicago*) **108**, 53 (1973).
311*a*. Katz, St. I., Falchuk, Z. H., Dahl, M. V., Rogentine, G. N. and Strober, W.: *J. clin. Invest.* **51**, 2977 (1972).
312. Katz, St. I., Halprin, K. M. and Inderbitzin, Th. M.: *J. invest. Derm.* **53**, 390 (1969).
313. Kärcher, K. H.: *Dermatologica* (*Basel*) **120**, 255 (1960).
313*a*. Kern, F.: *Derm. News* **7**/6, 1 (1974).
314. Khamaganova, A. V.: *Vestn. Derm. Vener.* (*Moscow*) **47**/8, 82 (1973).
314*a*. Kim, R. and Winkelmann, R. K.: *Arch. Derm.* (*Chicago*) **83**, 895 (1961).
315. Kimberling, W. and Dobson, R. L.: *J. invest. Derm.* **60**, 538 (1973).
316. Kint, A. and Geerts, M. L.: *Arch. belg. Derm.* **27**, 131 (1971).
317. Király, K., Fülöp, É. and Daróczy, J.: In *Abstr. XIVth Int. Congr. Derm., Padua-Venice 1972*. Ed. by Flarer, F., Paton, P. M., Rabito, C., Serri, F. and Kleinman, R. L. Int. Congr. Series No. 248. Excerpta Medica Foundation, Amsterdam 1972, p. 69.
318. Király, K., Fülöp, É. and Vajda, Mrs. T.: *Bőrgyógy. Vener. Szle.* (*Budap.*) **46**, 241 (1970).
319*a*. Kislyakova, L. N.: *Vestn. Derm. Vener.* (*Moscow*) **45**/7, 34 (1971).
319*b*. ibid., **45**/10, 12 (1971).
319*c*. Klein, E.: *Geriatrics* **23**, 154 (1968).
319*d*. id., *N. Y. State J. Med.* **68**, 900 (1968).
319*e*. id., *Cancer Res.* **29**, 2351 (1969).
320. Klein, E. and Cochran, A. J.: In *Immunological Aspects of Allergy and Allergic Diseases*. Vol. 2. Ed. by Rajka, E. and Korossy, Akadémiai Kiadó, Budapest 1974, p. 727.
320*a*. Klein, E., Holtermann, O. A. and Case, R. W.: *Amer. J. clin. Path.* **62**, 281 (1974).
321. Klein, E. and Klein, G.: *Triangle* **11**, 15 (1972).
322. Klein, G.: In *Clinical Immunobiology*. Vol. I. Ed. by Bach, F. H. and Good, R. A. Academic Press, New York 1972, p. 219.
323. Klein, G., Clifford, P., Klein, E. and St. Jernward, J.: *Proc. nat. Acad. Sci.* (*Wash.*) **55**, 1628 (1966).
324. Koester, H. and Fikentscher, R.: *Derm. Mschr.* **159**, 230 (1973).
325*a*. Kohn, J.: In *Chromatographic and Electrophoretic Techniques*. Vol. II. Ed. by Smidt, I. Heinemann, London 1968, Chapt. 3.
325*b*. id., *Postgrad. Med.* **48**, 335 (1972).
326. Koizumi, Y.: *Jap. J. Derm.* **72**, 923 (1962).
327. Kokoschka, E. M., Kraft, D., Spängler, E., Bettelheim, H. and Zehetbauer, G.: *Hautarzt* **25**, 227 (1974).
328. Kolker, I. I.: *Fed. Proc.* **24**, 507 (1965).
329. Konopik, J.: *Hautarzt* **21**, 95 (1970).
330. Kopf, A. W., Siberberg, I. and Cooper, N. S.: *J. invest. Derm.* **47**, 83 (1966).
331. Koplon, B. S. and Shapiro, L.: *Arch. Derm.* (*Chicago*) **98**, 631 (1968).
332. Korossy, S., Böszörményi, J., Gózony, M. and Fehér, E.: *Bőrgyógy. Vener. Szle.* (*Budap.*) **35**, 75 (1959).
333. Korossy, S., Csákány, G., Bozsóky, S. and Bakos, L.: *Rheum. Balneol. Allerg.* (*Budap.*) **2**, 134 (1961).
334. Koumans, R. K. J. and Burke, J. F.: *Surgery* **66**, 89 (1969).
335*a*. Krain, L. S.: *Brit. J. Derm.* **90**, 397 (1974).
335*b*. id., *J. invest. Derm.* **62**, 67 (1974).

336. Krain, L. S., Landau, J. W. and Newcomer, V. D.: *Arch. Derm. (Chicago)* **106**, 657 (1972).
337. Krain, L. S., Terasaki, P. I., Newcomer, V. D. and Mickey, M. R.: *Arch. Derm. (Chicago)* **108**, 803 (1973).
338. Kremer, H. and Weitzel, H.: *Geburtsh. Frauenheilk.* **32**, 791 (1972).
339. Kreysel, H.-W. and Memmesheimer, A. R.: *Brit. J. Derm.* **85**, 519 (1971).
340. Krieger, B. L.: *Arch. Derm. (Chicago)* **100**, 247 (1969).
341a. Krogh, H. K.: *Int. Arch. Allergy* **37**, 104 (1970).
341b. ibid., **37**, 649 (1970).
341c. ibid., **38**, 78 (1970).
342a. Krogh, H. K., Maeland, J. A. and Tönder, O.: *Int. Arch. Allergy* **42**, 493 (1972).
342b. ibid., **47**, 839 (1974).
343a. Krogh, H. K. and Tönder, O.: *Int. Arch. Allergy* **34**, 170 (1968).
343b. id., *Clin. exp. Immunol.* **10**, 623 (1972).
344a. Krueger, G. G., Weston, W. L., Thorne, E. G., Mandel, M. J. and Jacobs, R. L.: *J. invest. Derm.* **60**, 282 (1973).
344b. id., *Scand. J. Immunol.* **2**, 45 (1973).
345. Kulcsár, G., Sallay, K., Nász, I., Dán, P. and Geck, P.: *Zbl. Bakt. I. Abt. Orig.* **213**, 455 (1970).
346. Kuramoto, A., Steiner, M. and Baldini, M. G.: *New Engl. J. Med.* **282**, 475 (1970).
347. Kushniruk, W.: *C. M. A. Journal* **108**, 1143 (1973).
348. La Chapelle, J.-M. and De la Brassinne, M.: *Brit. J. Derm.* **89**, 137 (1973).
349. Lachman, P. J., Müller-Eberhardt, H. J., Kunkel, H. G. and Paronetto, F.: *J. exp. Med.* **115**, 63 (1962).
350. Lai A Fat, R. F. M., Cormane, R. H. and van Furth, R.: *Brit. J. Derm.* **90**, 123 (1974).
351. Lai A Fat, R. F. M., Suurmond, D., Radl, J. and van Furth, R.: *Brit. J. Derm.* **88**, 107 (1973).
352. Lancaster-Smith, M., Kumar, P., Marks, R., Clark, M. L. and Dawson, A. M.: *Brit. J. Derm.* **89**, Suppl. 9, 13 (1973).
353. Landau, J. W., Gross, D. G., Newcomer, V. D. and Wright, E. P.: *Arch. Derm. (Chicago)* **91**, 607 (1965).
354. Landing, B. H. and Shirkey, H. S.: *Pediatrics* **20**, 431 (1957).
355a. Landry, M., Sams, W. M., jr. and Jordon, R. E.: *J. invest. Derm.* **60**, 247 (1973).
355b. ibid., **61**, 348 (1973).
356. Langhof, H., Feuerstein, M. and Schabinski, E.: *Hautarzt* **16**, 209 (1965).
357. Lapière, C.-M. and Salmon, J.: *Bull. Soc. franç. Derm. Syph.* **77**, 389 (1970).
358. Lassus, A., Apajalahti, A., Blomqvist, K., Mustakallio, M. and Kiistala, U.: *Acta derm.-venereol.* **52**, 229 (1972).
359. Lazarus, G. S., Goldsmith, L. A., Rocklin, R. E., Pinals, R. S., de Buisseret, J.-P., David, J. R. and Draper, W.: *Arch. Derm. (Chicago)* **105**, 46 (1972).
359a. Leading article: *Brit. med. J.* **iii**, 643 (1974).
360. Leguit, P., jr., Feltkamp, T. E. W., van Rossum, A. L., van Loghem, E. and Eijsvoogel, V. P.: *Int. Arch. Allergy* **45**, 392 (1973).
360a. Leguit, P., jr., Meinesz, A., Zeijewaker, W. P., Schellekens, P. T. A. and Eijsvoogel, V. P.: *Int. Arch. Allergy* **44**, 101 (1973).
361. Leguit, P., jr., Reerink-Brongers, E. and Eijsvoogel, V. P.: *Int. Arch. Allergy* **44**, 706 (1973).
362a. Lehner, Th.: *Lancet* **ii**, 7370 (1964).
362b. id., *I. A. D. R. Abstract, Thirteenth Meeting*, 1965.
362c. id., *Immunology* **13**, 159 (1967).
362d. id., *Proc. roy. Soc. Med.* **61**, 515 (1968).
362e. id., *Arch. Oral. Biol.* **14**, 843 (1969).
362f. id., *J. Pathol.* **97**, 481 (1969).
363. Lehner, Th. and Sagebiel, R. W.: *Brit. dent. J.* **121**, 454 (1966).
363a. Leinikki, P. and Salo, O. P.: *Acta derm.-venereol.* **53**, 65 (1973).
364. Leme, Cid de Abreu: *Hospital (Rio de Janeiro)* **76**, 583 (1969); Ref. *Zbl. Haut-Geschl.Kr.* **126**, 434 (1970).
365. Lemholt, K. and Nyfors, A.: *Ugeskr. Laeg.* **135**, 2377 (1973).
366. Letterer, V. E., Caesar, R. and Vogt, A.: *Dtsch. med. Wschr.* **85**, 1909 (1960).

367. Levene, G. M.: *Brit. J. Derm.* **86,** Suppl. 8, 62 (1972).
368*a*. Lever, W. F.: *Pemphigus and Pemphigoid.* Thomas, Springfield 1965.
368*b*. id., In *Dermatology in General Medicine.* Ed. by Fitzpatrick, Th. B., Arndt, K. A., Clark, W. H., jr., Eisen, A. Z., Van Scott, E. J. and Vaughan, J. H. McGraw-Hill, New York 1971, p. 609.
368*c*. id., *Arch. Derm. (Chicago)* **106,** 491 (1972).
369. Lever, W. F. and Hashimoto, K.: *J. invest. Derm.* **53,** 373 (1969).
370. Levin, A. S., Spitler, L. E., Stities, D. P. and Fudenberg, H. H.: *Proc. Nat. Acad. Sci. USA* **67,** 821 (1970).
371. Levy, N. L., Mahaley, M. S., jr. and Day, E. D.: *Int. J. Cancer* **10,** 244 (1972).
371*a*. Lewis, H. M.: *Cutis (New York)* **12,** 863 (1973).
372*a*. Lewis, M. G.: *Lancet* **ii,** 921 (1967).
372*b*. id., *Rev. Inst. Pasteur Lyon* **4,** 309 (1971).
372*c*. id., *Ser. Haematol. (Kbh).* **5,** 44 (1972).
373. Lewis, M. G. and Copeman, P. W. M.: *Abstr. Brit. Ass. Derm. Summer Meeting, 1971.*
374. Lewis, M. G., Ikonopisov, R. L., Nairn, R. C., Phillips, T. M., Hamilton Fairley, G., Bodenham, D. C. and Alexander, P.: *Brit. med. J.* **iii,** 547 (1969).
375. Lewis, M. G. and Kiryabwire, J. W. M.: *Cancer* **21,** 876 (1968).
376. Lewis, M. G. and Phillips, T. M.: *J. nat. Cancer Inst.* **49,** 915 (1972).
377. Lewis, M. G., Phillips, T. M., Cook, K. B. and Blake, J.: *Nature* **232,** 52 (1971).
377*a*. Lewis, W. R., Kraemer, K. H., Klinger, W. G., Peck, G. L. and Terry, W. D.: *Cancer Res.* **33,** 3036 (1973).
377*b*. Lippelt, H. and Söltz-Szöts, J.: *Arch. ges. Virusforsch.* **9,** 127 (1959).
378. Litt, M.: *Ann. N. Y. Acad. Sci.* **116,** 964 (1964).
379. Long, P. I. and Uesu, C. T.: *J. Amer. med. Ass.* **187,** 336 (1964).
380. Lorincz, A. L. and Pearson, R. W.: *Arch. Derm. (Chicago)* **85,** 2 (1963).
381. Lyell, A.: *Brit. J. Derm.* **81,** 228 (1969).
382. Lynch, F. W. and Albrecht, E. J.: *Arch. Derm. (Chicago)* **93,** 446 (1966).
382*a*. MacCallum, F. O. and Juel-Jensen, B. E.: *Brit. med. J.* **ii,** 805 (1966).
383. Mach, K.: *Arch. klin. exp. Derm.* **222,** 325 (1965).
384*a*. Macher, E.: *Med. Welt* **21,** 451 (1970).
384*b*. id., *Hautarzt* **21,** 558 (1970).
385. Mackay, I. R.: *Austr. J. Derm.* **9,** 113 (1967).
386. Mackie, R. M., Spily, W. G. S., Thomas, C. E. and Cochrane, A. J.: *Brit. J. Derm.* **87,** 523 (1972).
387. Macland, J. A., Krogh, H. K. and Tönder, O.: *Int. Arch. Allergy* **46,** 619 (1974).
388. MacVicar, D. N., Graham, J. H. and Bargoon, C., jr.: *J. invest. Derm.* **41,** 289 (1963).
389. Maggiora, A.: *Dermatologica (Basel)* **137,** 263 (1968).
390. Mahler, D. and Batchelor, J. R.: *Transplantation* **12,** 409 (1971).
390*a*. Malek-Mansour, S.: *Lancet* **ii,** 503 (1973).
391*a*. Marghescu, S.: *Wien. med. Wschr.* **120,** 179 (1970).
391*b*. id., *Med. Klin.* **67,** 320 (1972).
392. Marghescu, S. and Braun-Falco, O.: *Arch. klin. exp. Derm.* **238,** 417 (1970).
393. Marill, F.-G. and Ysmail-Dahlouk, M.: *Bull. Soc. franç. Derm. Syph.* **79,** 634 (1972).
394. Marks, J. and Shuster, S.: *Arch. Derm. (Chicago)* **100,** 136 (1969).
395. Marks, J., Shuster, S. and Watson, A. J.: *Lancet* **ii,** 1280 (1966).
395*a*. Marks, J., Young, S., Scott, S., Rajak, S. M. and Losowsky, M. S.: *J. invest. Derm.* **64,** 292 (1975).
396. Master, S. P., Taylor, J. F., Kyalwazi, S. K. and Ziegler, J. L.: *Brit. med. J.* **i,** 600 (1970).
396*a*. Matras, A.: *Wien. klin. Wschr.* **66,** 753 (1954).
397. Matter, P., Chambler, K., Bailey, B., Lewis, S. R., Blocker, T. G., jr. and Blocker, V.: *Ann. Surg.* **157,** 725 (1963).
398. Matthews, R. S. and Shirodaria, P. V.: *Lancet* **i,** 689 (1973).
399. Mauer, A. M.: *J. invest. Derm.* **60,** 522 (1973).
399*a*. Mc Bride, C. M., Bowen, J. M. and Dmochowski, L. L.: *Surg. Forum* **23,** 92 (1972).

400. McCarthy, J. T., Osserman, E. F., Lombardo, P. C. and Takatsuki, K.: *Arch. Derm. (Chicago)* **89**, 446 (1964).
401. McCarthy, M. D.: *Proc. Soc. exp. Biol. (N. Y.)* **117**, 693 (1964).
402. McCarthy, M. D. and McCarthy, M. D.: *Ann. Surg.* **157**, 446 (1963).
403. McClelland, D. B. L., Basnetson, R. St. C., Parkin, D. M., Warwick, R. R. G., Heading, R. C. and Shearman, D. J. C.: *Lancet* **ii**, 1108 (1972).
403*a*. Meinel, H.: *Z. inn. Med.* **28**, 633 (1973).
404. Mellors, R. C. and Ortega, L. C.: *Amer. J. Pathol.* **32**, 445 (1956).
405*a*. Mészáros, Cs. and Vadász, E.: *Bőrgyógy. Vener. Szle. (Budap.)* **46**, 262 (1970).
405*b*. id., *Z. Haut-Geschl.Kr.* **47**, 95 (1972).
406. Michailov, P. and Berowa, N.: *Allergie und Asthma* **12**, 217 (1966).
406*a*. Michel, B. and Ko, C. S.: *J. invest. Derm.* **62**, 541 (1974).
407. Michel, B., Sy, E. K., David, K. and Haserick, J. R.: *J. invest. Derm.* **54**, 428 (1970).
408. Miller, D. G.: *Ann. intern. Med.* **66**, 507 (1967).
409. Miller, R. W.: *J. nat. Cancer Inst.* **40**, 1079 (1968).
410. Misgeld, V.: *Hautarzt* **24**, 511 (1973).
411. Misgeld, Y., Schmidt, H. and Wogenstein, M.: *Z. Hautkr.* **48**, 585 (1973).
412. Mitchell, D. M.: *Brit. med. J.* **ii**, 1324 (1966).
413. Moller, G. and Moller, E.: In *Immune Cytotoxicity and Immunological Enhancement of Antibodies to Biologically Active Molecules*. Pergamon Press, Oxford 1964, p. 349.
414. Montemagno, U., Cardone, A. and Mastrantonio, P.: *Arch. Ostet. Ginec.* **76**, 65 (1971).
415. Morison, W. L.: *Brit. J. Derm.* **90**, 531 (1974).
415*a*. Morton, D. L., Eilber, F. R., Malmgreen, R. A. and Wood, W. C.: *Surgery* **68**, 158 (1970).
416. Morton, D. L., Malmgreen, R. A., Holmes, E. C. and Ketcham, A. S.: *Surgery* **64**, 233 (1968).
417. Moschella, S. L.: *Arch. Derm. (Chicago)* **95**, 121 (1967).
418. Mosonyi, L., Halmy, L. and Csiky, T.: *Allergie u. Asthma* **13**, 156 (1967).
418*a*. Movassaghi, N.: *Clin. Pediat.* **12**, 299 (1973).
418*b*. Movshev, B. E. and Averchenko, V. I.: *Bull. exp. Biol. Med.* **75**, 142 (1973).
419. Mowbray, J. F., Hoffbrand, A. V., Holborow, E. J., Seah, P. P. and Fry, L.: *Lancet* **i**, 400 (1973).
419*a*. Mukherji, B., Nathanson, L. and Clark, D. A.: *Yale J. Biol. Med.* **46**, 681 (1973).
420. Muller, H. K., Kalnins, R. and Sutherland, R. C.: *Brit. J. Derm.* **88**, 443 (1973).
421. Muller, H. K., Sutherland, R. C., Jamieson, W. J. and de Boer, W. G. R. M.: *Med. J. Austr.* **58**, 429 (1971).
422. Muna, N. M., Marcus, S. and Smart, C.: *Cancer* **23**, 88 (1969).
423. Munster, A. M., Eurenius, K., Mortensen, R. F. and Mason, A. D.: *Transplantation* **14**, 106 (1972).
424. Mustakallio, K. K., Blomqvist, K. and Laiho, K.: *Ann. clin. Res.* **2**, 13 (1970).
425. Nadler, S. H. and Moore, G. E.: *Surg. Forum* **16**, 229 (1965).
426. Nagel, G. A.: *Schweiz. med. Wschr.* **100**, 995 (1970).
426*a*. Nahmias, A. J. and Roizman, B.: *New Engl. J. Med.* **289**, 781 (1973).
426*b*. Nairn, R. C.: In *Immunological Aspects of Skin Diseases*. Ed. by Fry, L. and Seah, P. P. Medical and Technical Publ., Lancester 1974, p. 153.
427. Nathanson, L.: *Cancer Chemother. Rep.* **56**, 659 (1972).
428. Nellhaus, G.: *Nemology* **20**, 965 (1970).
429. Nesterenko, G. B., Lukovsky, L. A. and Bashmakov, G. V.: *Vestn. Derm. Vener. (Moscow)* **44**/8, 19 (1970).
430. Nicolau, Şt. Gh., Bădănoiu, A. and Băluş, L.: *Oncologia* **17**, 134 (1964).
431. Nicolau, Şt. Gh., Bădănoiu, A. and Gavrilescu, M.: *Arch. klin. exp. Derm.* **220**, 492 (1964).
431*a*. Niedworok, J., Denys, A. and Tchórzewski, H.: *Ann. Immunol. (Warsaw)* **5**, 59 (1973).
432. Nieland, M. L.: *J. invest. Derm.* **60**, 61 (1973).
432*a*. Nishikawa, T., Harada, T., Hatano, H., Ogawa, H. and Miyazaki, H.: *Acta derm.-venereol.* **54**, 275 (1974).

432*b*. Nishikawa, T., Harada, T., Hatano, H., Ogawa, H. and Miyazaki, H.: *Acta derm.-venereol.* **55**, 21 (1975).
433. Oettgen, H. F., Aoki, T., Old, L. J., Boyse, E. A., De Harven, E. and Mills, G. H.: *J. nat. Cancer Inst.* **41**, 827 (1968).
434. Oguchi, Y. and DeGroot, L. J.: *Ann. intern. Med.* **71**, 935 (1969).
435. Ohashi, M., Sawada, Y. and Makita, R.: *Acta derm.-venereol.* **53**, Suppl. 73, 43 (1973).
436. Ohshiro, A.: *Jap. J. clin. Derm.* **23**, 1145 (1969).
437. Old, L. J., Clarke, D. A. and Benacerraf, B.: *Nature* **184**, 291 (1959).
438. Olson, K., Biberfeld, G. and Fagraeus, A.: *Acta derm.-venereol.* **52**, 389 (1972).
439. Oppenheim, J. J., Blaese, R. M. and Waldmann, T. A.: *J. Immunol.* **104**, 835 (1970).
440. Osserman, E. F. and Takatsuki, K.: *J. clin. Invest.* **42**, 962 (1963).
441. Ott, J. and Käser, H.: *Schweiz. med. Wschr.* **103**, 1421 (1973).
442. Pack, G. T. and Miller, T. R.: *J. Amer. med. Ass.* **176**, 55 (1961).
443. Page, D. L., Isersky, C., Harada, M. and Glenner, G. G.: *Res. exp. Med.* **159**, 75 (1972).
443*a*. Palosuo, T.: *Scand. J. infect. Dis.* **4**, 83 (1972).
444. Pambor, M. and Höfs, W.: *Arch. klin. exp. Derm.* **232**, 127 (1968).
445*a*. Parish, W. E.: In *Immunology and the Skin.* Ed. by Montagna, W. and Billingham, R. E. Appleton-Century-Crofts, New York 1971, p. 233.
445*b*. id., In *Textbook of Dermatology.* Vol. I. 2nd ed. Ed. by Rook, A., Wilkinson, D. S. and Ebling, F. J. Blackwell, Oxford 1972, p. 219.
446. Parish, W. E. and Rook, A. J.: in *Clinical Aspects of Immunology.* Ed. by Gell, P. G. H. and Coombs, R. R. A. Blackwell, Oxford 1963, p. 895.
447. Parish, W. E., Rook, A. J. and Champion, R. H.: *Brit. J. Derm.* **77**, 479 (1965).
448. Parker, Ch. W.: In *Dermatology in General Medicine.* Ed. by Fitzpatrick, Th. B., Arndt, K. A., Clark, W. H. jr., Eisen, A. Z., van Scott, E. J. and Vaughan, J. H. McGraw-Hill, New York 1971, p. 699.
449. Pashkov, B. M., Mashkilleison, A. L., Abramova, E. I., Antonova, T. N. and Kundel, L. M.: *Vestn. Derm. Vener.* (*Moscow*) **47**/11, 3 (1973).
450. Pasricha, J. S., Mathur, N. K. and Kandhari, K. C.: *Arch. Derm.* (*Chicago*) **106**, 19 (1972).
451*a*. Pass, F., Janis, R. and Marcus, D. M.: *J. invest. Derm.* **54**, 428 (1970).
451*b*. ibid., **56**, 305 (1971).
452. Pass, F. and Maizel, J. V. jr.: *J. invest. Derm.* **60**, 307 (1973).
453. Pass, F. and Marcus, D. M.: *J. invest. Derm.* **60**, 301 (1973).
454. Pasternak, L. and Pasternak, G.: *Derm. Mschr.* **156**, 372 (1970).
454*a*. Pastinszky, I.: *Bőrgyógy. Vener. Szle.* (*Budap.*) **49**, 141 (1973).
455. Pastinszky, I. and Kovács, M.: *Honvédorvos* (*Budapest*) **23**, 243 (1971).
456. Pearse, A. G., Ewen, S. W. and Polak, J. M.: *Virchows Arch.* (*Zellpathol.*) **10**, 93 (1972).
457. Pearson, R. W.: *Arch. Derm.* (*Chicago*) **85**, 130 (1962).
458. Peck, S. M., Osserman, K. E. and Rule, A. H.: *J. invest. Derm.* **58**, 133 (1972).
459. Peck, S. M., Osserman, K. E., Samuels, A. J., Berger, B. W. and Osserman, R. S.: *Arch. Derm.* (*Chicago*) **103**, 441 (1971).
460. Penneys, N. S., Eaglstein, W. H., Indgin, S. and Frost, Ph.: *Arch. Derm.* (*Chicago*) **108**, 56 (1973).
461. Petrányi, Gy.: In *Autoimmune Diseases.* Ed. by Petrányi, Gy. Akadémiai Kiadó, Budapest 1974.
462. Pettit, J. E., Hoffbrand, A. V., Seah, P. P. and Fry, L.: *Brit. med. J.* **ii**, 438 (1972).
463*a*. Phillips, T. M.: *Rev. Inst. Pasteur Lyon* **4**, 59 (1971).
463*b*. ibid., **4**, 331 (1971).
464. Phillips, T. M., Everall, J. and Viza, D.: *Brit. J. Derm.* 9, **89**, Suppl. 12 (1973).
465. Phillips, T. M. and Lewis, M. G.: *Rev. europ. Ét. clin. biol.* **15**, 106 (1970).
466. Piérard, J. and Whimster, I.: *Brit. J. Derm.* **73**, 253 (1961).
467. Piessens, W. F.: *Cancer* **26**, 1212 (1970).
468. Pillemer, L., Ecker, E. E. and Wells, J. R.: *J. exp. Med.* **69**, 191 (1939).
468*a*. Pindborg, J. J.: In *Textbook of Dermatology.* Vol. II. 2nd ed.Ed. by Rook A. J., Wilkinson, D. S. and Ebling, F. J. G. Blackwell, Oxford 1972, p. 1703.

469. Piper, W., Hardmeier, Th. and Schäfer, E.: *Schweiz. med. Wschr.* **97,** 829 (1967).
470. Podányi, B., Dénes, M. and Horváth, E.: *Bőrgyógy. Vener. Szle.* (*Budap.*) **49,** 249 (1973).
471. Pototsky, I. I. and Grebennikov, V. A.: *Vestn. Derm. Vener.* (*Moscow*) **44**/1, 14 (1970).
472. Pototsky, I. I., Rodin, Yu. A. and Gerasimova, E. M.: *Vestn. Derm. Vener.* (*Moscow*) **46**/1, 9 (1972).
473. Pöttgen, W., Davaris, P. S., Hausamen, T. U. and Kindler, U.: *Dtsch. med. Wschr.* **96,** 1793 (1971).
474. Pras, M. and Reshef, T.: *Biochim. Biophys. Acta* **271,** 192 (1972).
475. Prehn, R. T. and Lappé, M. A.: *Transplant. Rev.* **7,** 26 (1971).
476. Price, W. R., Wood, M. and Childers, D.: *Amer. J. Surg.* **118,** 871 (1969).
476*a*. Provost, T. T. and Tomasi, T. B.: *J. clin. Invest.* **52,** 1779 (1973).
477. Pulvertaft, R. J. V.: In *Modern Trends in Pathology.* Ed. by Collins, D. H. Butterworth, London 1959, p. 19.
478. Quie, P. G., Kaplan, E. L., Page, A. R., Gruskey, F. L. and Mahwista, S. E.: *New Engl. J. Med.* **278,** 976 (1968).
479. Quie, P. G., White, J. G., Holmes, B. and Good, R. A.: *J. clin. Invest.* **46,** 668 (1967).
480. Quinn, R. W. and Singh, K. P.: *Proc. Soc. exp. Biol.* (*N. Y.*) **95,** 290 (1957).
481. Quismorio, F. P., Bland, S. L. and Friou, G. J.: *Clin. exp. Immunol.* **8,** 701 (1971).
482. Rapaport, T. F. and Converse, J. M.: In *Research in Burns.* Ed. by Wallace, A. B. and Wilkinson, A. W. Livingstone, Edinburgh 1966, p. 407.
483. Raque, C. J., Stein, K. M. and Samitz, M. H.: *Arch. Derm.* (*Chicago*) **102,** 371 (1970).
483*a*. Rawls, W. E., Adam, E. and Melnick, J. L.: *Proc. 2nd Int. Congr. Virol., Budapest 1971.* Ed. by Melnick, J. L. Karger, Basel 1972.
484. Rebrik, M. S., Pashkov, B. M. and Beletskaya, L. V.: *Vestn. Derm. Vener.* (*Moscow*) **47**/7, 26 (1973).
485. Reinert-Dietkey, J.: *Z. Haut-Geschl.Kr.* **45,** 241 (1970).
486. Riches, D. J., Martin, B. G. H., Seah, P. P. and Fry, L.: *Brit. J. Derm.* **88,** 323 (1973).
487*a*. Rimbaud, P., Meynadier, J., Guilhou, J.-J. and Clot, J.: *Nouv. Presse méd.* **1,** 2836 (1972).
487*b*. id., *Arch. Derm.* (*Chicago*) **108,** 371 (1973).
488. Rimbaud, P., Meynadier, J., Guilhou, J.-J., Clot, J. and Barthélémy, Mme J.: *Bull. Soc. franç. Derm. Syph.* **80,** 477 (1973).
489. Ritzenfeld, P.: *Arch. klin. exp. Derm.* **216,** 521 (1963).
490. Ritzmann, S. E., Daniels, J. C. and Larson, D. L.: *Amer. J. clin. Pathol.* **60,** 135 (1973).
491. Rizzetto, M. and Doniach, D.: *J. clin. Path.* **26,** 841 (1973).
492. Rocklin, R. E., Roson, F. S. and David, J. R.: *New Engl. J. Med.* **282,** 1340 (1970).
493*a*. Rodin, Yu. A.: *Vestn. Derm. Vener.* (*Moscow*) **43**/12, 31 (1969).
493*b*. ibid., **47**/7, 19 (1973).
493*c*. ibid., **48**/9, 8 (1974).
494. Rodnan, G. P., McEwen, C. and Wallace, St. L.: *J. Amer. med. Ass.* **224,** Suppl. to No. 5, 721 (1973).
494*a*. Roed-Petersen, B., Roed-Petersen, J. and Bendixen, G.: *Int. J. Cancer* **12,** 66 (1973).
495. Roenigk, H. H., jr. and Doedhar, Sh.: *Arch. Derm.* (*Chicago*) **107,** 353 (1973).
495*a*. Roenigk, H. H., jr., Doedhar, Sh., Jacques, R. St. and Burdick, K.: *Arch. Derm.* (*Chicago*) **109,** 668 (1974).
496. Roenigk, H. H., Ryan, J. G. and Bergfield, W. F.: *Arch. Derm.* (*Chicago*) **103,** 1 (1971).
496*a*. Rogers III, R. S. and Movius, D. L.: *J. invest. Derm.* **64,** 287 (1975).
497. Rogers, R. S., Sams, W. M., jr. and Shoter, R. G.: *Arch. Derm.* (*Chicago*) **109,** 361 (1974).
498. Rothbard, S. and Watson, R. F.: *J. exp. Med.* **116,** 337 (1962).
498*a*. Royston, A. L. and Aurelian, L.: *Proc. nat. Acad. Sci. USA* **67,** 204 (1970).

499. Rowell, N. R., Waite, A. and Scott, D. G.: *Brit. J. Derm.* **81,** 753 (1969).
500. Rowson, K. E. K. and Mahy, B. W. J.: *Bact. Rev.* **31,** 110 (1967).
501. Röckl, H.: *Hautarzt* **7,** 248 (1956).
502. Rudzki, E., Lagerlöf, B. and Nilzén, Å.: *Acta derm.-venereol.* **46,** 477 (1966).
503*a*. Rudzki, E. and Nilzén, Å.: *Acta derm.-venereol.* **46,** 368 (1966).
503*b*. ibid., **46,** 377 (1966).
503*c*. Russel, A. S.: *Amer. J. clin. Pathol.* **60,** 826 (1973).
503*d*. Russel, A. S., Maini, R. A., Bailey, M. and Dumonde, D. C.: *Clin. exp. Immunol.* **14,** 181 (1973).
503*e*. Sabin, A. B. and Tarro, G.: *Proc. nat. Acad. Sci. USA* **70,** 3225 (1973).
504. Sachs, A.: *Lancet* **ii,** 959 (1970).
505*a*. Saikia, N. K.: *Brit. J. Derm.* **86,** 411 (1972).
505*b*. ibid., **88,** 407 (1973).
506. Saikia, N. K. and Macconnell, L. E. S.: *Brit. J. Derm.* **87,** 1 (1972).
507. Saito, Y.: *Kitakanto med. J.* **21,** 228 (1971).
508. Sakai, H., Lynch, J. B., Lewis, S. R. and Ritzmann, S. E.: Meeting of Burn Association, California 1972.
509*a*. Sallay, K.: A recidiváló aphthás szájgyulladás kóreredetének vizsgálata és a therapia kérdése (On the Pathogenesis and Therapy of Recurrent Aphthous Stomatitis). Thesis. Budapest 1970.
509*b*. id., *Acta stomat. belg.* **67,** 273 (1970).
510. Sallay, K., Dán, P., Geck, P., Kulcsár, G. and Nász, I.: *Arch. derm. Forsch.* **241,** 15 (1971).
511. Sallay, K., Hajós, M. K. and Bánóczy, J.: *Allergie Immunologie* **17,** 17 (1971).
512. Sallay, K., Kulcsár, G., Dán, P., Nász, I. and Geck, P.: *Orv. Hetil.* **114,** 1874 (1973).
513. Salvin, S. B. and Smith, R. F.: *J. exp. Med.* **111,** 465 (1960).
514. Sams, W. M., jr.: *Arch. Derm. (Chicago)* **102,** 485 (1970).
515. Sams, W. M., jr. and Jordon, R. E.: *J. invest. Derm.* **56,** 474 (1971).
516*a*. Sams, W. M., jr. and Schur, P. H.: *J. invest. Derm.* **58,** 256 (1972).
516*b*. id., *J. Lab. clin. Med.* **82,** 249 (1973).
517. Sams, W. M., jr. and Smith, J. G., jr.: *Arch. Derm. (Chicago)* **90,** 137 (1964).
518*a*. Sanderson, K. V.: In *Textbook of Dermatology.* Vol. I. 2nd ed. Ed. by Rook, A. J., Wilkinson, D. S. and Ebling, F. J. G. Blackwell, Oxford 1972, p. 157.
518*b*. ibid., Vol. II, p. 1921.
519. Sarkany, I. and Gaylarde, P. M.: *Brit. J. Derm.* **87,** 81 (1972).
520. Sasai, Y. and Fujiyama, T.: *Tohoku J. exp. Med.* **99,** 9 (1969).
521. Schaumburg-Lever, G., Orfanos, C. E. and Lever, W. F.: *Arch. Derm. (Chicago)* **106,** 662 (1972).
522. Schnyder, U. W. and Hardmeier, T.: In *XIIIth Int. Congr. Derm., München 1967.* Vol. III. Ed. by Jadassohn, W. and Schirren, C. G. Springer, Berlin 1968, p. 137.
523. Schroeter, A. L., Copeman, P. W. M., Jordon, R. E., Jordon, W. M., jr. and Winkelmann, R. K. W.: *Arch. Derm. (Chicago)* **104,** 254 (1971).
524. Schroeter, A. L., Sams, W. M., jr. and Jordon, R. E.: *Arch. Derm. (Chicago)* **100,** 736 (1969).
525. Schultz, R. T., Calkins, E. and Milgrom, F.: *Amer. J. Pathol.* **50,** 957 (1967).
526. Scoggins, R. B.: In *Dermatology in General Medicine.* Ed. by Fitzpatrick, Th. B., Arndt, K. A., Clark, W. H., jr., Eisen, A. Z., Van Scott, E. J. and Vaughan, J. H. MacGraw-Hill, New York 1971, p. 1640.
527. Seah, P. P., Fry, L., Hoffbrand, A. V. and Holborow, E. J.: *Lancet* **i,** 834 (1971).
528. Seah, P. P., Fry, L., Mazaheri, M. R., Mowbray, J. F., Hoffbrand, A. V. and Holborow, E. J.: *Lancet* **ii,** 175 (1973).
529. Seah, P. P., Fry, L., Rossiter, M. A., Hoffbrand, A. V. and Holborow, E. J.: *Lancet* **ii,** 681 (1971).
530. Seah, P. P., Fry, L., Stewart, J. S., Chapman, B. L., Hoffbrand, A. V. and Holborow, E. J.: *Lancet* **i,** 611 (1972).
531. Seah, P. P., Mazaheri, M. R. and Fry, L.: *Brit. J. Derm.* **89,** Suppl. 9, 12 (1973).
531*a*. Segall, A., Weiler, O., Gemin, J., Lacour, J. and Lacour, F.: *Int. J. Cancer* **9,** 417 (1972).

532. Seiger, H. F., Shingleton, W. W., Metzgar, R. S. and Buckley, C. E.: *Ann. Surg.* **178**, 352 (1973).
533. Serre, H., Simon, L., Mandin, J., Clot, J. and Sany, J.: *Presse méd.* **79**, 2110 (1971).
534. Shelly, W. B., Preucel, R. W. and Spoont, S. S.: *J. Amer. med. Ass.* **190**, 35 (1964).
535. Shiner, M. and Ballard, J.: *Lancet* **i**, 1202 (1972).
535*a*. Shingleton, W. W., Seigler, H. F., Stocks, L. H. and Downs, R. W., jr.: *Med. News* **228**, 1358 (1974).
536. Shochat, S., Abulata, N. and Knight, S.: *Cytolios (Cambridge)* **6**, 21 (1972).
537. Shore, R. N. and Shelley, W. B.: *Arch. Derm. (Chicago)* **109**, 400 (1974).
538. Shrivastava, P. K.: *Dermatologica (Basel)* **144**, 310 (1972).
539. Silberberg, I., Kopf, A. W., Sasagawa, S. and Morill, S. D.: *J. invest. Derm.* **47**, 99 (1966).
540. Simon, N., Dobozy, A. and Hunyadi, J.: *Arch. derm. Forsch.* **247**, 367 (1973).
541. Simon, N., Husz, S. and Berkó, Gy.: *Z. Hautkr.* **49**, 407 (1974).
542. Singh, I. and Garg, B. R.: *Indian J. Derm.* **16**, 11 (1970).
543. Singh, I., Sharma, N. N., Seth, H. N. and Gaind, M. L.: *Dermatologica (Basel)* **146**, 55 (1973).
544. Skog, E. and Linder, O.: *Acta derm.-venereol.* **45**, 461 (1965).
545. Sluis, I. v. d.: *Dermatologica (Basel)* **132**, 409 (1966).
546. Smith, J. L. and Stehlin, J. S.: *Cancer* **18**, 1399 (1965).
547. Smith, R. T.: *New Engl. J. Med.* **287**, 439 (1972).
548. Sood, V. D. and Pasricha, J. S.: *Brit. J. Derm.* **90**, 575 (1974).
549. Southam, Ch. M.: In *Immunological Diseases*. Vol. I. 2nd ed. Ed. by Samter, M. Little-Brown, Boston 1971, p. 743.
549*a*. Sophocles, A. M. and Nadler, S. H.: *Surg. Gynec. Obstet.* **133**, 321 (1971).
549*b*. Söltz-Szöts, J.: *Arch. klin. exp. Derm.* **220**, 105 (1964).
549*c*. id., *Z. Haut-Geschl.Kr.* **38**, 123 (1965).
550*a*. Sönnichsen, N.: *Hautarzt* **22**, 222 (1971).
550*b*. id., *Bőrgyógy. Vener. Szle. (Budap.)* **49**, 135 (1973).
551. Sönnichsen, N., Klug, H., Thormann, Th., Ziegler, H., Beckmann, I. and Lisewski, G.: *Derm. Mschr.* **158**, 773 (1972).
551*a*. Sparks, F. C., Silverstein, M. J., Hunt, J. S., Haskell, Ch. M., Pilch, Y. H. and Morton, D. L.: *New Engl. J. Med.* **289**, 827 (1973).
552. Spier, H. W.: *Hautarzt* **21**, 94 (1970).
553. Sri Ram, J., Delellis, R. A. and Glenner, J. J.: *Int. Arch. Allergy* **34**, 269 (1968).
554. Stastny, P., Stembridge, V. A. and Ziff, J.: *J. exp. Med.* **118**, 635 (1963).
555. Steffen, C.: *Allgemeine und experimentelle Immunologie und Immunpathologie sowie ihre klinische Anwendung*. Thieme, Stuttgart 1968, p. 411.
556. St. Geme, J. W., jr., Prince, J. T., Burke, B. A., Good, R. A. and Krivit, W.: *New Engl. J. Med.* **273**, 229 (1965).
557. Stillman, M. A. and Baer, R. L.: *Acta derm.-venereol.* **52**, 393 (1972).
557*a*. Stjernsward, J. and Levin, A.: *Cancer (Phil.)* **28**, 628 (1971).
558. Stringa, S. G., Bianchi, C., Casala, A. and Bianchi, O.: *Arch. Derm. (Chicago)* **105**, 541 (1972).
559. Stutman, O. and Good, R. A.: In *Immunology and the Skin*. Ed. by Montagna, W. and Billingham, R. E. Appleton-Century-Crofts, New York 1971, p. 357.
560. Summer, W. C. and Foraker, A. G.: *Cancer* **13**, 79 (1960).
561. Summerlin, W. T. and Jordon, R. E.: *J. invest. Derm.* **62**, 342 (1974).
562. Su-Yu, Sh. and Beutner, E. H.: *J. invest. Derm.* **61**, 270 (1973).
563. Szabó, É.: Az immunofluoreszcens eljárás optikai standardizálása és alkalmazásának lehetőségei a bőrgyógyászatban. (Optical standardization of the immunofluorescence and its possible use in the dermatology.) Thesis, Szeged 1973, p. 141.
564. Szabó, É., Berkó, Gy., Husz, S. and Simon, N.: *Acta. morph. Acad. Sci. hung.* **21**, 155 (1973).
565*a*. Szabó, É., Czakó, F., Husz, S., Török, L. and Simon, M.: *Bőrgyógy. Vener. Szle. (Budap.)* **49**, 145 (1973).
565*b*. id., *Derm. Mschr.* **159**, 608 (1973).
566. Szabó, É., Husz, S., Berkó, Gy. and Simon, N.: *Acta morph. Acad. Sci. hung.* **21**, 165 (1973).

567. Szegedi, Gy., Bobory, J., Kakuk, Gy., Leövey, A. and Petrányi, Gy.: *Magyar Belorv. Arch. (Budapest)* **10,** Suppl., 189 (1973).
568. Takasuki, M. and Klein, E.: *Immunology* **21,** 675 (1971).
569. Tan, J. S., Watanakunakorn, C. and Phair, J. P.: *J. Lab. clin. Med.* **78,** 316 (1971).
570. Taylor, J.: *Lancet* **i,** 883 (1973).
571. Témime, P., Latourelle, P. and Sally, J.-C.: *Ann. Derm. Syph.* **98,** 509 (1971).
572. ten Have-Opbroeck, A. A. W.: *Dermatologica (Basel)* **132,** 109 (1966).
573. Terasaki, P. I. and Chamberlain, C. C.: *J. exp. Med.* **115,** 439 (1962).
574. Terner, K.: *Fogorv. Szle. (Budapest)* **61,** 289 (1968).
575. Thé, T. M., Eilergen, R., Lomberts, H. B., Oldnoff, J., Ploeg, E., Schrafford-Koops, H. and Nieweg, H. O.: *Acta. med. scand.* **192,** 141 (1972).
576. Theiss, B., Schnyder, U. W. and Boni, A.: *Arch. klin. exp. Derm.* **239,** 70 (1970).
576*a*. Thies, W.: *Arch. klin. exp. Derm.* **227,** 541 (1966).
576*b*. Thies, W. and Klaschka, F.: *Arch. klin. exp. Derm.* **237,** 51 (1970).
577. Thio, Th. H., Cormane, R. H. and Szabó, É.: *Sth. Afr. med. J.* **45,** Special Issue, 57 (1971).
578. Thio, Th. H., Leynse, B., Feltkamp, T. E. W. and Neumann, H.: *Sth. Afr. med. J.* **45,** Special Issue, 199 (1971).
579*a*. Thivolet, J. and Beyvin, A.-J.: *Hautarzt* **18,** 412 (1967).
579*b*. id., *Bull. Soc. franç. Derm. Syph.* **74,** 300 (1967).
579*c*. id., *Experientia (Basel)* **24,** 945 (1968).
579*d*. id., *Bull. Soc. franç. Derm. Syph.* **78,** 369 (1971).
580*a*. Thivolet, J., Beyvin, A.-J. and André, D.: *Presse méd.* **77,** 1973 (1969).
580*b*. id., *Dermatologica (Basel)* **140,** 310 (1970).
580*c*. id., *Ann. Derm. Syph.* **97,** 534 (1970).
581. Thivolet, J., Beyvin, A.-J., Perrot, H. and André, Mlle: *Bull. Soc. franç. Derm. Syph.* **76,** 463 (1969).
582. Thivolet, J., Bondet, P., Perrot, H. and Claudy, A.: *Bull. Soc. franç. Derm. Syph.* **78,** 263 (1971).
583. Thivolet, J., Perrot, H. and Beyvin, A.-J.: *Bull. Soc. franç. Derm. Syph.* **76.** 587 (1969).
584. Thomas, H. C., Ferguson, A., McLennan, J. G. and Mason, D. K.: *J. clin. Path.* **26,** 371 (1973).
585. Thunold, S.: *Spectrum* **17,** 37 (1973).
586. Tillmann, W. B.: *Brit. med. J.* **i,** 1471 (1950).
587. Tolman, M. M.: *Arch. Derm. (Chicago)* **77,** 462 (1968).
588. Tromovitch, T. A. and Heggli, W. F.: *Calif. Med.* **106,** 211 (1967).
589*a*. Ueki, H.: *Arch. Derm. (Chicago)* **100,** 610 (1965).
589*b*. id., *Jap. J. Derm. Ser. B.* **77,** 45 (1967).
590. Ueki, H., Nakagawa, Sh. and Komoto, A.: *Jap. J. Derm. Ser. B.* **80,** 150 (1970).
590*a*. Utsuki, Y., Kawaoi, A. and Hamashima, Y.: *Acta path. jap.* **22,** 207 (1972).
591. Vaerman, J. P. and Heremans, J. F.: *Immunology* **18,** 27 (1970).
592. Van de Staak, W. J. B. M. and Bergers, A. M. G.: *Dermatologica (Basel)* **144,** 294 (1972).
593. Van de Staak, W. J. B. M., Van Tongeren, J. H. M., Schillings, P. H. M. and Doomernik, L.: *Dermatologica (Basel)* **140,** 231 (1970).
594*a*. Van der Meer, J. B.: *Brit. J. Derm.* **81,** 493 (1969).
594*b*. id., *Dermatitis herpetiformis: A Specific (Immunopathological?) Entity.* N. V. Drukkerij v. h. Batteljee and Terpstra. Leiden 1972.
595. Van Dijk, T. J. A. and Van Velde, J. L.: *Dermatologica (Basel)* **147,** 179 (1973).
596*a*. Van Joost, Th., Cormane, R. H. and Pondman, K. W.: *J. invest. Derm.* **56,** 450 (1971).
596*b*. id., *Brit. J. Derm.* **87,** 466 (1972).
597. Vavelzidis, A. and Theodoris, A.: *Brit. J. Derm.* **85,** 14 (1971).
598. Vazquez, J. J. and Dixon, F. J.: *J. exp. Med.* **104,** 727 (1956).
599. Verhagen, H., De Cree and Brugmans, J.: *Lancet* **ii,** 842 (1973).
600. Vetters, J. M., Saikia, N. K., Wood, J. and Simpson, J. A.: *Brit. J. Derm.* **88,** 437 (1973).
601. Voelter, W. W., Newell, G. B., Schwartz, St. L., Bean, S. F. and Mullins, J. F.: *Arch. Derm. (Chicago)* **108,** 93 (1973).

602. Voisin, G. and Maurer, P.: *Sem. Hôp. (Paris)* **31,** 1909 (1955).
602*a*. Vul, S. M. and Grigorieva, M. A.: *Vestn. Derm. Vener. (Moscow)* **48**/10, 34 (1974).
603. Waisman, M., Dundon, B. C. and Michel, B.: *Arch. Derm. (Chicago)* **107,** 200 (1973).
604. Waldmann, T. A., Pilmar, S. H., Balestra, S. T., Jost, M. C., Bruce, R. M. and Terry, W. D.: *J. Immunol.* **109,** 304 (1972).
605. Walzer, R. A., Einbinder, J. and Nelson, C. T.: *Arch. Derm. (Chicago)* **90,** 583 (1964).
606. Wanger, N. S. and Hashimoto, K.: *J. invest. Derm.* **56,** 402 (1971).
607. Wassermann, H. P. and Van der Walt, J. J.: *Sth. Afr. med. J.* **47,** 7 (1973).
608. Welke, S., Jost, H. and Schwarz, J. A.: *Z. Hautkr.* **48,** 943 (1973).
609. Wells, G. C. and Rimington, C.: *Brit. J. Derm.* **65,** 337 (1953).
610. Wells, J. V., Fudenberg, H. H. and Epstein, W. L.: *J. Immunol.* **108,** 977 (1972).
611. Wesbach, H. W., Lischka, G. and Tritsch, H.: *Arch. derm. Forsch.* **245,** 346 (1972).
612. Whimster, I. W.: *Brit. J. Derm.* **90,** 111 (1974).
613. White, A. G., Barnetson, R. St. C., DaCosta, J. A. G. and McClelland, D. B. L.: *Lancet* **i,** 108 (1973).
614*a*. Whitefield, A.: *Lancet* **ii,** 122 (1921).
614*b*. id., *Brit. J. Derm.* **34,** 331 (1922).
614*c*. id., In *C. R. VIII. Congr. Int. Derm., Copenhague 1930*. Engelsen et Schrøder, Copenhague 1931, p. 142.
615. Whittingham, S. and Mackay, I. R.: *Brit. J. Derm.* **84,** 1 (1971).
616. Wick, G. and Beutner, E. H.: *Immunology* **16,** 149 (1969).
617. Wilgram, G. F., Caulfield, J. B. and Lever, W. F.: *J. invest. Derm.* **36,** 373 (1961).
618. Wilhelmj, C. M., jr., Kierland, R. R. and Owen, C. A., jr.: *Arch. Derm. (Chicago)* **86,** 161 (1962).
619. Wilkinson, R. D., Elie, J. D., Miot, M.-J. and Wakkary, J. A.: *J. invest. Derm.* **57,** 401 (1971).
620. Wilson, R. E., Hager, E. B., Hampers, C. L., Corson, J. M., Merril, J. P. and Murray, J. E.: *New Engl. J. Med.* **278,** 479 (1968).
621. Windhorst, D. B.: In *Dermatologic Allergy*. Ed. by Criep, L. H. W. B. Saunders, Philadelphia 1967, p. 457.
622. Windhorst, D. B., Holmes, B. and Good, R. A.: *Lancet* **i,** 737 (1967).
623. Windhorst, D. B., Page, A. R., Holmes, B., Quie, P. G. and Good, R. A.: *J. clin. Invest.* **47,** 1026 (1968).
624. Winkelmann, R. K. and Gleich, G. J.: *J. Amer. med. Ass.* **225,** 378 (1973).
624*a*. Winkelmann, R. K. and Roth, H. L.: *Arch. Derm. (Chicago)* **82,** 390 (1960).
625. Witebsky, E., Rose, N. R., Terplan, K., Paine, J. R. and Egan, R.: *J. Amer. med. Ass.* **164,** 1439 (1957).
626. Wolff, K. and Schreiner, E.: *Nature* **229,** 59 (1971).
627. Wolff, K., Tappeiner, K. and Schreiner, E.: *Arch. klin. exp. Derm.* **232,** 325 (1968).
627*a*. Yang, J. P. S., Gale, J. L. and Lee, G. C. Y.: *Proc. Soc. exp. Biol. (N. Y.)* **143,** 28 (1973).
628. Ziegler, J. L., Lewis, M. G., Luyomba, J. M. S. and Kiryabwire, J. W. M.: *Brit. J. Cancer* **23,** 729 (1969).
629. Zombai, E. and Kelényi, G.: In *Abstr. XIVth Int. Congr. Derm., Padua–Venice 1972*. Ed. by Flarer, F., Paton, P. M., Rabito, C., Serri, F. and Kleinmann, R. L. Int. Congr. Series No. 248. Excerpta Medica Foundation, Amsterdam 1972, p. 78.
630. Zondek, B. and Bromberg, V.: *J. Allergy* **16,** 1 (1945).
631. Zucker-Franklin, D. and Franklin, E. C.: *Amer. J. Pathol.* **59,** 23 (1970).

CHAPTER 41

IMMUNOLOGICAL FACTORS IN INFERTILITY. SPERMAL IMMUNITY AND AUTOIMMUNITY

by

J. MOLNÁR

INTRODUCTION

In the last few decades a new branch of immunoallergology dealing with sperm immunity has developed. In the medical practice it is of interest from two points of view: (*i*) anti-sperm antibodies in the female organism may explain the infertility of some marriages; (*ii*) sperm autoimmunity in the male organism is a newly recognized factor of male infertility.

In 1899 the pioneers of the field, Metchnikoff [78*a*] and Landsteiner [65], described independently that semen and spermatozoa may act as antigen. Similar findings were published by Metalnikoff [78*b*] and by Moxter [79] in the subsequent year and by others [32, 47] later. All these authors successfully immunized male animals with semen spermatozoa or testicular tissue. The immunized animals (*i*) developed antibodies; (*ii*) the spermatozoa injected into their peritoneal cavity agglutinated and became immobile; (*iii*) the spermatogenesis of the animals became severely damaged. The antibodies proved to be organ-specific.

A preparation isolated from human testis, containing protein and carbohydrates, showed antigenic potency in guinea pigs. The resulting antibodies demonstrated by precipitation, Schultz–Dale reaction and immunoelectrophoresis cross-reacted with guinea pig testicular antigen [56*b*]. Guinea pig testicular cells continuously propagated *in vitro* for 5 months produced an antigen which sensitized guinea pigs upon being injected with the culture and caused in them ileal anaphylactic contracture and aspermatogenesis [59].

Ahlgren [1] examined *post coitum* Douglas punctates from 127 infertile women including 13 who had proved to be positive for seminal agglutinins according to the Kibrick test. Spermatozoa were found in the punctates from 2 of the Kibrick-positive women and in 17 of the remaining 114. Ahlgren suggested that the presence of spermatozoa in the abdominal cavity plays no major role in the induction of anti-sperm antibodies.

The possible role of the human testis in the immunological response to autoimmunization or isogeneic sensitization was substantiated during attempts to induce allergic orchitis. In Günther's [41*b*] experiments the deferent duct and the epididymis of guinea pigs were laid open surgically on one side and placed in the abdominal cavity. Spermatozoa migrating into the abdominal cavity were resorbed there and caused isogeneic immunization which was stimulated by simultaneous parenteral administration of complete Freund's adjuvant. Three to 4 weeks thereafter agglutinating antibodies to spermatozoa appeared in the serum of half of the animals. Some of the animals developed bilateral testicular damage in the form of an autoimmune aspermatogenesis. Katsh [56*d*] carried out serial experiments to induce allergic orchitis in volunteers with prostate carcinoma before therapeutic castration. Only few of the volunteers developed low-titre antibodies and positive skin reaction; testicular biopsies showed numerous foci of lesions with sloughing and cytolysis of germinal cells.

Immunization per vaginam may occur in females [63]. Increased amounts of IgG have been found in vaginal fluids [23, 49] and the secretory piece has been detected in cervical glandular epithelial cells suggesting that local antibody formation may occur in these cells. The antigens of spermatozoa and seminal plasma are normally broken down by the enzymes of the uterine mucosa. If some local or systemic factor interferes with this mechanism, immunization might occur.

SPERM IMMUNITY

ANTIGENS

Some of the immunizing antigens come from the spermatozoa, others from the seminal plasma.

Sperm-specific antigens have been detected with fluorescent antibody technique in the rabbit genital tract at the spermatid stage of spermatogenesis [54]. These antigens were associated primarily with the acrosome and the cytoplasmic droplet, and to a lesser degree with the midpiece and tail. The gradual loss of immunofluorescence by the cytoplasmic droplet during passage through the epididymis was paralleled by the appearance of similarly detectable antigens in the epithelium of the epididymis, especially in the cauda epididymidis. This was more pronounced in sexually rested bucks than in sexually active bucks, suggesting loss of antigens from the spermatozoa and absorption by the epididymal epithelium. In addition, antigens common to accessory gland tissue and seminal plasma were detectable on spermatozoa throughout the genital tract. These antigens were removed by absorption with liver powder.

The head of the human spermatozoon is covered by what is called 'spermatozoa-coating antigens' [118], which are procuced by the seminal vesicles and coat the spermatozoa migrating out of the testis. The acrosome of the spermatozoon head has also been found to contain antigen and antigens have been demonstrated in the midpiece [40] and in the tail [124]. In testicular sperm cells only one type of antigen has so far been demonstrated [71*b*]. The spermatozoal antigens are thermostable, non-dialysable and organ-specific.

In the seminal plasma 8 or 9 antigenic fractions have been found [9*b*, 10]. Of these 4 or 5 appear to be identical with spermatozoal components, 2 or 3 originate from the prostate and one from the epididymis.

Recently 23 antigens have been demonstrated in the human seminal plasma using an immunoelectrophoretic technique [28]. Of these, five have been found to be identical with antigens occurring in the female genital tract and another five, with antigens of other secretions and tissues of the female organism. It has been suggested that immunization of females is prevented by the seminal plasma because the antigens of the latter are recognized as self by the female organism. The major antigenic component of human seminal plasma is a protein. It is specific, highly immunogenic and probably not prostatic in origin [111].

The testicular tissue antigens are organ-specific, but cross-reactions with heterologous spermatozoa as well as liver, spleen, kidney and pancreas antigens, etc. may occur.

Examined with rabbit antiserum, guinea pig epididymal sperm showed two antigens that were also demonstrable in epididymal and testicular extracts and in seminal sperm [46].

The human prostate and prostatic secretions contain [11] (*i*) antigens which are shared by other organs and tissues; (*ii*) the major antigens which are specific to the prostate and are also found in the secretions and excretions of the male urogenital tract. Cross-reactions may be obtained with monkey (Macacus) prostatic tissue, but not with those of nonprimate species.

Attempts have been made to clarify the chemical composition of seminal antigens [60]. By immunoelectrophoresis albumin, IgG, IgA, IgM, transferrin and 6 further plasma proteins have been distinguished, viz. [98]:

	per cent
albumin	6.3
α-globulin	15.9
β-globulin	41.1
γ-globulin	23.2
O fraction	12.7
Non-identifiable	0.8

According to a more recent publication [48], the P_1 fraction of the seminal plasma contains several different proteins including α_2-globulins, the β_1 globulin belongs to the P_2 fraction and the fractions P_3–P_8 correspond to the serum proteins. The antigens in the lipid fraction of the spermatozoa are different from those in the polysaccharide-polypeptide fraction (containing 18 to 20 amino acid molecules and 20–30 per cent carbohydrate) inducing antibodies which give rise to midpiece-to-midpiece and tail-to-tail agglutination, respectively [40]. The head-to-head agglutination [97] is attributed to a lipoprotein which, being present in the spermatozoon-free semen as well, cannot be considered to be a spermatozoal component. When immunizing rabbits with an isolated human sperm inhibitor, the production of an antiserum could be observed, which gave a strong precipitation reaction with isolated antigen. It seemed to be lactoferrin. Fluorescence was only obtained in the head of human spermatozoa: the inhibitor appears to be bound to the protease of the head [48*a*].

ANTIBODIES

The mode of action of the antibodies inducible by the above antigens is variable. First of all, the different types of spermatozoan agglutination [96*d*], viz. head-to-head, tail-to-tail and end-piece-to-end-piece agglutination may be mentioned. The mobile agglutinins are to be found in the blood serum, partly bound to lymphocytes [20]; fixed antibodies most frequently occur in lymph nodes [68] and in the female genital organs. The agglutinated spermatozoa may retain some sluggish mobility *in loco* for several hours, but they do not change their place, wherefrom they are not suitable for fertilization. False spermatozoon agglutination may frequently occur. (*i*) The most common false reaction is the so-called heteroagglutination, a phenomenon based on the attachment of spermatozoa to larger, e.g. epithelial cells, in a manner analogous to taxis, i.e. to their affinity to the ovum. Grouped bacteria or *Trichomonas vaginalis* organisms may also give rise to this phenomenon and perhaps this is why treatment of cervicitides in infertile women was followed by pregnancy in several cases. (*ii*) The spermatozoon agglutination that occurs in the liquefied semen prior to testing must also be considered as a false reaction. (*iii*) According to immunologists physiological substances necessary for fertilization, e.g. fertilizin and antifertilizin, may bring about a phenomenon similar to spermatozoon agglutination. (*iv*) Dilution of the semen with saline may also stimulate spermatozoon agglutination. This is especially important from the point of view of artificial insemination of animals. To avoid this phenomenon, sperm used for such purposes is diluted and stored in a buffered phosphate–egg yolk–glycerol medium.

Anti-seminal antibodies have been found in three immunoglobulin classes: antibodies cytotoxic for spermatozoa were found to be IgG; those harmless for spermatozoa and capable of combining with seminal plasma antigens absorbed to the cell surface were IgM or IgA [86]. Using the three-layer immunofluorescence technique [44], it was revealed that the antibodies against the antigen in the front part of the acrosome were primarily IgG. Antibodies against antigens in the equatorial segment and the postnuclear cap showed a varying predominance of these two immunoglobulins. Spermatozoal antibody of IgA nature was found in small amounts. Antibodies against seminal plasma and prostate may cause agglutination of seminal spermatozoa and higher haemagglutination titres than antibodies against testis, epididymis, seminal vesicle or spermatozoa [73*b*]. The immobilizing, agglutinating, and cytotoxic activities of the anti-seminal-plasma antibodies appear to be more intensive than those of the anti-spermatozoal and anti-testis antibodies [35]. It is therefore reasonable to assume that the testis contributes a few antigens to semen which appear to be sperm-specific because they are present in washed epididymal and seminal spermatozoa but not in seminal plasma, whereas the prostate and the seminal vesicles provide the major part of secondary sperm antigens. Specific agglutination of homologous spermatozoa could not be produced with human anti-A and anti-B immune serum. However, human spermatozoa can be immobilized and agglutinated with rabbit anti-human-seminal-plasma serum. It appears that spermatozoa are able to adsorb anti-ABO antibodies, moreover to a higher degree than red blood cells [35*a*].

IMMUNOLOGICAL TESTS

Of the numerous procedures having been developed to demonstrate anti-seminal antibodies the best-known ones are described in the following.*

1. The macro-agglutination test of Kibrick et al. [62] (direct spermatozoon agglutination test). Liquefied semen from a highly fertile man is left to sediment and the supernatant is removed by a pipette and mixed with Baker's solution to obtain a dilution containing approximately 40 million spermatozoa with satisfactory mobility per ml. This suspension is mixed with an equal volume of 10 per cent gelatine solution and incubated at 37 °C for 10 min. A halving dilution series from 1 : 2 to 1 : 1,024 is prepared from the serum to be tested in precipitation tubes in 0.3 ml volumes of diluent. Then 0.3 ml of the incubated spermatozoon suspension is added to each dilution. The mixtures are incubated for two hours at 37 °C. Any turbidity in dilutions over 1 : 16 is considered positive. This is an advantageous method [52], approximately 100 times as sensitive as Baskin's micro-test (Fig. 41-1). The capillary method if used in animal experiments may be as sensitive as the Kibrick test, but with human spermatozoa and antiserum raised against them in rabbits, the latter method proved superior [104].
2. Baskin's micro-agglutination test [12]. One drop of diluted semen (40 million spermatozoa per ml) prepared as described above is mixed on a slide with one drop of the serum under testing. The preparation is examined under the microscope at 15-min intervals within a period of 6 hours. This procedure is suitable first of all for screening [9*b*]; earlier it was also used as a quantitative test.
3. Double gel diffusion precipitation (Ouchterlony) test [83]. Diffusion in agar plate of spermatozoon suspension on the one hand and of anti-seminal antibodies on the other, results in precipitation lines the number of which depends on the speed of the diffusion of different antigens. Cross agar diffusion reaction showed that seminal plasma has higher common antigenicity with prostate and seminal vesicle than with seminal spermatozoa, testis or epididymis [9*a*]. Several antigens could be revealed by gel diffusion studies, using well-washed but not ruptured spermatozoa, indicating that intentional cell breaking is not essential for demonstrating these antigens [46].
4. The passive haemagglutination test [21] is based on the phenomenon that red blood cells are able to bind soluble antigens on their surface ('coating'). Pretreatment with tannic acid facilitates coating and increases the agglutinability of the coated red blood cells with antibodies against the coating antigen. Under appropriate conditions the test can be read in 30 min. Several authors [9*a*, 107]

* The reliability of all methods can be enhanced by adopting the precautionary measures suggested by Shulman [101*b*]: (*i*) to use serum at a minimal dilution of 1 : 4; (*ii*) to make repeated tests on each serum; (*iii*) to use at least two different test methods; (*iv*) to include in every test a positive control serum and a negative control serum, both of human origin.

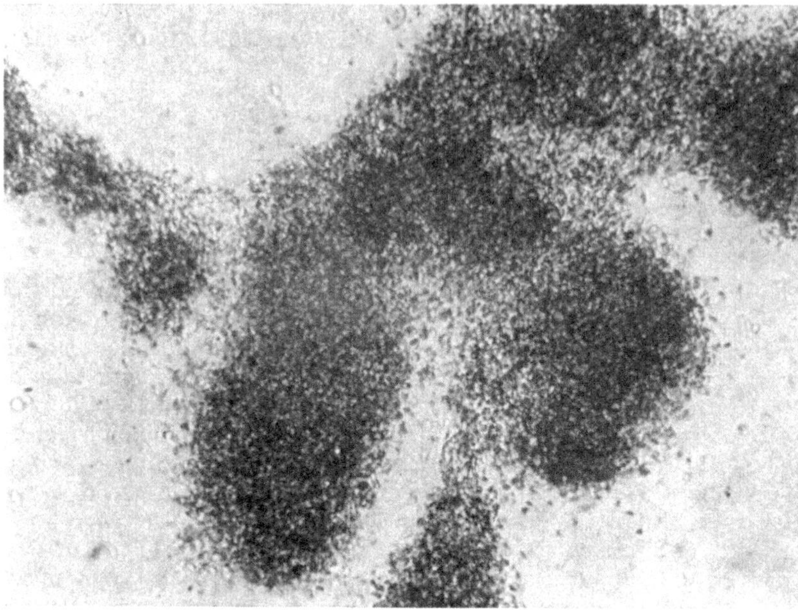

a

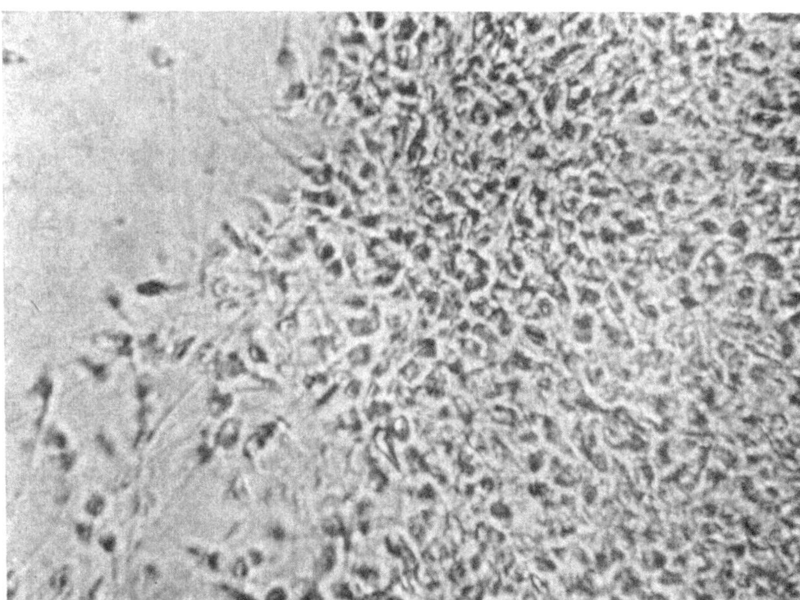

b

Fig. 41-1. Agglutinated spermatozoa (*a* ×100; *b* ×450)

have recommended this test for titration of anti-seminal antibodies. It was found 10 times as sensitive as the spermatozoon agglutination and immobilization tests [50]. However, blood group isoantigen present in sperm cells or in the seminal fluid may induce false positive results [3]. Recently this test has been considered of little practical importance [9*b*].

5. Immobilization or cytotoxicity test is a simple procedure. On the effect of antibodies spermatozoa lose their mobility either without any morphological change or accompanied by swelling of the middle piece and, in certain cases, complete lysis of spermatozoa [52].

6. Recently the immunofluorescence technique has acquired importance [9*b*, 34, 70, 86]. Antibodies are labelled with fluorescein isothiocyanate and the pattern of fluorescence is observed in seminal smears or in testicular sections. The acrosomes of the head of spermatozoa and the perinuclear area of the spermatids [34, 71*a*, 74], occasionally also the mid-portion of the tail [45], stain intensively. It has been claimed [52] that even non-agglutinating (incomplete, i.e. univalent) antibodies can be revealed by the immunofluorescence technique. Both anti-seminal plasma and anti-vesicular fluid antisera failed to stain guinea pig sperm cells. In contrast with the normal serum, the immunofluorescent staining with rabbit or guinea pig antiserum is thermostable [46].

The indirect double-layer immunofluorescence technique [44] is suitable for studying different antigens of human spermatozoa. A three-layer technique with monospecific antisera against human immunoglobulins as the second layer was employed with fractionation of sera on Sephadex G-200 or DEAE cellulose, followed by testing of the concentrated pools by a double-layer immunofluorescence technique.

7. The mixed antiglobulin reaction is suitable for the demonstration of both antigens and antibodies adsorbed on the cell surface. To the cell suspension under test red blood cells coated with antiglobulin are added. The antiglobulin will be bound to the immunoglobulin on the test cells so that a mixed aggregate of test cells and red blood cells is formed [33, 85, 86].

8. Species-specific anti-semen and anti-adnexal gland antibodies are demonstrable by the C fixation test as well [73*b*]. Using the C consumption test, positive result was obtained in 9 per cent of the cases tested.

9. Immunoelectrophoresis has been used for the analysis of complex mixtures such as seminal plasma proteins, which are thus separable on the basis of their electrophoretic mobility and antigenic character [48]. By this method one of the prostate antigens was identified as acid phosphatase and that of the seminal vesicle as lactoferrin; the latter is said to be the most potent sperm-coating antigen [45].

10. Radioimmunoassay is a method of measuring antibody or antigen concentration by employing radioactive reactant(s) [50, 81].

11. The microtest of Franklin and Dukes [37] can be employed for the demonstration of antibodies or antigenic components of the seminal plasma [19]. The value of this test as compared with Kibrick's macro-method has been recently challenged [101*b*].

12. Kremer's capillary mucus-penetration test [64] reveals the behaviour of spermatozoa penetrating in the cervical mucus.

13. The intracutaneous test (or scratch test) is considered to be a test of unsatisfactory accuracy [42].

14. The leukocyte migration inhibition test using soluble sperm extract antigens is a valuable method for the *in vitro* detection of delayed hypersensitivity to human sperm [106*a*].

ROLE OF ANTI-SEMINAL ANTIBODIES IN THE INFERTILITY OF FEMALES

The role of anti-seminal antibodies in the infertility of females has been suggested by several observations. (*i*) The low frequency of pregnancy and the high incidence of abortion in prostitutes cannot always be explained by gynaecological abnormalities, such as cervicitis, adnexitis, obliteration of tube, etc. In a group of prostitutes studied for sperm-agglutinating antibodies the incidence of positive reaction was 75 per cent compared with the 25 per cent in a group of unmarried women [14*b*]. (*ii*) Wives who earlier had been unable to conceive became pregnant when their husbands had returned after prolonged absence, e.g. from the war or POW camps. This might be attributed to a fall in anti-seminal antibody titres. (*iii*) Women divorced after an infertile marriage became pregnant in the second marriage, although there appeared to be no abnormality in the first husband which might have explained the infertility of the marriage. It has been suggested that following unprotected coitus substances having antigenic properties might be absorbed from the semen through the vagina, uterus, tubes or peritoneum and induce an antibody response. The antibodies thus produced may immobilize the spermatozoa and, consequently, prevent conception. C fixing anti-seminal antibodies were demonstrated [7*a*] in serum samples from women, healthy or suffering from gynaecological disease, and the antibody titres were in direct relation with the frequency of sexual intercourses. The probability of conception seemed to be inversely related to the antibody titre, but there was no correlation with the increased rate of spontaneous abortion. In sera from intact girls such C fixing antibodies could not be demonstrated. High-titre (1 : 64 or higher) anti-seminal agglutinins were detected in 16 per cent of 70 infertile wives [80]. Such antibodies were found in 6 per cent in fertile women, but these antibodies reacted with the spermatozoa of only one donor; those from other donors did not agglutinate. With the immunofluorescent technique tissue-fixed serum antibodies were demonstrated in the cervical and endometrial tissues of patients with high-titre circulating anti-seminal antibodies. Serum samples from apparently normal, yet infertile, women contained significantly more antibodies reacting with spermatozoa of their husbands than sera from fertile control women. Anti-sperm reaction was observed in 23 per cent of wives living in infertile marriage [84]. Other investigators [31] found sperm agglutinins in 25 per cent of 404 infertile women in contrast to the 8 per cent positivity for 83 women capable of conceiving. 236 infertile couples were examined using a modified variety of the Franklin–Dukes microtest [43]; iso-agglutinins were found in the sera of 4.5 per cent of the women and autoagglutinins in 2.6 per cent of the men. This finding failed to show significant correlation with subsequent pregnancies, abortions, ABO constellation in men and women and with the results of the Sims–Huhner postcoital test. Günther [41*a*] has summarized some related data in an instructive table (Table 41-I).

TABLE 41-I

Spontaneous incidence of anti-seminal antibodies in women (after Günther, completed) [35*a*]

Author	Test applied	Women examined	Of these positive
Ardelt [7*b*]	C fixation test for humoral antibodies	229 healthy or with gynaecological disease Virgins	12–18% 0%
Aszódi, Szántó [8]	C fixation test (humoral)	33 women 34 pregnant 37 virgins	19 18 None
Behrman [14*a*]	Immunofluorescence in cervical tissue	15 prostitutes	15
Bocci, Notarbartolo [17]	*a.* Intracutaneous test *b.* Kibrick test	25 women	*a.* 5 *b.* 25
Bodnár, Kamniker [18]	Agglutination and immobilization (humoral)	1 pregnant Virgins	1 None
Donat [29]	*a.* Haemagglutination *b.* Indirect immuno-fluorescence	24 infertile	16.6%
Dukes [30]	Sperm agglutination (humoral)	67 idiopathically sterile 44 fertile 39 control	67% 9% 7%
Dukes, Franklin [31]	Sperm agglutination	404 infertile 83 fertile	25% 8%
Franklin, Dukes [37]	Macro-agglutination (humoral)	19 sterile 17 fertile	15 2
Hanafiah et al. [43]	Franklin–Dukes micro-test	236 infertile	4.5%
Katsh et al. [60, 61]	Precipitation (humoral)	54 sterile 50 fertile	30% 14%
Nakabayashi et al. [80]	*a.* Kibrick test *b.* Haemagglutination Spermatozoon agglutination	514 sterile 70 infertile wives 20 fertile wives	*a.* 3.5% *b.* 3.3% 15.7% 6.0%
Papasov, Entschev [84]	Intracutaneous test	56 sterile	23%
Rommer [95]	Intracutaneous test with the husband's sperm	144 women	2.8%
Rümke [96*b*]	Sperm agglutination	177 infertile	0.56%

Table 41-I (cont'd)

Author	Test applied	Women examined	Of these positive
Shulman [101*b*]	*a*. Kibrick test *b*. Franklin–Dukes test *a*. Kibrick test *b*. Franklin–Dukes test	150 infertile 100 fertile	*a*. 23.0% *b*. 16.0% *a*. 0% *b*. 0%
Southam [107]	Haemagglutination (humoral)	95 women 61 pregnant	12.6% 50.8%
Southerland, Landing [108]	Immunofluorescence sperm	Prostitutes	None
[illegible] 11	Sperm agglutination	43 sterile 12 fertile	32.5% 0%

In contrast to the above findings, Rümke [96*a*] failed to demonstrate anti-spermatozoon antibodies in any of 124 childless women; he succeeded in demonstrating such antibodies in one of further 53 women.

According to other investigation [36*a*], the antibodies produced by male rabbits to human spermatozoa (or human seminal plasma) reduce the capacity of spermatozoa to penetrate the cervical mucus as demonstrable by Kremer's capillary mucus penetration test [64]. Supposedly the high-titre immobilizing antibodies in human blood are of similar effect and thus may reduce fertility. Jeffery and Parish [52] suggest that most of the women who have been in contact with semen containing organ-specific antigens produce anti-seminal antibodies which do not influence conception. In some women, however, these antibodies immobilize and sometimes destroy spermatozoa.

Statistical analysis has, nevertheless, failed to confirm the immunological explanation of infertility of women. Allo-immunization could not be proved by a number of authors investigating the cervical mucus and serum [23, 89]. Günther [41*a*] believes that spermatozoa may pass through the cervical mucosa, especially if it is diseased, and then, undergoing phagocytosis, induce antibody response. Bacterial infection may enhance antibody production and after recovery from the inflammatory process the appearance of anti-seminal antibodies only depends on the subsequent exposures to sperm.

These partly contradictory results have been discussed in many papers, attributing the controversies to technical errors among others. The majority of the authors believe that sperm immunity induced by the resorbed sperm in the wife plays but a minor role in the infertility of marriages. In the course of allogeneic artificial insemination the sperm injected into the uterus does not penetrate the abdominal cavity except for cases of high insemination (injection into the fundus area of the uterus by means of a long buttoned cannula); anaphylactic reaction has not been published even in such cases. An astonishing case may be mentioned [42]: severe anaphylaxis occurred in a 29-year-old woman after the first coitus; repeated copulations were followed by dyspnoea, collapse and loss of consciousness. The sensitizing antigen was in connection with a glucoprotein in the seminal plasma, undetectable in the blood serum and in spermatozoa. In another case immediate-type allergic reaction to human seminal plasma [106] occurred following the husband's ejaculation during sexual intercourse manifested in vaginal oedema, diffuse severe urticaria, angioedema, and rhinitis starting 15 to 120 min after intercourse and persisting for 1 to 6 days. Positive intracutaneous immediate-type reaction could be elicited to the husband's ejaculate, and to semen from 3 different normal males and to that from 12 males with vasectomies. Sephadex G-200 fractionation of pooled seminal plasma showed activity corresponding to a fraction with 10,000 to 15,000 Dalton's mol. weight with a UV-spectrum resembling protein. The patient's serum did not agglutinate washed sperm but agglutinated sperm in whole ejaculate. Recently, several cases of such reactions have been reported [78*c*].

Connection between HL-A haplotypes and unexplained infertility has also been studied [69]. In fertile couples haplotypes showed negative associations between the first (LA) locus alleles; on the contrary in a group of infertile individuals the second (FOUR) HL-A locus alleles seemed to occur more frequently than in the control group.

The therapeutic possibilities are poor. Sexual abstinence, coitus interruptus or coitus condomatus practiced for about six months seems to be a useful advice that may be given to such couples. During this time the anti-seminal antibodies may decline in titre, or may even disappear and conception may occur thereafter [30, 63]. In the course of a study the antibodies disappeared in this way in 25 out of 29 women [30].

SPERM AUTOIMMUNITY

Sperm autoimmunity is a relatively new immunological entity; unlike sperm immunity, it develops in males against their own spermatozoa. High-titre antibodies in the seminal plasma agglutinate, immobilize and degenerate normal spermatozoa in the ejaculate, thus rendering them incapable of penetrating cervical mucus. In this way, sperm autoimmunity may cause infertility in men [96*b*]. In most of the infertile patients of this type autoantibodies are present in both the serum and the seminal plasma, but not in proportional concentrations.

Another type of autoimmune infertility has been demonstrated in experimental animals. Severe damages, viz. autoimmune orchitis with consequent autoimmune aspermatogenesis, developed in animals to which their own semen, spermatozoa or testicular homogenate had been administrated in repeated injections with complete Freund's adjuvant. In this case the germinal epithelium was destroyed by autoimmune processes. The consequent testicular atrophy may become complete as soon as within the first month [117]. Such animal experiments were first published by Voisin et al. [113] in 1951 and subsequently by Freund et al. [38*a*] in 1953.

A variety of heterologous animal testicular tissues have proved to be antigenic for experimental animals. Allergic response to testicular tissue developed in two to eight weeks. This was characterized [73*b*] by (*i*) congestion and serous oedema in most of the intertubular spaces of the gonad and foci of perivascular cellular infiltration mostly including plasmacytes and lymphocytes; (*ii*) vacuolization and sloughing of the germ cells, beginning with spermatids, finally involving spermatocytes and spermatogonia (Sertoli cells showed striking vacuolization, but their nuclei remained intact); (*iii*) absence of damage in Leydig's interstitial cells and other connective tissue cells, such as fibroblasts and scattered mast cells; (*iv*) appearance of humoral anti-spermatic and cell-mediated antibodies concurrent with the testicular lesion; (*v*) azoospermia due to germ cell destruction which rendered the animal sterile for several months; (*vi*) signs of complete recovery of fertility, apparent about 165 days after immunization, and evidence of normal motile spermatozoa in the ejaculate after about five months of azoospermia; (*vii*) failure of injections of adjuvant alone, immature testis, or immunologically damaged testis to evoke the reaction [15, 38*b*, 58, 66]. In addition to guinea pigs, less susceptible species, such as inbred mouse strains and adult rats, may respond to similar autoimmunization or homoimmunization. According to some authors, not all species are equally suitable for the experimental study of autoimmune aspermatogenesis, for instance, no decrease in fertility has been found to be caused by the presence of anti-spermal antibody in mice [63]. Autoimmune orchitis has been also produced in primates [4]. Animal experiments of contrary results have also been reported. For instance, according to Kantor and Dixon [55] the fertility of male guinea pigs did not change in response to immunization with testicular antigen in Freund's incomplete adjuvant, although γ-globulin could be demonstrated in the semen.

The antigens of testicular homogenate are of heterogeneous nature as revealed serologically by the presence of other tissue antigens common to kidney, liver and serum proteins [2]. The immunofluorescent technique and the periodic acid-Schiff reaction of the acrosome support the view that particularly the acrosome of spermatids and of spermatozoa share the antigenicity of testis [13, 56*c*, 75, 76, 110].

The antigenicity of the germinal epithelium has been demonstrated in tissue cultures as well [59]. However, no correlation was found between the antibody titre and the degree of testicular injury. The peculiarity of autoimmune aspermatogenesis consists in its manifestation in an organ which matures and begins to function long after birth [16]. If an emulsion prepared from testicular tissue of sexually mature animals is administered together with complete Freund's adjuvant to newborn animals, these will not develop a pathological reaction of germinal epithelium until their sexual maturation. In such cases the damage of the spermatogenetic cells is not a primary one; it does not ensue until spermatids and even spermatozoa have developed. In contrast, autoimmunity cannot be induced with homogenates of still inactive testicles removed from newborn animals, although the early spermatogenetic cells already contain substances of antigenic nature [38*a*, 56*a*]. Other investigators [114] succeeded in inducing autoimmune aspermatogenesis by partially purified epididymal spermatozoa, termed S, T, Z and P autoantigens. Of these S occurs on the acrosomes of mature spermatozoa, T on the surface of immature spermatogenetic cells, and P as a β-protein on the acrosomes of spermatozoa. It was found [114] that several different spermatozoon autoantigens can induce autoimmune aspermatogenic orchitis by immunotoxic reactions, delayed hypersensitivity reactions and also serum-mediated hypersensitivity reactions (such as Arthus-type phenomenon). These different mechanisms might play a role in the development of autoimmune aspermatogenic orchitis induced with testis homogenates, whole spermatozoa or even unpurified extracts [114].

Experimental allergic aspermatogenesis can be induced in another way, too.

Antigen has been obtained from isolated spermatozoal heads and acrosomes as well as from tails of spermatozoa and lipoprotamines prepared from spermatozoal head membranes [22]. In each case Freund's complete adjuvant was necessary for immunization. Wilson et al. [119] succeeded in inducing varying degrees of seminiferous epithelial damage, including aspermatogenesis, by transfer of immune serum. Aspermatogenesis was consistently produced in recipient guinea pigs pre-treated with Freund's complete adjuvant in saline intradermally 7 days prior to transfer of serum from donor guinea pigs immunized 7 days previously with testicular homogenate in Freund's complete adjuvant. Aspermatogenesis was also induced by transfer of cells of lymph node, spleen or peritoneal exudate from the same immune animals. Katsh et al. [57] made experiments aimed at the purification and partial characterization of 'aspermatogenic antigen'. Antigen was obtained from guinea pig testes and epididymides, purified by digestion with pepsin and fractionation on Sephadex G-50 followed by precipitation with antibody and elution from the antigen–antibody complex. This material induced autoimmune aspermatogenesis in guinea pigs when injected with Freund's complete adjuvant. The antigen with mol. wt. of approx. 12,600 was a glycopeptide containing approx. 13 per cent of carbohydrate.

The antigenicity of the seminal plasma has been proved in heterologous or homologous immunization experiments [73*b*]. Antigens common to seminal plasma, spermatozoa and secretions of prostate and seminal vesicles have been demonstrated [73*b*]. At the same time, conflicting results have also been published [120]: while intensive autoimmunization of rabbits could be induced with native or chemically modified seminal plasma incorporated with complete Freund's adjuvant (autoantibodies against the homologous material and against testicular antigens, as well as testicular lesions were observed in most animals), when using accessory gland extract as the immunizing material, repeated injections failed to induce anti-testicular antibodies or to cause testicular damage. Semen analysis during immunization showed the presence of immature cells from the seminiferous epithelium. According to other reports, rabbit male accessory glands showed the presence of strictly organ-specific autoantigens [121]. It is well known that seminal plasma shares most antigens with male accessory glands in rabbits [105, 123]. A detailed study of the problem is necessary.

Two types of autoantibodies against testicular tissue have been described in the immunized guinea pig. The humoral antibodies, mainly of IgM and IgG class [24] with *in vitro* cytotoxic properties, viz. immobilization and agglutination of motile spermatozoa and lytic effect on the acrosome of the spermatid and spermatozoon reach low titre if any; there is no strict correlation between them and the degree of gonadal lesions [73*b*]. The IgM fraction from serum contains homologous cytotoxic antibodies [91].

Cell-mediated antibodies appear around the sixth day (humoral antibodies can be detected about three days later) [20, 21]. It has widely been accepted [73*b*] that cell-mediated immunity may induce allergic orchitis, which therefore may be considered as a delayed-type hypersensitivity reaction. The use of complete adjuvant is essential. Delayed hypersensitivity to human and guinea pig sperm was demonstrated in guinea pigs of the Rockefeller strain by immunization with H37Ra adjuvant [77]. The sensitivity was not only directed towards the sensitizing antigen, but also showed cross-reactivity. Thus, peritoneal exudate cells derived from guinea pigs sensitized to human sperm were inhibited by guinea pig sperm. In addition, supernatants obtained after incubation of the sensitized lymph node cells with specific antigen were found to be spermatotoxic.

The testicular tissue alone or with incomplete adjuvant may only elicit systemic or local anaphylaxis, passive cutaneous anaphylaxis and immunofluorescent antibodies [21, 25]. Mononuclear cells from lymph nodes of immunized animals are capable of passively inducing delayed-type dermal hypersensitivity or testicular lesions in normal recipients [20, 64]. In contrast, humoral antibodies do not induce aspermatogenesis passively, except in recipient guinea pigs pretreated with Freund's complete adjuvant [10]. In addition, some authors [21, 25] refer to protective antibodies. Experimental allergic aspermatogenesis was prevented by thymectomy early in the postnatal period [115] or by the administration of suppressive drugs prior to immunization [116]. Immunotolerance failed to be induced: germ cells were destroyed as the animals had reached puberty [16].

Animal experiments suggest that autoimmune aspermia (*i*) comes about by sloughing off of spermatogenetic cells from the convoluted seminiferous tubules, (*ii*) it is based mainly on a cell-mediated delayed hypersensitivity reaction passively transferable with lymphocytes and (*iii*) it is easily inducible by injecting isogeneic or allogeneic antigens, but its induction by xenogeneic antigen is difficult.

These observations on experimental animals are of no practical value for man. In man only isogeneic immunization may play a role in autoimmunity. There is little if any evidence that isogeneic immunization might lead to an atrophy of the germinal epithelium. In the andrological practice symptoms suggestive of an immune response to spermatozoa cannot be excluded [41*c*] but orchitis of immunological origin has not been observed. Mancini et al. [72, 73*a*] semicastrated four patients suffering from prostatic carcinoma. Subsequently, two of the patients were immunized with an isogeneic, the others with a xenogeneic, testicular homogenate, using Freund's adjuvant. Two to 4 months later the heterolateral testicles showed signs of immunological atrophy, viz. a morphological picture characteristic of a complete depopulation of the convoluted seminiferous tubules. Based on these, Schirren and Rossberg [99] and Günther [41*a*] have suggested that the Sertoli cell syndrome in man may not only be the result of primary germinal aplasia or postnatal testicular injury but also a consequence of clinically inapparent autoimmune orchitis. Although anti-spermal serum antibodies were not found in cases of Sertoli syndrome, their earlier presence and subsequent disappearance cannot be excluded. On the other hand, based on testicular biopsies, Rümke [97] believes that the spermatogenesis in man is not damaged by direct immunological factors.

Therefore, in man mainly immunological damages due to autoimmune serum agglutinins and immobilizins may play a role [96*d*], similarly as in animals immunized without adjuvant. Sperm agglutinating autoantibodies have been found in about 3–6 per cent of infertile men [39]. A titre of more than 1 : 32 of autoantibodies in the serum of men may be a cause of infertility [39]. The autoantibodies were of two main types: head-to-tail and head-to-head sperm agglutinating ones [39]. Head-to-tail autoantibodies may pass from the serum into the seminal plasma and cause autoagglutination of the sperm in the ejaculate. Agglutinated spermatozoa cannot penetrate an ovulatory cervical mucus and this is probably the cause of infertility in patients with head-to-tail autoantibodies in the serum.

Head-to-head autoantibodies cannot pass from the serum into the seminal plasma. No autoagglutination is observed in the ejaculate and the spermatozoa show normal penetration of the cervical mucus [39]. The reason for infertility in these patients is obscure. Fractionation of sera from infertile men in Sephadex G-200 and Sephadex DEAE columns shows that head-to-tail autoantibodies are of the IgG type [39], while head-to-head autoantibodies are of the IgM type. Of 2,015 infertile husbands 3.3 per cent had serum agglutinins demonstrable by macroscopic agglutination up to a dilution of 1 : 32 or higher [97]. In contrast, none of 416 fertile men had a titre higher than 1 : 16. Ejaculates from 17 men positive for serum agglutinins were also examined and agglutinins were detected in 11. Fjällbrant [36*a*] examined 400 infertile and 500 fertile husbands for spermatozoon agglutinin by the Kibrick test. The percentage incidence of high-titre and low-titre agglutinin was as follows.

	High-titre (1 : 64)	Low-titre (1 : 32)	Total positive per cent
	serum agglutinin per cent		
Sterile marriages	4.4	2.4	6.8
Fertile marriages	0.8	1.8	2.6

Statistically significant positive correlations were demonstrated between sterility on the one hand and (*i*) anti-seminal antibody level in the serum, (*ii*) spermatozoon immobility and agglutination and (*iii*) the penetrating ability of the spermatozoa in cervical mucus, on the other. Furthermore, in the men positive for anti-seminal antibodies the serum IgG and IgM levels were significantly higher than in control men. However, the mean IgA level was lower in the antibody-positive men than in the control group. More recently the same author [36*b*] found sperm agglutinins in 11 per cent of 800 infertile husbands using the Kibrick test, but the titre reached 1 : 64 only in 4 per cent. Rümke [96*c*] followed up 284 infertile male patients positive for sperm agglutinins. Thirty-four patients became fertile within 14 years, although 16 of these had an unchanged agglutinin titre over the years.

The factors responsible for the spontaneous production of autoantibodies to spermatozoa and testicular spermatogenetic cells are only partially known. It might be supposed that the autoantibodies react either directly or, if secreted into the seminal plasma, indirectly, with spermatozoa thus giving rise to infertility. It has been suggested [101*a*] that these autoantibodies belong to the general group of the autoallergic phenomena, rather than to those of histocompatibility. A few cases of exception to this rule have also been found, in which there was a difference in the reactivity against donor semen, and these cases indicate possibilities of heterogeneity of the sperm cells with regard to the sperm antigens.

The problem of the mode of penetration of spermatozoal antigens into the host organism was raised a long time ago. It first had been supposed [34, 44] that due to seminal duct obstruction, disintegrating spermatozoa may be absorbed via the interstitial tissue [39], the lymph vessels and the blood capillaries. By use of immunofluorescence and fluorescent protein tracing techniques [53] vascular permeability to serum protein was studied in the tests [53]. A very low permeability to serum protein and to spermatozoal antibody was found in the peritubular and periductular membranes, but with a 'weak point' at the rete testis through which a little serum protein may enter and then reflux back into the seminiferous tubules. Rümke and Hellinga [97] found bilateral obstruction in 16 out of 67 infertile men with high serum antibody titre and succeeded in demonstrating anti-spermatozoon antibodies in one of four emergency-sterilized men. Coombs et al. [26] examined seminal plasma and serum samples from infertile vasectomized men for anti-spermatozoon antibodies. They found no such antibodies of the IgG class in the serum samples. In a few cases IgA-type antibodies occurred in the seminal plasma, but not in the serum. It is nevertheless probable that spermatozoa or their components can penetrate, and thus may immunize, the organism as a result of epididymitis, accidental ligation of the vas deferens during herniorrhaphy or deliberate ligation of the vas deferens as a family limitation procedure, traumatic swelling of the testis, local cold or warm stimuli, germ cell destruction in inflammatory conditions of the gonads with mumps orchitis, infection of the vas deferens or epididymis in oligospermic or azoospermic patients, etc. [5, 41*b*, 71*a*, 82, 93, 96*b*]. After surgical relief of the obstruction some patients induced conception in spite of having persistent positive sperm agglutinin titres. Ansbacher studied the changes in sperm agglutinating and sperm immobilizing antibodies in vasectomized men. The Kibrick test was positive in only 2.0 per cent prior to vasectomy, while the Isojima test was invariably negative [6*a*]. The initiation of anti-sperm antibody activity in the serum within 7 to 11 days after bilateral ligation was demonstrated [6*b*]. Six months after vasectomy spermatozoon agglutinating antibodies were found in 54.2 per cent and spermatozoon immobilizing antibodies in 31.3 per cent [6*a*]. Sperm-agglutinating activity of the serum peaked at 18 months postvasectomy in incidence and level of the titre; two years later it was still found in 62 per cent [6*b*]. Sperm immobilizing antibodies were present in 30 per cent of men 12 months postvasectomy, but there was a marked drop in incidence to 9.5 per cent at 18 months and in titre at 24 month [6*b*].

Experimental cryoimmunization deserves special mention. It has been demonstrated that cryostimulation (repeated freezings) of the genital organs of experimental animals is able to induce haemagglutinating and precipitating autoantibodies [122]. Cryosurgery of rabbit male accessory glands induce homocytotropic antibodies as part of humoral response [94]. Tissue injury provoked by cryosurgery of the rabbit male accessory glands is able to induce organ-specific autoantibody response, as demonstrated by passive haemagglutination and immunodiffusion assays [102]. Eighty per cent of the animals stimulated on the coagulating gland produced an immune response of anamnestic character (measured by the method of passive haemagglutination), in the form of antibody peaks of increasing intensity, after the successive episodes of freezing. The animals stimulated on the seminal vesicle produced in 75 per cent of the cases a similar though weaker response [125]. Cryosurgery of rabbit male accessory glands induced the formation of not only organ-specific haemagglutinating, but also skin sensitizing antibodies. The latter antibodies appeared to fulfill the criteria for homocytotropic antibodies since they fixed to homologous skin, showed heat lability and were clearly differentiable from IgG and IgM antibodies (chromatographically). Using Sephadex G-100 rabbit seminal plasma fractions it was possible to prove that autoantigens and autoallergens are confined in different fractions [121].

An increasing number of authors believe that both in case of long-standing obstruction of the efferent seminiferous ducts and in case of undisturbed sperm transport there must be some local chronic inflammation loosening the tissues, and thus enabling sperm components to be absorbed. Extravasation of sperm in the epididymis results in infiltration with macrophages, lymphocytes and plasma cells. It has been suggested that some patients who resorb their own spermatozoa may secondarily respond by formation of autoantibodies. Testicular biopsies performed in patients with aspermia due to complete obstruction of the efferent ducts were found normal [110], indicating that sperm antibodies are not capable of preventing spermatogenesis. The spermatozoon-resorption granulomata found beside the canal of epididymis in cases with local inflammation (in Oberndorfer's textbook) speak for the absorption theory which has also been substantiated by experimental evidence [41*b*]. Epididymitis spermiostatica granulomatosa, granulomatous orchitis and chronic epididymitis may also loosen the meatus walls and thus support the sperm components in penetrating the adjacent tissues and, therefrom, the lymph and capillary circulation. Bandhauer [9*a*] definitely supports this view, especially in connection with chronic epididymitides. Among his 29 patients with sperm agglutinins 19 suffered from non-specific or specific epididymitis. Autoimmunization was less frequently demonstrable in cases of prostatovesiculitis. Fjällbrant [36*a*] diagnosed prostatovesiculitis in 37 per cent of 43 men having anti-spermatozoon antibodies in their sera. The agglutination was of the tail-to-tail type in the majority of the cases and the percentage of mobile spermatozoa was reduced. There was a significant correlation between the percentage of mobile spermatozoa and the immobilizing activity of the serum as also between the spermatozoon agglutinin titre of the serum and the degree of agglutination of the spermatozoa in the semen. Bandhauer [9*b*] demonstrated autoimmunization in inflammatory diseases of the epididymides, less frequently in those of the prostate and of the seminal vesicle. The appearance of sperm-agglutinins accompanying in some cases the transurethral resection of the prostate might be attributed to disturbed resorption.

In spite of the above hypotheses supported by clinical observations and experimental evidence, it remains unclear how autoimmunity develops in cases where no special inducing factor is at work. The blame may be put on the diagnostic procedures, which may be insufficient for revealing latent inflammations in part of the cases.

In general, the existence of autoimmune processes in some sterile men is acceptable if not, as suggested by some authors, proved. Antibodies may be produced to specific antigens of spermatozoa, seminal plasma and testicular parenchyma. As a specific autoimmune reaction, degeneration of the germinal epithelium of testicular tubules may develop. Although active germinal cell breakdown in the testis or spermiostasis in the efferent duct has been observed, a simultaneous inflammatory process and an abnormal immune system seem to be necessary to initiate the autoimmune response to sperm [73*b*].

THERAPEUTICAL POSSIBILITIES

No effective treatment is known, which would reduce the titre of autoantibodies in serum and restore fertility in each case [39]. Unsuccessful experiments have been carried out with ACTH and glucocorticoids [9*b*, 97]. Queseda et al. [92] administered antibiotics to 59 infertile patients suffering from genital tract infection. The sperm agglutinin titres declined and four patients induced conception. A reconstitution of the normal resorption conditions and the elimination of endogenous foci should be achieved [9*a*, 96*a*]. Schoysman [100] induced rebound phenomenon with a large dose of testosterone. This was followed by azoospermia in 17 patients and in 14 of them the sperm agglutinin titre fell below 1 : 32. Interruption of the hormone therapy was followed in half of the patients by normospermia prior to the repeated rise in the sperm agglutinin titre. Five patients even induced conception. Rümke [96*a*] failed to reproduce these results by long-acting testosterone. He succeeded in inducing temporary azoospermia in 12 patients and a decline in the sperm agglutinin level of the seminal plasma in 6 cases; in 3 cases also the serum agglutinin level could be lowered. In the rest of the patients the titres remained unchanged. Although the wives of two patients conceived, Rümke does not accept that the behaviour of the sperm agglutinin titre had any role in this. Thus, the therapeutical possibilities are extremely poor, even no guiding principle being recommendable.

Investigations into sperm immunity and autoimmunity are in progress. Obviously, this branch of science is well-grounded, but the practical value of the experimental and statistical data and the importance of immunological factors in the explanation of infertile marriages have remained to be determined.

REFERENCES

1. Ahlgren, M.: *II. Int. Symp. Immun. Reprod., Varna 1971.* Cited by Herrmann, W. P.: *Hautarzt* **23**, 461 (1972).
2. Alonso, A., Bueno, M. P., Scacciati, J. M., Gonzalez, N. and Mancini, R. E.: *Acta Europ. Fertil.* **1**, 28 (1969).
3. Amano, Y. and Behrman, S. J.: *Int. J. Fertil.* **12**, 291 (1967).
4. Andrada, J. A., Andrada, E. C. and Witebsky, E.: *Proc. Soc. exp. Biol.* (*N. Y.*) **130**, 1106 (1969).
5. Andrada, J. A., Mengone, A., Lavieri, J. C. and Mancini, R. E.: *J. Reprod. Fertil.* (In press).

6*a*. Ansbacher, R.: *Fertil. Steril.* **22**, 629 (1971).
6*b*. ibid., **24**, 788 (1973).
7*a*. Ardelt, F.: *Zbl. Gynäk.* **55**, 3028 (1931).
7*b*. ibid., **58**, 273 (1934).
8. Aszódi, A. and Szántó, G.: *Z. ges. exp. Med.* **97**, 485 (1936).
9*a*. Bandhauer, K.: *Urol. Int.* **21**, 247 (1966).
9*b*. id., *Derm. Mschr.* **158**, 729 (1972).
10. Bandhauer, K., Marberger, E. and Marberger, H.: *Urologe* **3**, 222 (1964).
11. Barnes, G. W.: *Biol. Reproduct.* **6**, 384 (1972).
12. Baskin, M. J.: *Amer. J. Obstet. Gynec.* **24**, 892 (1932).
13. Baum, J., Boughton, B., Mongat, L. and Schild, O. H.: *J. Immunol.* **4**, 95 (1961).
14*a*. Behrman, S. J.: *Int. J. Fertil.* **8**, 829 (1963).
14*b*. id., In *Progress in Infertility*. Little-Brown, Boston 1968, p. 678.
15. Bishop, D. W. and Carlson, G. L.: *Ann. N. Y. Acad. Sci.* **124**, 247 (1965).
16. Bishop, D. W., Narbaitz, R. and Lessof, H.: *Develop. Biol.* **3**, 444 (1961).

17. Bocci, A. and Notarbartolo, R.: *Zbl. Haut-Geschl.Kr.* **107,** 270 (1960).
18. Bodnár, L. and Kamniker, H.: *Dtsch. med. Wschr.* **51,** 2119 (1925).
19. Boettcher, B. and Kay, D. J.: *Nature* **223,** 737 (1969).
20. Boughton, B. and Schild, H. O.: *Immunology* **5,** 522 (1962).
21. Boyden, S. V.: *J. exp. Med.* **93,** 107 (1951).
22. Brown, P. C., Glynn, L. E. and Holborow, E. J.: *J. Path. Bact.* **86,** 505 (1963).
23. Chodirker, W. B. and Tomasi, T. B.: *Science* **142,** 1080 (1963).
24. Chutna, J. and Pokorna, Z.: *Folia biol.* (*Praha*) **13,** 68 (1967).
25. Chutna, J. and Rychlikova, M.: *Folia biol.* (*Praha*) **10,** 177 (1964).
26. Coombs, R. A., Rümke, Ph. and Edwards, R. G.: *II. Int. Symp. Immun. Reprod., Varna 1971.* Cited by Herrmann, W. P.: *Hautarzt* **23,** 461 (1972).
27. Cronquist, S.: *Acta path. microbiol. scand.* **26,** 786 (1949).
28. de Fazio, S. R. and Ketchel, M. M.: *J. Reproduct. Fertil.* **30,** 125 (1972).
29. Donat, H.: *Zbl. Gynäk.* **93,** 321 (1973).
30. Dukes, C. D.: *Proc. Wld. Congr. Fertil. Steril., Stockholm.* Congr. Series 109. Excerpta Medica Foundation, Amsterdam 1966.
31. Dukes, C. D. and Franklin, R. R.: *Fertil. Steril.* **19,** 263 (1968).
32. Eastman, N. J.: *J. Contracept.* **4,** 147 (1939).
33. Edwards, R. G., Ferguson, L. C. and Coombs, R. A.: *J. Reprod. Fertil.* **7,** 153 (1964).
34. Feltkamp, T. E. W., Kruyff, K., Ladiges, N. C. J. J. and Rümke, Ph.: *Ann. N.Y. Acad. Sci.* **124,** 702 (1965).
35. Fernández-Collazo, E.: *Acta XIV Reunión Soc. Arg. Invest. Clinica, Medicina* **30,** 61 (1970).
35*a*. Fern–ndez-Collazo, E. and Thierer, E.: *Fertil. Steril.* **23,** 376 (1972).
36*a*. Fjällbrant, B.: *Acta Obstet. gynec. scand.* Suppl. (1968).
36*b*. id., *II. Int. Symp. Immun. Reprod., Varna 1971.* Cited by Herrmann, W. P.: *Hautarzt* **23,** 461 (1972).
37. Franklin, R. R. and Dukes, C. D.: *Amer. J. Obstet. Gynec.* **89,** 6 (1964).
38*a*. Freund, J., Lipton, M. M. and Thompson, G. E.: *J. exp. Med.* **97,** 711 (1953).
38*b*. id., *Proc. Soc. exp. Biol.* (*N. Y.*) **87,** 408 (1954).
39. Friberg, C. J.: *T. Norske Laegeforen* **92,** 987 (1972).
40. Gutierrez, J. T. G., Jimenez, R. N. and Vazquez, J. J. G.: *Proc. Wld. Congr. Fertil. Steril., Stockholm.* Congr. Series 109. Excerpta Medica Foundation, Amsterdam 1966.
41*a*. Günther, E.: *Z. ärztl. Fortbild.* **63,** 747 (1969).
41*b*. id., *Derm. Mschr.* **157,** 381 (1971).
41*c*. ibid., **158,** 730 (1972).
41*d*. id., *Andrologie* **4,** 157 (1972).
42. Halpern, B. N., Ky, T. and Robert, B.: *Immunology* **12,** 247 (1967).
43. Hanafiah, M. J., Epstein, J. A. and Sobrero, A. J.: *Fertil. Steril.* **23,** 493 (1972).
44. Hansen, K. B.: *Clin. exp. Immunol.* **10,** 243 (1971).
45. Heckman, A. and Rümke, Ph.: *Fertil. Steril.* **20,** 313 (1969).
46. Heckman, A. and Shulman, S.: *Clin. exp. Immunol.* **9,** 147 (1971).
47. Henle, W., Henle, G. and Chambers, L. A.: *J. exp. Med.* **68,** 335 (1938).
48. Herrmann, W. P. and Schirren, C.: *Z. Haut-Geschl. Kr.* **34,** 134 (1963).
48*a*. Hirschhäuser, C. and Baudner, S.: *Fertil. Steril.* **23,** 393 (1972).
49. Hulka, J. F. and Omran, K. F.: *Amer. J. Obstet. Gynec.* **104,** 440 (1969).
50. Isojima, S., Li, T. S. and Ashitaka, Y.: *Amer. J. Obstet. Gynec.* **101,** 677 (1968).
51. Isojima, S. and Tsuzuku, O.: *Amer. J. Obstet. Gynec.* **102,** 304 (1969).
52. Jeffery, W. and Parish, W. E.: *Clin. Allergy* **2,** 261 (1972).
53. Johnson, M. H.: *Fertil. Steril.* **23,** 383 (1972).
54. Johnson, W. L. and Hunter, A. G.: *Biol. Reprod.* **6,** 13 (1972).
55. Kantor, G. L. and Dixon, F. J.: *Clin. exp. Immunol.* **13,** 225 (1973).
56*a*. Katsh, S.: *Amer. J. Obstet. Gynec.* **78,** 946 (1959).
56*b*. id., *J. Urol.* **87,** 896 (1960).
56*c*. id., *Int. Arch. Allergy* **16,** 241 (1960).
56*d*. id., Unpublished data.
57. Katsh, S., Aguirre, A. A., Leaver, F. W. and Katsh, G. F.: *Fertil. Steril.* **23,** 644 (1972).

58. Katsh, S. and Bishop, D.: *J. Embryol. exp. Morph.* **6,** 94 (1958).
59. Katsh, S. and Jordan, R. T.: *Int. Arch. Allergy* **21,** 163 (1962).
60. Katsh, S. and Katsh, G. F.: *Fertil. Steril.* **12,** 522 (1961).
61. Katsh, S., Talmage, D. W. and Katsh, G. F.: *Science* **143,** 41 (1964).
62. Kibrick, S., Belding, D. L. and Merrill, B.: *Fertil. Steril.* **3,** 430 (1952).
63. Krebs, D.: *Urologe, B* **12,** 44 (1972).
64. Kremer, J.: *The in vitro Spermatozoal Penetration Test.* Rijksunivers, Groningen 1968.
65. Landsteiner, K.: *Zbl. Bakt. I. Abt. Orig.* **25,** 546 (1899).
66. Laurence, K. A., Carpuk, B. A., Lefevre, A. and Mauldin, D.: *Int. J. Fertil.* **10,** 341 (1965).
67. Laurence, K. A., Carpuk, B. A. and Perlbachs, M.: *Int. J. Fertil.* **10,** 13 (1965).
68. Laurence, K. A. and Perlbachs, M.: *Bact. Proc.* **62,** 88 (1962).
69. Lindblom, J. B., Friberg, J., Högman, C. F. and Genzell, C.: *Tissue Antigens* **2,** 352 (1972).
70. Lüders, G. and Adam, W.: *Z. Haut-Geschl. Kr.* **47,** 479 (1972).
71*a*. Mancini, R. E.: *Proc. 3rd Int. Pharmacol. Meeting* **2,** 75 (1966).
71*b*. id., *Actas Congr. Arg. Esterilidad* **1,** 53 (1968).
71*c*. id., *II. Int. Symp. Immun. Reprod., Varna 1971.* Cited by Herrmann, W. P.: *Hautarzt* **23,** 461 (1972).
72. Mancini, R. E., Alonso, A., Barquet, J., Alvarez, B. and Nemirovsky, M.: *J. Reprod. Fertil.* **8,** 325 (1964).
73*a*. Mancini, R. E. and Andrada, J. A.: *J. clin. Endocrin. Metabol.* **25,** 859 (1965).
73*b*. id., In *Immunological Diseases.* 2nd ed. Vol. II. Ed. by Samter, M. Little-Brown, Boston 1971, p. 1240.
74. Mancini, R. E., Andrada, J. A., Saraceni, A., Bachmann, A. E., Laviesi, J. C. and Nemirovsky, M.: *J. clin. Endocr.* **25,** 859 (1965).
75. Mancini, R. E., Davidson, O. W., Nemirovsky, M. and Bueno, D. C.: *Proc. Soc. exp. Biol. (N. Y.)* **8,** 435 (1962).
76. Mancini, R. E., Davidson, O. W., Vilar, O., Nemirovsky, M. and Bueno, M. P.: *Fertil. Steril.* **25,** 695 (1964).
77. Marcus, Z. H., Soffer, Y. and Ben David, A.: *Europ. J. Immunol.* **3,** 75 (1973).
78*a*. Metchnikoff, N.: *Ann. Inst. Pasteur* **13,** 737 (1899).
78*b*. Metalnikoff, S.: *Ann. Inst. Pasteur* **14,** 577 (1900).
78*c*. Mikkelsen, E. J., Henderson, L. L., Leiferman, K. M. and Gleich, G. J.: *Ann. Allergy* **34,** 239 (1975).
79. Moxter, D. V.: *Dtsch. med. Wschr.* **26,** 61 (1900).
80. Nakabayashi, N. T., Tyler, E. T. and Tyler, A.: *Fertil. Steril.* **12,** 544 (1961).
81. Noyes, R. W.: *Fertil. Steril.* **20,** 43 (1969).
82. Ostrovsky, F. M. and Sokolovskaja, J. I. (1971): *II. Int. Symp. Immun. Reprod., Varna 1971.* Cited by Herrmann, W. P.: *Hautarzt* **23,** 461 (1972).
83. Ouchterlony, C.: *Acta path. microbiol.* **26,** 507 (1949).
84. Papasov, B. and Entschev, E. M.: *Zbl. Gynäk.* **85,** 1542 (1963).
85. Parish, W. E., Carron-Brown, J. A. and Richards, C. B.: *J. Reprod. Fertil.* **13,** 469 (1967).
86. Parish, W. E. and Ward, A.: *J. Obstet. Gynec. Brit. Cwlth.* **75,** 1089 (1968).
87. Petter, O. and Zimmermann, H.: *Allergie u. Asthma* **15,** 162 (1969).
88. Phadke, A. M. and Padukone, K.: *J. Reprod. Fertil.* **7,** 163 (1964).
89. Pillot, J., Cohen, J. and Krulik, D.: *Path. Microbiol. (Paris)* **21,** 69 (1973).
90. Piskazeck, K.: *Derm. Mschr.* **158,** 731 (1972).
91. Pokorna, Z.: *Folia biol. (Praha)* **16,** 320 (1970).
92. Queseda, E. M., Dean Dukes, C., Deen, G. H. and Franklin, R.: *J. Urol.* **99,** 106 (1968).
93. Raytsina, S. S., Davidova, A. J. and Gladkova, N. S.: *II. Int. Symp. Immun. Reprod., Varna 1971.* Cited by Herrmann, W. P.: *Hautarzt* **23,** 461 (1972).
94. Riera, C. M., Faillaci, M. G. and Yantorno, C.: *J. Immunol.* **111,** 647 (1973).
95. Rommer, J. J.: *West. J. Surg. Obstet. Gynec.* **55,** 278 (1947).
96*a*. Rümke, Ph.: *Verh. Dtsch. Ges. inn. Med.* **68,** 455 (1962).
96*b*. id., *Proc. roy. Soc. Med. (London)* **61,** 275 (1968).

96*c*. id., *II. Int. Symp. Immun. Reprod., Varna 1971*. Cited by Herrmann, W. P.: *Hautarzt* **23,** 461 (1972).
96*d*. id., *Andrologie* **4,** 191 (1972).
96*e*. id., *Vox sang.* (*Basel*) **4,** 135 (1972).
97. Rümke, Ph. and Hellinga, G.: *Amer. J. clin. Path.* **32,** 357 (1959).
98. Schirren, C.: *Fertilitätsstörungen des Mannes*. Enke, Stuttgart 1961.
99. Schirren, C. and Rossberg, I.: *Arch. klin. exp. Derm.* **221,** 584 (1965).
100. Schoysman, R.: *Proc. VIth World Congr. Fertil. Steril. Tel-Aviv*. Excerpta Medica Foundation, Amsterdam 1968.
101*a*. Shulman, S.: *J. Allergy clin. Immunol.* **51,** 102 (1973).
101*b*. id., *J. Amer. med. Ass.* **225,** 993 (1973).
102. Shulman, S., Brandt, E. J. and Yantorno, C.: *Immunology* **14,** 149 (1968).
103. Shulman, S. and Heckman, A.: *Clin. exp. Immunol.* **9,** 137 (1971).
104. Shulman, S., Heckman, A. and Pann, Ch.: *J. Reproduct. Fertil.* **27,** 31 (1971).
105. Shulman, S., Riera, C. and Yantorno, C.: *J. Immunol.* **100,** 682 (1968).
106. Siraganian, R. P., Schenkein, I. and Levine, B. B.: *J. Allergy clin. Immunol.* **51,** 102 (1973).
106*a*. Soffer, Y., Marcus, Z. H. and Nebel, L.: *Harefuah* **84,** 523 (1973).
107. Southam, A. L.: *J. Reprod. Fertil.* **5,** 458 (1963).
108. Southerland, J. M. and Landing, B. H.: *Lancet* **ii,** 56 (1961).
109. Stavitsky, A. B. and Arquilla, E. R.: *J. Immunol.* **74,** 306 (1955).
110. Svenson Beck, J., Edwards, R. G. and Young, M. R.: *J. Reprod. Fertil.* **4,** 103 (1962).
111. Tien Shun Li and Beling, C. G.: *Fertil. Steril.* **24,** 134 (1973).
112. Tyler, A.: *Clin. Obstet. Gynec.* **7,** 829 (1964).
113. Voisin, G. A., Delaunay, A. and Barber, M.: *Ann. Inst. Pasteur* **81,** 48 (1951).
114. Voisin, G. A. and Foullet, F.: *Folia allergol.* **18,** 310 (1971).
115. Vojtisková, M. and Pokorna, Z.: *Lancet* **i,** 644 (1964).
116. Vojtisková, M., Vikliky, V., Jirsakova, A., Nouza, K. and Pokorna, Z.: *Folia biol.* (*Praha*) **11,** 364 (1965).
117. Waksman, B. H.: *J. exp. Med.* **109,** 311 (1959).
118. Weil, A. J. and Finkler, A. E.: *Proc. Soc. exp. Biol.* (*N. Y.*) **102,** 624 (1959).
119. Willson, J. T., Jones, N. and Katsh, S.: *Int. Arch. Allergy* **43,** 172 (1972).
120. Yantorno, C., Debanne, M. T. and Vottero-Cima, E.: *J. Reproduct. Fertil.* **27,** 311 (1971).
121. Yantorno, C., Riera, C. M., Faillaci, M. G. and Vides, M. A.: *Int. Arch. Allergy* **46,** 351 (1974).
122. Yantorno, C., Soanes, W. A., Gonder, M. J. and Shulman, S.: *Immunology* **12,** 395 (1967).
123. Yantorno, C., Vides, M. A. and Vottero-Cima, E.: *J. Reprod. Fertil.* **29,** 229 (1972).
124. Zak, K. and Zak, O.: *Proc. Wld. Congr. Fertil. Steril., Stockholm 1966*.
125. Zappi, E., Orsini, F. and Shulman, S.: *Invest. Urol.* **10,** 171 (1972).
126. Zettergen, L.: *Acta chir. scand.* **114,** 150 (1957).

CHAPTER 42

IMMUNOALLERGIC LUNG PURPURA

by

B. STEINER

Immunoallergic lung purpura (IALP) is a new term for the disease known in the literature as idiopathic pulmonary haemosiderosis. We have omitted the attribute 'idiopathic' because the disease proved to be of immunoallergic origin. Purpura being the primary process, it seems to be a better term than haemosiderosis.

The first description of this disease was due to Virchow [22] in 1864 who called it 'brown induration of the lung'. The pathologic features were first summarized by Ceelen [7]. Glanzmann and Walthard [13], and Waldenström [23] were the first to diagnose the disease *in vivo*. The characteristic symptoms are shown in Table 42-I. The diagnosis is usually easy in typical cases, however, lung biopsy may be required in doubtful cases. The first and subsequent crises may often be extremely severe leading to death in some cases. They are usually introduced by tachycardia, haemoptoe or haematemesis.

TABLE 42-I

	Classic IALP	Formes frustes
Recurrent lung haemorrhage	+++	±
Sideropenic anaemia of unknown origin	+++	±
Radiological signs (symmetrical pulmonary foci)	+++	±
Cardiorespiratory crisis	+++	±
Cor pulmonale	+++	±
Haemosiderin-containing macrophages	+++	±
Lung biopsy	+++	+++

The radiogram shows symmetric foci in the lungs, due to which pneumonia is often thought to be present [6]. Medical advice is, as a rule, first sought because of dyspnoea, high pulse rate, marked abdominal pain. More or less severe anaemia is a constant finding which, in the absence of other signs like chronic pulmonary infiltration and cor pulmonale, may suggest IALP. Reticulocytosis of variable degree, sometimes attaining 20 per cent, is almost invariably present. The radiological findings will be dealt with separately below. Positive Coombs' test is rarely found in such patients. Lung biopsy reveals characteristic histological changes: abundant free iron is deposited in the alveoli and there are macrophages loaded with much haemosiderin; the alveolar wall is thickened, the elastic fibres are broken or disappear completely.

PATHOLOGY

Characteristic findings include initial recurring haemorrhage in the pulmonary tissue and alveoli. Progressive siderosis of the elastic fibres might be observed mainly in the blood vessels. As a result, their elasticity is impaired, the vessels are dilated, and circulation is slowed down. Aneurysm-like dilatations of the vessels develop associated with destruction of the vascular wall. This is followed by haemorrhage per diapedesim and per rhexim and progression of siderosis [6]. It has been shown by electron-optical methods that the deposition of iron in the elastic fibres is irreversible [16]. Red blood cells were labelled with ^{59}Fe and the activity in circulation and in the lung was measured. At normal red cell life-span activity was found to slowly increase in circulation and to decrease in the lungs.

In the opinion of Ceelen [7], the disease is caused by the decay and local hypertrophy of the elastic fibres, which he attributed to an inborn defect of connective tissue elements. Subsequent investigations, however, have revealed that the damage of the elastic fibres is not invariably present and can, therefore, be regarded as a consequence and not as a cause of the disease.

It has been suggested that the spleen might play a key role in the pathogenesis of IALP. Based on this assumption, numerous attempts were made to cure the disease by splenectomy. In fact, many of the patients survived significantly longer, but often it failed to bring improvement. The intermittent character of the symptoms suggested allergic mechanism. One case was described who recovered on a milk-free diet [2]. In 1954, the present author [18*a*, *b*] expressed his view about the autoimmune origin of IALP, assuming that the crucial events were the capillary dilatation, consequent congestion, diapedesis and rhexis which occurred in the lung as the shock organ. At that time, only indirect proofs were available in support of this hypothesis, viz. eosinophilia, about 8 per cent on the average but often in excess of 20 per cent, increased prevalence of plasma cells in the RES and around the bronchi and pulmonary vessels, the presence of mast cells in the lungs of some patients, demonstration of cold agglutinin in about half of the patients, and in some cases a positive Coombs' tests.

This concept was supported by the demonstration of complete and incomplete autoantibodies in one of our patients [19] and by the results obtained with immunosuppressive treatment [18*e*, *f*, 20].

The theories relating to the initial pulmonary haemorrhage fall into three groups [5]: (*i*) Primary occurrence of acid mucopolysaccharides in the ground substance of the elastic fibres of small pulmonary blood vessels. Elasticity is lost and the resultant circulatory changes lead to diapedetic haemorrhage, deposition of iron in the connective tissue and perivascular accumulation of haemosiderophages. (*ii*) Damage of the elastic fibres is secondary to haemosiderosis. The primary factor would be circulatory changes due to capillary sinus proliferation, some infective or toxic process or to some anomaly of bronchopulmonary arteriovenous anastomosis. (*iii*) Allergic origin: the lung would be the centre of an antigen–antibody reaction. Allergic condition would be due to sensitization or auto-sensitization (to products of red cell lysis?) [18*d*, 25]. The immuno-allergic theory is supported by the favourable results obtained with corticosteroid and immunosuppressive treatment as well as by the partial results of splenectomy. This latter concept challenged the existence of primary or acquired degeneration of the elastic fibres. As a proof, peracute cases were described without involvement of the elastic fibres. Combined incidence with Henoch–Schönlein syndrome served as a further proof of the allergic concept. On the other hand, the theory was opposed on strength of the success rate of only 50 per cent of corticosteroid treatment, the considerable number of remissions in response to blood transfusion and iron substitution without corticosteroids, as well as of the presence of extrapulmonary vascular anomalies and angiodysplasias.

The symptoms are not regarded as a disease entity from the aetiopathogenetic aspect by some authors [9], although the manifestations do not exclude one another [9]. Inflammatory renal lesion occurs in 7.7 per cent of the cases [9]. The following explanation has been offered for this finding [6]. As a result of primary or secondary damage of the pulmonary elastic fibres, acid mucopolysaccharide deposition and increased Fe binding in the fibres ensue. The allergic-hyperergic mechanism is at the same time activated. The altered pulmonary tissue may acquire antigenic properties. Traces of the antigen are carried by circulation to the kidneys, where it is deposited in the basement membrane of the glomerular capillaries. The antibodies formed as a result are deposited at the same site and bound by the antigen. In this way the symptoms of focal nephritis (Goodpasture's syndrome) may develop [18*e*].

MONO- AND POLYSYSTEMIC FORMS

In the majority of cases the pathological changes are confined to the lung. In other cases, the condition may be associated with rheumatoid arthritis, anaphylactoid purpura (Henoch–Schönlein syndrome), glomerulonephritis, occasionally lupus erythematosus, or retinal haemorrhage. Association of IALP with Goodpasture's syndrome has already been referred to. It has been shown [8, 12] that the pulmonary and glomerular antigens are structurally related, and nephrotoxic sera give rise to lung purpura [11]. In animal experiments, Sturgill and Westervelt [21] demonstrated human γ-globulins in the interalveolar septa and the glomerular basement membrane in Goodpasture's syndrome. Beirne et al. [4] found IgG and β_1C-globulin in the alveolar septa, and on the alveolar capillary and glomerular basement membrane in Goodpasture's syndrome. They suggested that these might have been deposited autoantibodies.

Chronic cor pulmonale is a frequent finding in IALP [18*c*]. In some cases the diagnosis may be easily established on the basis of clinical symptoms, although detailed spirometric and cardiac catheterization studies may be required occasionally. In the adult, years or even decades are necessary for the full development of cor pulmonale while in childhood several months or a few years may be sufficient. Autopsy usually reveals that the lungs contain much iron. There is grave anaemia in the majority of the cases. The urinary excretion of hyaluronic acid is increased [15].

DIAGNOSIS

The diagnosis of IALP may be difficult or even impossible if (*i*) physical examination yields negative results; (*ii*) chest radiography is negative even on repeated examinations at intervals of several years; (*iii*) anaemia is not traceable for months or, occasionally during the whole course of the disease [24]; (*iv*) the patient is completely free of symptoms in the periods between crises; (*v*) the characteristic recurrence of crises is not observed and the patient dies during the first attack [3]. The recognition of formes frustes cases will be more successful if IALP is thought of in cases of anaemia of unknown origin. Lung purpuras with cardiac involvement should be differentiated when establishing the leading symptom. Miliary tuberculosis is often suspected on the basis of the chest radiogram, but the negativity of bacteriologal examinations and lack of calcification help to exclude this disease.

IALP has to be distinguished from sarcoidosis, cancer and mycosis of the lungs, haemorrhagic diseases, bronchiectasia, bronchial adenoma, interstitial pneumonia, Gaucher's lipoidosis, etc.

RADIOLOGIC FEATURES OF IALP

The chest radiogram usually shows diverse abnormalities. During symptom-free intervals it may be negative, while at the time of the attacks the picture is similar to that seen in severe miliary tuberculosis. Confluent foci frequently imitate pneumonia. It is important that severe radiologic abnormalities are usually associated with vague physical signs; on auscultation the lung may appear normal. The pulmonary infiltration is usually bilateral, however, the appearance of the infiltration on one side may be followed subsequently by the infiltration of the other lung. In some cases the upper lobe may be cleared, while the infiltration in the lower lobes shows no regression. After repeated crises haemosiderosis and fibrosis of the lungs predominate the picture. In such cases small foci of higher density and with well defined outlines may obscure the usual radiologic pattern of the lungs. The hilar and mediastinal lymph nodes are less marked than in sarcoidosis. At this stage of the disease, the chest radiogram resembles that of silicosis; spots of lower density are interspersed with infiltrations simulating lobar pneumonia (pumice stone). The severity of changes partly depends on the extent and frequency of lung purpuras. In one of our patients the radiologic appearance of the lung was completely normal 9 years after splenectomy, however, the diagnosis could be confirmed with lung biopsy. Thus, the radiologic features of IALP are diverse, cloudy, soft foci; miliary dispersion as well as solid infiltrates may be observed, and the picture may be similar to the changes observed in pulmonary infarction or pneumonia.

The radiologic changes are caused not only by intra-alveolar bleeding but also by the haemosiderin deposited in the interalveolar septa. The size of the foci varies between 2 and 3 mm in diameter. During attacks, the pulmonary alterations are usually of the exudative type, while in the symptomless intervals proliferative changes predominate. Hodson and Gordon [14] mention three criteria of the chest radiographic changes in IALP, viz. multiple pulmonary infiltrates which tend to clear within a week, variable confluence of the foci, and reticular pattern.

TREATMENT

In some cases with splenectomy and steroid treatment transitory improvement can be achieved, but the long-term result of therapy is uncertain. Therefore azathioprine (Imuran) administration has been recommended as an effective immunosuppressive measure. The initial daily dose should be 2.5 mg per kg of body weight [18*f*]; this dose should be given for at least 3–4 weeks. If there is no response, the dose should be increased to 5 mg per kg of body weight. Leukocyte count should be checked during the treatment, because fatal leukopenia may develop even after withdrawal of the drug [9]. There is no uniform attitude as to how long immunosuppressive treatment should be continued. In our first case treated with Imuran intermittent administration could be started after a year, and after two years the drug could be completely withdrawn. Nevertheless, five years after the first symptoms had appeared, siderophages could again be detected in the gastric juice [18*f*]. With the introduction of—mostly prolonged—immunosuppressive treatment, which is occasionally combined with corticosteroid, IALP has ceased to be a fatal condition.

REFERENCES

1. Apt, L., Pollycove, M. and Ross, J. F.: *J. clin. Invest.* **36,** 1150 (1957).
2. Archer, J. M.: *Proc. roy. Soc. Med.* **64,** 1217 (1971).
3. Avery Jones, F., Lennard-Jones, J. E., Hinton, J. M. and Reeves, W. C.: *Brit. med. J.* **1,** 1418 (1966).
4. Beirne, G. J., Octaviano, G. N., Kopp, W. L. and Burns, R. O.: *Ann. intern. Med.* **69,** 1207 (1968).
5. Brünesholz, K.: Die idiopathische Lungenhämosiderose der Erwachsenen. Inaug. Diss. Homburg/Saar. 1962.
6. Büsing, C. M., Fölsch, U. R. and Wanke, M.: *Med. Welt* **24,** 231 (1973).
7. Ceelen, W.: In *Handbuch der speziellen pathologischen Anatomie und Histologie.* Vol. III/3. Ed. by Henke, F. and Lubarsch, O. Springer, Berlin 1931.
8. Da Silva, W. D., Vieira, M. N. R. and Diniz, C. R.: *Clin. exp. Immunol.* **6,** 395 (1970).
9. Döring, P.: *Ergebn. inn. Med. Kinderheilk.* **14,** 482 (1960).
10. Döring, P. and Gothe, H. D.: *Klin. Wschr.* **35,** 1105 (1967).
11. Durrell, R. G., Esber, H. J., Hagadorn, J. E. and Andrews, C. E.: *Amer. Rev. Resp. Dis.* **94,** 743 (1966).
12. Gell, P. S. H. and Coombs, R. R. A.: In *Clinical Aspects of Immunology.* 2nd ed. Ed. by Gell, P. S. H. and Coombs, R. R. A. Blackwell, London 1968, p. 841.
13. Glanzmann, E. and Walthard, B.: *Mschr. Kinderheilk.* **88,** 1 (1941).
14. Hodson, C. J. and Gordon, I.: *J. fac. Rad.* **5,** 50 (1953).
15. Kaiser, E., Klujber, L. and Sulyok, E.: *Acta paediat. Acad. Sci. hung.* **11,** 253 (1970).
16. Propst, A.: *Virchows Arch. Abt. A. path. Anat. Physiol.* **326,** 633 (1955).
17. Smith, W. E. and Fienberg, R.: *New Engl. J. Med.* **289,** 808 (1958).

18*a*. Steiner, B.: *Orv. Hetil.* **95,** 1100 (1954).

18*b*. id., *Arch. Dis. Child.* **29,** 391 (1954).
18*c*. id., *Magyar Belorv. Arch.* (*Budapest*) **12,** 14 (1959).
18*d*. id., *Acta paediat. Acad. Sci. hung.* **7,** 157 (1966).
18*e*. id., In *A Korányi Sándor Társaság tudományos ülései* (Scientific sessions of the Sándor Korányi Society). Vol. VI. Ed. by Rajka, E. Akadémiai Kiadó, Budapest 1967. p. 249.
18*f*. id., *Helv. paediatr. Acta* **24,** 413 (1969).
19. Steiner, B. and Backhausz, R.: *Gyermekgyógyászat* **8,** 86 (1957).
20. Steiner, B. and Nábrády, J.: *Orv. Hetil.* **105,** 2322 (1964).
21. Sturgill, B. C. and Westervelt, F. B.: *J. Amer. med. Ass.* **194,** 914 (1965).
22. Virchow, R.: In *Die krankhaften Geschwülste.* Vol. II. Hirschwald, Berlin 1864, p. 470.
23. Waldenström, J.: *Acta radiol.* (*Stockh.*) **25,** 194 (1944).
24. Weippl, G. and Wolf, H. G.: *Neue öst. Z. Kinderheilk.* **3,** 327 (1958).
25. Zollinger, H. and Hegglin, R.: *Schweiz. med. Wschr.* **88,** 4 (1958).

INDEX

GPSR Compliance

The European Union's (EU) General Product Safety Regulation (GPSR) is a set of rules that requires consumer products to be safe and our obligations to ensure this.

If you have any concerns about our products, you can contact us on ProductSafety@springernature.com

In case Publisher is established outside the EU, the EU authorized representative is:

Springer Nature Customer Service Center GmbH
Europaplatz 3
69115 Heidelberg, Germany

Batch number: 10683525

Printed by Printforce, the Netherlands